Pediatric
Nephrology
for Primary Care

Amin J. Barakat and Russell W. Chesney
Editors

American Academy of Pediatrics
141 Northwest Point Blvd
Elk Grove Village, IL 60007-1098

AAP Department of Marketing and Publications

Maureen DeRosa, MPA, Director, Department of Marketing and Publications
Mark Grimes, Director, Division of Product Development
Diane Lundquist, Senior Product Development Editor
Sandi King, MS, Director, Division of Publishing and Production Services
Kate Larson, Manager, Editorial Services
Theresa Wiener, Manager, Editorial Production
Peg Mulcahy, Graphic Designer
Jill Ferguson, Director, Division of Marketing
Linda Smessaert, Manager, Clinical and Professional Publications Marketing
Robert Herling, Director, Division of Sales

Library of Congress Control Number: 2008941470

ISBN: 978-1-58110-297-0

MA0441

The recommendations in this publication do not indicate an exclusive course of treatment or serve as a standard of medical care. Variations, taking into account individual circumstances, may be appropriate.

9-200/1108

Last digit is the print number: 9 8 7 6 5 4 3 2 1

Contributors

Alfred Z. Abuhamad, MD
Professor and Chairman, Department of Obstetrics and Gynecology,
Eastern Virginia School of Medicine, Norfolk, VA

Uri S. Alon, MD
Professor of Pediatrics, Director of Bone and Mineral Disorders Clinic,
Section of Pediatric Nephrology, Children's Mercy Hospital and Clinics,
University of Missouri Kansas City School of Medicine, Kansas City, MO

Sharon P. Andreoli, MD
Byron P. and Frances D. Hollett Professor of Pediatrics, Department of
Pediatrics, James Whitcomb Riley Hospital for Children, Indiana
University Medical Center, Indianapolis, IN

Billy S. Arant, Jr, MD, FAAP
Professor, Department of Pediatrics, University of Tennessee College of
Medicine, Chattanooga, TN

Bettina H. Ault, MD
Associate Professor, Department of Pediatrics, University of Tennessee
Health Science Center, Memphis, TN

Amin J. Barakat, MD, FAAP
Clinical Professor, Department of Pediatrics, Georgetown University
School of Medicine, Washington, DC

Eliza M. F. Berkley, MD
Assistant Professor, Division of Maternal Fetal Medicine, Department
of Obstetrics and Gynecology, Eastern Virginia Medical School,
Norfolk, VA

Eileen D. Brewer, MD, FAAP
Professor and Head, Pediatric Renal Section, Baylor College of Medicine,
and Chief, Renal Service at Texas Children's Hospital, Houston, TX

Douglas A. Canning, MD
Chief, Division of Urology, University of Pennsylvania School of Medicine,
Children's Hospital of Philadelphia, Philadelphia, PA

Andy Yu-How Chang, MD
Assistant Professor, Division of Pediatric Urology, Children's Hospital Los Angeles, Keck School of Medicine, University of Southern California, Los Angeles, CA

Russell W. Chesney, MD, FAAP
Le Bonheur Professor and Chair, Department of Pediatrics, The University of Tennessee Health Science Center, Memphis, TN

Noel M. Delos Santos, MD
Assistant Professor of Pediatrics and Pediatric Nephrology, University of Tennessee Health Science Center, Memphis, TN

Agnes B. Fogo, MD
Professor of Pathology, Medicine and Pediatrics, and Director of the Renal/ Electron Microscopy Laboratory, Vanderbilt University Medical Center, Nashville, TN

John Foreman, MD, FAAP
Professor and Chief, Division of Pediatric Nephrology, Duke University Medical Center, Durham, NC

Aaron Friedman, MD, FAAP
Professor and Chairman, Department of Pediatrics, Brown Medical School, Hasbro Children's Hospital, Providence, RI

Uttam Garg, PhD
Professor of Pathology, Director of Clinical Chemistry and Toxicology, Department of Pathology and Laboratory Medicine, Children's Mercy Hospital and Clinics, University of Missouri Kansas City School of Medicine, Kansas City, MO

M. Colleen Hastings, MD
Assistant Professor, Departments of Pediatrics and Internal Medicine, University of Tennessee Health Sciences Center, Children's Foundation Research Center at Le Bonheur Children's Medical Center, Memphis, TN

Iekuni Ichikawa, MD
Professor of Pediatrics and Medicine, Vanderbilt University School of Medicine, Nashville, TN, and Professor of Bioethics, Tokai University School of Medicine, Isehara, Japan

Deborah P. Jones, MD
Professor of Pediatrics, University of Tennessee Health Science Center, Children's Foundation Research Center at Le Bonheur Children's Medical Center, Memphis, TN

Fumio Niimura, MD
Associate Professor of Pediatrics, Tokai University School of Medicine, Isehara, Japan

H. Norman Noe, MD, FAAP, FACS
Professor of Urology and Chief, Division of Pediatric Urology, University of Tennessee, Memphis College of Medicine, Le Bonheur Children's Medical Center, Memphis, TN

Victoria F. Norwood, MD
Professor of Pediatrics and Chief, Pediatric Nephrology, University of Virginia Children's Hospital, Charlottesville, VA

H. Gil Rushton, MD, FAAP
Professor of Urology and Pediatrics, The George Washington University School of Medicine, and Chief, Division of Pediatric Urology, Children's National Medical Center, Washington, DC

Nina Salhab, MS, RD/LD
Pediatric Renal Dietician, Department of Pediatrics, University of Texas Southwestern Medical School at Dallas, Children's Medical Center of Dallas, Dallas, TX

S. Sedberry-Ross, MD
Chief Resident, Department of Urology, George Washington University School of Medicine, Washington, DC

Mouin G. Seikaly, MD, FAAP
Professor of Pediatrics, University of Texas Southwestern Medical School at Dallas, and Chief of Solid Organ Transplant Program, Children's Medical Center of Dallas, Dallas, TX

Tarak Srivastava, MD
Assistant Professor of Pediatrics, Section of Pediatric Nephrology, Children's Mercy Hospital and Clinics, University of Missouri Kansas City School of Medicine, Kansas City, MO

Mark A. Williams, MD, FAAP, FACS

Assistant Professor, Department of Urology, University of Tennessee College of Medicine, Le Bonheur Children's Medical Center, Memphis, TN

Robert J. Wyatt, MD

Chief, Division of Pediatric Nephrology, University of Tennessee Health Science Center, Children's Foundation Research Center at Le Bonheur Children's Medical Center, Memphis, TN

Aida Yared, MD, FAAP

Assistant Professor of Pediatrics, Vanderbilt University School of Medicine, Nashville, TN

To our children, our grandchildren, and the children of the world, who inspire us to work harder for a better life for all.

Contents

Foreword

One cannot write a foreword without first looking back. Russell Chesney and I were Keith Drummond's fellows in Montreal in the 1970s. We were excited by the great advances in the diagnosis and classification of glomerular diseases and the emerging understanding of the tubulopathies at that time. So much has changed since I began my training. Chronic hemodialysis and successful renal transplantation for children were in their infancy. Chronic peritoneal dialysis had not been invented. The 1970s were a period during which many now well-known conditions, such as immunoglobulin A nephropathy, focal segmental glomerulosclerosis (FSGS), and atypical hemolytic-uremic syndrome (HUS), were being discovered and defined.

So much has changed. The advent of molecular biology has yielded exciting insights and posed new nosologic challenges. Our understanding of phenotypes is undergoing a radical change; mutations on different chromosomes may produce similar phenotypes—for example, *PKD1* and *PKD2* both produce polycystic kidney disease—and apparently similar mutations can produce phenotypic variability. This is exemplified by the Venn diagram in Amin Barakat's paper on Denys-Drash syndrome.[1] Charles Scriver demonstrated the increasing importance of genetic forms of rickets compared with acquired nutritional rickets; an apparent increase in the former coincided with increasing recognition and prevention of the latter. Similar observations have been made in HUS and FSGS. The most dramatic advances have been in dialysis and renal transplantation for infants and children. However, these advances are not without their costs. The scourges of osteodystrophy, rickets, and the adverse cosmetic effects of antirejection medications have been overcome, but the goal posts are constantly being shifted. Patients, parents, physicians, and society are no longer satisfied with saving a life. All want the optimum quality of life. Unfortunately, new success also comes with new consequences. Post-transplant lymphoproliferative disease, BK virus, and transplant glomerulopathy are blights on the radiant successes of transplantation.

We have also witnessed an erosion of the roles of nephrologists as interventionists, surgeons, or interventional radiologists insert peritoneal dialysis catheters and dialysis lines and perform renal biopsies. Intensive care specialists are doing hemodiafiltration. Rheumatologists are treating the glomerulonephritides caused by systemic lupus erythematosus, Wegener granulomatosis, and Henoch-Schönlein purpura. Acute renal emergencies are more often being treated by intensive care specialists in the intensive care unit. Where does that leave pediatric nephrology? Nephrology is a cognitive specialty—we have truly evolved from *Homo habilis* (man the toolmaker) to *Homo sapiens*. Most of our practice is devoted to the care of persons with chronic diseases. Patients with renal transplants are now becoming the biggest group of patients with chronic kidney disease. Patients with chronic kidney disease cannot be cared for by one physician; these patients need a team of caregivers. The care of these patients and families raises profound ethical, psychological, social, economic, and nutritional issues. These are exciting challenges that are covered in *Pediatric Nephrology and Urology*.[2]

What roles do pediatricians play in the diagnosis, evaluation, and management of pediatric renal diseases? The tone and approach of this volume takes its lead from the initial chapter by Amin Barakat. The approach is careful and sober and emphasizes a sound clinical approach. There is emphasis on the importance of understanding basic concepts in the use and interpretation of laboratory tests and imaging studies. Common and important conditions are emphasized. Pediatricians have the unenviable task of finding needles in haystacks. It is their duty to diagnose without overinvestigating. This is a fine balance because they cannot and should not do extensive studies on every child with hypertension or microscopic hematuria or proteinuria, and yet they cannot miss the important diagnosis of hypertension or glomerulonephritis. This text is easy to read and is recommended to every pediatrician and to pediatric residents as a primer in pediatric nephrology.

Bernard S. Kaplan, MB BCh
Chief of Pediatric Nephrology
Laffey-Connolly Professor of Pediatric Nephrology
The Children's Hospital of Philadelphia
University of Pennsylvania

1. Barakat AY, Papadopoulou ZL, Chandra RS, Hollerman CE, Calcagno PL. Pseudohermaphroditism, nephron disorder and Wilms' tumor: a unifying concept. *Pediatrics.* 1974;54:366–369

2. Kaplan BS, Meyers KEC. *Pediatric Nephrology and Urology.* Philadephia, PA: Elsevier Mosby; 2005

Preface

In this era of health care management, it has become evident that pediatricians and other primary care physicians who care for children need at their disposal a book that helps them in the diagnosis and management of kidney disease. The purpose of this book is to provide primary care physicians, pediatricians, residents, medical students, and all health care professionals who deal with children with a brief but complete discussion of renal disease in children. The book covers the complete scope of pediatric nephrology problems and can serve as a desk reference and a bedside clinical manual for physicians in diagnosing and treating children with uncomplicated kidney problems. It is not designed for use as a textbook.

The book offers an overview approach, with clinical "pearls" interspersed throughout; allows discussion of the clinical course, pathogenesis, etiology, and management of different renal conditions; and helps the practitioner understand the scope of the problem. The book is replete with tables, algorithms, and appendices that will assist readers in the differential diagnosis and workup of patients with renal disease. It consists of 21 chapters that cover aspects of pediatric nephrology pertinent to primary care physicians who deal with children. Among these are approaches to diagnosing and treating children with renal disease and to the evaluation of patients with hematuria and proteinuria, either together or alone. Timely chapters on the role of the clinical laboratory and the use of imaging of both the kidneys and the urinary tract are beneficial. Other chapters cover key renal and genitourinary issues, including urinary tract infection, renal stones, acid-base disorders, hypertension, and fluid and electrolyte disorders. Prenatal diagnosis and prevention are also discussed. Because of space limitations, an exhaustive list of references is not provided; rather, a limited number of specific references and a few key articles are included to allow the interested reader to pursue certain issues in depth. Cross-referencing is used to avoid repetition and redundancy. Detailed appendices are provided that include (1) reference ranges, (2) nomograms, (3) formulas, and (4) a table presenting various diseases and syndromes associated with renal and urinary tract abnormalities.

Knowledge concerning the nosology, etiology, pathology, pathogenesis, and treatment of renal and urologic diseases in children has risen exponentially over the past 4 decades. Improvements in renal and urinary tract imaging, knowledge of genetic abnormalities in numerous childhood renal disorders, a greater knowledge of the embryology of the genitourinary tract, and more precise use of urinary biomarkers to define the type and degree of renal injury are included recent advances. Two changes in our approach to childhood kidney disease, however, stand out. First, experts in pediatric nephrology and pediatric urology have come together to design and conduct multicenter, pan-national or international clinical studies, often employing a prospective and evidence-seeking approach. Second, the offshoots of these trials allow the creation of algorithms, clinical guidelines and, in some instances, evidence-based approaches to diagnosis and management. Additions to the therapeutic armamentarium include anti-inflammatory, immunomodulating, and antihypertension drugs. Approaches to glomerulonephritic conditions and the management of renal transplantation are also accelerating. An emphasis on the testing of drugs and the dosage definition for drugs in children has made possible the use of newer, more targeted agents. These developments are presented to make primary care physicians aware of advances in pediatric nephrology.

We have made every effort to present the material in a simple and practical manner and to clearly discuss controversial issues. When serious controversy exists, such as that regarding the investigation and treatment of urinary tract infection, we have presented various opinions and left it up to the reader to decide on the best course to follow.

We thank the authors for their valuable and authoritative contributions to this text. We are also thankful to Andrea Patters for her outstanding editorial assistance; to Diane Lundquist, senior product development editor; to Kate Larson, manager of editorial services; and the publishing and editorial staff of the American Academy of Pediatrics for their help and support. We do hope that our readers find this book useful and will profit from this concerted effort.

Amin J. Barakat

Russell W. Chesney

Chapter 1

Presentation of Patients With Renal Disease and Guidelines for Patient Referral

Amin J. Barakat

Abbreviations

CKD	Chronic kidney disease
DI	Diabetes insipidus
ESRD	End-stage renal disease
GN	Glomerulonephritis
NS	Nephrotic syndrome
RBC	Red blood cell
sg	Specific gravity
UTI	Urinary tract infection
VCUG	Voiding cystourethrogram

Introduction

Renal disease is a major cause of morbidity and mortality.[1-3] Primary care physicians should be familiar with the modes of presentation of various renal conditions and should have a high index of suspicion for patients with asymptomatic disease. The use of routine prenatal ultrasonography has increased the diagnosis of congenital renal anomalies and created a new challenge for practicing pediatricians. Pediatricians and primary care physicians who deal with newborns and children should have knowledge of the diagnosis, management, and prognosis of these conditions and should be able to confidently discuss them with parents. Early diagnosis and treatment of renal disease in children is important in the prevention of renal failure and ESRD (Chapter 21). In this chapter, the presentation of patients with renal disease, the role of primary care physicians in the workup and treatment of children with renal disease, guidelines for patient referral to a pediatric nephrologist or urologist, and the role of nephrologists in the workup of children with renal disease are discussed.

Presentation of Patients With Renal Disease

Patients with renal disease may present with (1) signs and symptoms of renal disease, (2) abnormal urinalysis, (3) UTI, (4) congenital abnormalities of the kidney or urinary tract, (5) electrolyte and acid-base disturbances, (6) glomerular disease, (7) tubular disease, (8) decreased renal function, (9) hypertension, and (10) renal involvement in systemic disease. These findings should prompt a thorough history and physical examination, including blood pressure determination (Chapter 2). A few laboratory and radiologic studies may suggest the diagnosis or lead to a prompt referral to a pediatric nephrologist or urologist. Often, renal disease may be asymptomatic; therefore, a urinalysis and blood pressure determination, in addition to a thorough abdominal examination, should be an integral part of the routine medical examination for children.

Signs and Symptoms of Renal Disease

Renal disease, particularly in children, may present in a subtle manner and may be detected during a routine physical examination. Failure to thrive, unexplained fevers, vague pains, gastrointestinal symptoms, anemia, abdominal mass, edema, hypertension, and metabolic acidosis may be the first indications of kidney disease. Anemia, growth failure, hypertension, and abnormal retinal changes may be the first signs of CKD. Patients with uremia may present with lassitude, anorexia, and vomiting. Failure to thrive may suggest CKD or renal tubular disease. Frequency, urgency, dysuria, hesitancy, and urinary retention suggest a UTI, obstructive uropathy, or urinary calculi. Abdominal, loin, or suprapubic pain may also be present.

Physicians should be familiar with the normal voiding pattern of children at various ages (Chapter 2 and Appendix I). *Frequency* is frequent urination suggesting UTI, whereas *polyuria* is the passage of a larger-than-normal amount of urine. Polyuria, which indicates a decrease in urine-concentrating ability, occurs in patients with diabetes mellitus, DI, and CKD. A child with polyuria and decreased random urine sg should be administered a fasting sg or water deprivation test (Chapter 11). A random urine sg of greater than 1.020 in the absence of glucosuria and proteinuria excludes a urine concentration defect. Decreased concentrating ability with evidence of other renal disease may be due to chronic pyelonephritis, hydronephrosis, renal cystic disease, or sickle cell nephropathy. Referral to a pediatric nephrologist may be necessary if these conditions are suspected. *Pollakiuria* (Greek *pollakis,* meaning "often") refers to daytime urinary frequency that has a sudden onset and tends to affect toilet-trained schoolchildren, especially boys. It is usually

▵ Pearl

Renal disease, particularly in children, may present in a subtle manner and may be detected during a routine physical examination.

an isolated symptom, which lasts from a few days to a few weeks. Results of physical examination, urinalysis, and urine culture are normal, and no further investigation is necessary.

Enuresis (nocturnal incontinence) is bed-wetting since birth and is usually idiopathic and associated with a positive family history. It initially requires no other investigation than a urinalysis and urine culture. Secondary incontinence, daytime incontinence, and enuresis beyond the age of 10 or 12 years require further evaluation with renal ultrasound, VCUG, and other studies as needed.

It is important to keep in mind that renal disease in children may present in a subtle manner. Urinary tract infection, for example, often presents with signs and symptoms not related to the urinary tract, such as unexplained fevers, gastrointestinal symptoms, and irritability. Physicians, therefore, should have a high index of suspicion and should perform urinalyses and urine cultures in any child with unexplained fevers. Younger children with UTI may have a normal urinalysis, and a urine culture is necessary to make the diagnosis.

Most renal diseases are painless. Flank pain may be due to infection or inflammation of the renal parenchyma or stretching of the renal capsule. When pain is associated with nausea, vomiting, and fever, acute pyelonephritis should be suspected. Renal calculi may present with hematuria and colicky abdominal or flank pain of rapid onset (Chapter 19). Passed stones are very valuable in diagnosis and should be analyzed.

Renal and bladder injury following trauma may also present with pain. Dysuria, or pain on urination, is a symptom of UTI or urethritis. The pain of cystitis or prostatitis is usually suprapubic and gradual in onset.

Abdominal masses of renal origin may be due to hydronephrosis; multicystic, dysplastic, or polycystic kidney disease; renal vein thrombosis; Wilms tumor; or neuroblastoma (Chapters 5 and 18). A pediatric nephrologist or urologist may be consulted if further workup is needed.

Abnormal Urinalysis

Patients with kidney disease may present with abnormal urinary findings. A routine urinalysis should be performed periodically in the office on every child (Chapter 3). The American Academy of Pediatrics recommends a urinalysis as a part of preventive pediatric health care at 5 years and mid-adolescence. The most common urinary abnormalities are hematuria and proteinuria (Chapters 7 and 8).

Hematuria may be gross or microscopic, discovered during a routine urinalysis. Persistent hematuria should be investigated. A primary care physician may easily initiate evaluation of a child with hematuria. This consists of history and physical examination including blood pressure determination; urinalysis with special emphasis on RBC morphology; urine culture; blood studies; quantitative urine protein determination; and, when indicated, creatinine clearance, audiogram, renal ultrasound, VCUG, and renal scan. The morphology of RBCs in the urine can help differentiate glomerular (dysmorphic RBC) from nonglomerular hematuria (normal RBC). Urinalysis and, when indicated, an audiogram should be performed on immediate family members because recurrent benign hematuria, Alport syndrome, immunoglobulin A nephropathy, and other forms of glomerular disease may be familial. In general, the presence of persistent and recurrent gross hematuria should prompt referral to a pediatric nephrologist. Immunoglobulin A nephropathy, membranoproliferative GN, Alport syndrome, recurrent benign hematuria, kidney stones, and various renal and urinary tract abnormalities may present with gross hematuria. Persistent proteinuria should be investigated. Primary care physicians may quantitate the proteinuria and exclude the orthostatic type. Significant proteinuria (>1 g/1.73 m^2/d) or proteinuria associated with abnormal RBC morphology, decreased renal function, hypertension, decreased serum complement level, or manifestations of systemic disease are suggestive of glomerular disease and are an indication for renal biopsy (Chapters 9 and 20).

Pyuria may originate from any part of the urinary tract and usually suggests UTI, but it may also be seen with any inflammatory process of the kidney and urinary tract, renal calculi, and abnormalities of the urinary tract. When pyuria is present, a urine culture should be performed. Persistence of pyuria after adequate treatment of the UTI should raise the rare possibility of infection with tuberculosis, anaerobes, or viruses.

ᵌ◈ *Pearl*

A routine urinalysis should be performed in the office on every child at 5 years and in midadolescence.

Trauma—as well as renal calculi, congenital abnormalities of the kidney or urinary tract with or without obstructive uropathy, and Kawasaki disease—should also be considered. Abnormal urine color and smell, crystalluria, and the significance of casts are discussed in Chapter 3.

Urinary Tract Infection

Urinary tract infection is common in children. Diagnosis of UTI requires a high degree of suspicion because of the nonspecific nature of the symptoms and is established only by a quantitative urine culture. Accurate and prompt diagnosis is important to reduce morbidity and prevent sequelae. Because UTI is frequently associated with congenital abnormalities of the kidney and urinary tract, imaging studies should be performed. Prompt and adequate treatment is of paramount importance to prevent renal scarring. Urinary tract infection and the controversial issues surrounding it are discussed in Chapter 6.

Congenital Abnormalities of the Kidney and Urinary Tract

Congenital abnormalities of the kidney and urinary tract reportedly occur in 5% to 10% of the population. They represent 25% of the total ultrasonographically diagnosed malformations that occur in 0.25% to 0.7% of fetuses. About one-third to two-thirds of ESRD in children is due to congenital abnormalities of the kidney and urinary tract. In addition, these abnormalities occur in 23% of patients with chromosomal aberrations and two-thirds of patients with abnormalities of other organ systems. Some of these abnormalities are minor and are discovered incidentally; others are

✎ Pearl

Urinary tract abnormalities should be suspected in any child with UTI, congenital anomalies of other organ systems, chromosomal aberrations, or malformation syndromes.

major, leading to obstruction, renal scarring, pyelonephritis, and ESRD. Urinary tract abnormalities should be suspected in any child with UTI, congenital anomalies of other organ systems (cardiovascular, gastrointestinal, central nervous system, and others), chromosomal aberrations, various malformation syndromes, and those with single umbilical artery or supernumerary nipples (Chapter 18 and Appendix IV). Prenatal diagnosis of these conditions by ultrasonography as early as 12 to 16 weeks' gestation will reduce the occurrence of renal damage and ESRD (Chapter 17).

Electrolyte and Acid-Base Disturbances

Electrolyte and acid-base disturbances are common in pediatrics. These abnormalities present with a very complex clinical picture, and treating physicians should be familiar with the intricacies of their diagnosis and management (Chapters 11 and 12). Symptoms include nausea, vomiting, diarrhea, decreased fluid intake, irritability, lethargy, weight loss, dry skin and mucous membranes, elevated pulse, seizures, and coma. Water deprivation results in dehydration, whereas extracellular fluid expansion produces edema. Severely affected patients should be referred immediately to a hospital that can provide expert care.

Glomerular Disease

Most children with GN present with proteinuria, hematuria, hypertension, edema, reduced renal function, or NS. Patients with systemic diseases associated with glomerular abnormalities may present with arthritis, rash, hypertension, hematuria, or proteinuria. Acute poststreptococcal GN is familiar to practicing physicians. Most children with acute GN have a benign course and can be easily treated by a primary care physician on an ambulatory basis. A nephrology consultation should be obtained for patients with oliguria, hyperkalemia, NS, cardiac overload, and renal insufficiency. Patients with prolonged oligoanuria, a persistently low serum complement for more than 8 to 12 weeks, or associated NS may require a kidney biopsy. Evaluation of patients with glomerular disease is discussed in Chapters 9 and 20.

Nephrotic syndrome is characterized by proteinuria of 40 mg/m^2/h (or 50 mg/kg/d) or higher and serum albumin less than 2.5 g/dL. The most common form of NS in children is minimal change NS, which is characterized by response to corticosteroids and good prognosis, although most patients have one or more relapses. A primary care physician may treat patients with this type of nephrosis. Those who are steroid-resistant or -dependent, those with a suspected structural glomerular abnormality, and those with systemic disease should be referred to a pediatric nephrologist because they usually require a kidney biopsy and a close follow-up.

> **ॐ Pearl**
>
> Children with GN present with proteinuria, hematuria, hypertension, edema, reduced renal function, or NS.

Tubular Disease

Primary care physicians should be familiar with renal tubular diseases such as renal glucosuria, Fanconi syndrome with or without cystinosis, cystinuria and other aminoacidurias, renal tubular acidosis, nephrogenic DI, Bartter syndrome, and others (Chapter 10). Affected patients may present with failure to thrive, acidosis, glucosuria, aminoaciduria, phosphaturia, rickets, and inability to concentrate urine. Renal tubular acidosis should be considered in patients with metabolic acidosis, persistently alkaline urine, and positive family history for the presence of these conditions (Chapter 12). Renal tubular diseases are rare and complex, and their management usually requires the help of a pediatric nephrologist.

> **ॐ Pearl**
>
> Renal tubular diseases are rare and complex, and their management usually requires the help of a pediatric nephrologist.

Decreased Renal Function

Azotemia is elevated serum urea nitrogen, *renal failure* is reduction in renal function, and *uremia* is the syndrome that encompasses the overt consequences of CKD such as anemia and osteodystrophy, and central nervous system, gastrointestinal, and other manifestations. *Acute kidney injury* is an abrupt severe reduction in glomerular filtration and is characterized by oliguria (urine <0.5 mL/kg/h) or anuria and azotemia (Chapter 13). A patient presenting with the preceding findings, hypertension, gross hematuria, electrolyte disturbances (particularly hyperkalemia) and acidosis, and volume overload should be referred to a pediatric nephrologist immediately. The etiology of acute kidney injury must be identified promptly because many causes of acute renal failure are reversible and because evaluation, management, and prognosis of this condition vary with the specific etiology.

The presence of growth retardation; anemia; history of underlying renal disease; renal osteodystrophy; or small, contracted kidneys suggests the presence of CKD, which is defined as the stage at which the kidneys are irreversibly damaged and unable to maintain the body homeostasis (Chapter 14). Once the diagnosis of CKD is suspected or documented, patients should be referred to a pediatric nephrologist because these patients invariably progress to ESRD, requiring long-term dialysis and renal transplantation (Chapter 14). Because many causes of ESRD in children are potentially preventable (hereditary and congenital abnormalities of the kidney and UTI), early diagnosis and treatment of these conditions is of utmost importance (Chapter 21). Physicians should adjust the dosage of various medications that are excreted by the kidney, including some antibiotics, analgesics, diuretics, and others, for patients with renal failure.

> ### ॐ Pearl
>
> The dose of various medications should be adjusted in patients with renal failure.

Hypertension

Blood pressure should be measured routinely in every child starting at 3 years or when indicated. Hypertension in children may be essential or secondary to renal, endocrine, cardiovascular, or neurologic causes. The 3 most common symptoms of hypertension in children are headache, difficulty sleeping, and tiredness, all of which improve with treatment. Severe persistent hypertension should be investigated promptly and thoroughly in children because treatable secondary causes are common in the pediatric age group (Chapter 15). A primary care physician may initiate the evaluation on children with persistent mild to moderate hypertension.

> ### ॐ Pearl
>
> Blood pressure should be measured routinely in every child starting at 3 years or when indicated.

Children presenting with severe or malignant hypertension requiring comprehensive evaluation and initiation of antihypertensive therapy should be referred to a pediatric nephrologist.

Renal Involvement in Systemic Diseases

Physicians should be aware of renal involvement in systemic diseases and various conditions and syndromes (Chapter 20 and Appendix IV). In general, renal involvement should be excluded in any individual with multisystem disease such as collagen disease, diabetes mellitus, and storage diseases. The diagnosis of renal involvement in systemic disease is based on clinical findings (hematuria, proteinuria, hypertension, decreased serum complement levels, decreased renal function, large kidneys, leukemia, lymphoma, amyloidosis, and others), as well as basic knowledge of renal histology. Renal biopsy contributes significantly to the diagnosis of collagen and other systemic diseases.

The Role of Primary Care Physicians and Guidelines for Patient Referral

In the present era of managed care, primary care physicians find themselves performing some duties that have traditionally been performed by specialists. It is difficult to clearly delineate the responsibilities of primary care physicians and to list indications for referral to a pediatric nephrologist. In general, primary care physicians may initiate evaluation to the extent that they feel comfortable. The most common reasons for referral to a pediatric nephrologist include fluid and electrolyte disorders and hematuria or proteinuria, followed by chronic GN, NS, UTI, hypertension, acute GN, and ESRD.[4]

✺ Pearl

The most common reasons for referral to a pediatric nephrologist are fluid and electrolyte disorders, hematuria, and proteinuria.

The role of primary care physicians in the workup and management of children with renal disease is outlined in Box 1-1. Guidelines for patient referral to a pediatric nephrologist are listed in Box 1-2, and the role of pediatric nephrologists in the workup and management of children with renal disease is presented in Box 1-3. An outline for screening children with suspected renal disease is presented in Chapter 21.

Box 1-1. Role of Primary Care Physicians in the Workup and Management of Children With Renal Disease

1. Keep a high index of suspicion for UTI and renal disease.
2. Take patient and family history and perform a complete physical examination, including blood pressure measurement.
3. Evaluate the general state of health and exclude systemic diseases.
4. Perform a urinalysis on the patient and, when indicated, on family members.
5. Perform a urine culture and antibiogram.
6. Laboratory tests should include blood urea nitrogen, creatinine, electrolytes, serum complement, quantitative proteinuria, creatinine clearance, and others as needed.
7. Order imaging studies, including renal ultrasound, voiding cystourethrogram, renal scan, and others on patients with UTI, suspected congenital abnormalities, and calculi.
8. Screen for orthostatic proteinuria, tubular disorders, and others.
9. Treat UTI, uncomplicated acute glomerulonephritis, conditions not associated with acute or progressive deterioration of renal function such as minimal change nephrotic syndrome, mild abnormalities, and others with which the physician is comfortable.
10. Follow-up for patients with whom the physician is comfortable.
11. Discuss and refer renal and urinary tract abnormalities diagnosed on routine prenatal ultrasound.

Abbreviation: UTI, urinary tract infection.

Box 1-2. Guidelines for Patient Referral to a Pediatric Nephrologist

1. Persistent unexplained hematuria, nonorthostatic proteinuria, and hypertension
2. Decreased renal function
3. Acute, chronic, and end-stage renal disease
4. Renal tubular disease
5. Nephrotic syndrome, particularly steroid-dependent or -resistant
6. Atypical or persistent GN
7. Unexplained acid-base and electrolyte abnormalities
8. Systemic diseases associated with progressive renal involvement such as SLE and diabetes mellitus
9. Genetic and congenital abnormalities likely to produce progressive renal damage
10. When invasive studies (eg, kidney biopsy) are indicated
11. Major renal and urinary tract abnormalities found on routine prenatal ultrasound
12. Renal disease that is likely to progress (eg, focal glomerulosclerosis, IgA nephropathy, and others)
13. Conditions associated with acute complications (eg, hypertension, calculi, and hemolytic uremic syndrome)
14. When teamwork is needed (urologist, geneticist, dietitian, social worker)
15. Parental anxiety

Abbreviations: GN, glomerulonephritis; SLE, systemic lupus erythematosus.

Box 1-3. Role of Pediatric Nephrologists in the Workup and Management of Children With Renal Disease

1. Repeat some of the steps listed in Box 1-1.
2. Perform renal function studies—glomerular, tubular, concentrating ability.
3. Request and interpret complicated imaging studies—CT, MRI, arteriogram.
4. Perform and interpret specialized studies such as renal biopsy.
5. Evaluate renin-angiotensin-aldosterone system.
6. Work closely with the urologist.
7. Treat and follow patients with chronic kidney disease, severe hypertension, renal transplantation, complicated urogenital abnormalities, and those conditions with which the primary care physician does not feel comfortable.
8. Treat and follow patients with complicated genetic renal disease.
9. Coordinate efforts between primary physician, urologist, transplant surgeon, geneticist, social worker, dietitian, and all those concerned with the care of the patient.

Abbreviations: CT, computed tomography; MRI, magnetic resonance imaging.

References

1. Kaplan BS, Meyers KEC. *Pediatric Nephrology and Urology.* St Louis, MO: Mosby; 2004
2. Avner ED, Harmon WE, Niaudet P. *Pediatric Nephrology.* 5th ed. Baltimore, MD: Lippincott Williams & Wilkins; 2003
3. Barakat AY, ed. *Renal Disease in Children: Clinical Evaluation and Diagnosis.* New York, NY: Springer-Verlag; 1990
4. Foreman JW, Chan JC. 10-year survey of referrals to a pediatric nephrology program. *Child Nephrol Urol.* 1990;10:8–13

Chapter 2

History and Physical Examination of the Child With Renal Disease

Aida Yared and Amin J. Barakat

Abbreviations

ADH	Antidiuretic hormone
ADPKD	Autosomal dominant polycystic kidney disease
APSGN	Acute poststreptococcal gomerulonephritis
ATN	Acute tubular necrosis
BP	Blood pressure
CKD	Chronic kidney disease
DI	Diabetes insipidus
GFR	Glomerular filtration rate
GN	Glomerulonephritis
NS	Nephrotic syndrome
PUV	Posterior urethral valve
RBC	Red blood cell
RTA	Renal tubular acidosis
SIADH	Syndrome of inappropriate anti-diuretic hormone
SLE	Systemic lupus erythematosus
UTI	Urinary tract infection

Introduction

In pediatric patients, especially younger children, serious renal disease may present with nonspecific findings unrelated to the urinary tract such as irritability, diarrhea, or failure to thrive. Thus health care professionals should always be highly suspicious of the presence of occult renal disease whenever assessing a child with symptoms or signs of unclear etiology.

⊰ Pearl

Patient history and physical examination are the most important clues to the presence of renal disease.

Patient history and physical examination are the most important clues to the presence of renal disease.[1-4] A simple urinalysis performed on a freshly voided urine specimen is very important in the diagnosis of renal disease (Chapter 3).

Clinical Presentation of Renal Disease

A child with renal disease usually presents with, or is referred for evaluation of, (1) abnormal voiding pattern, (2) abnormal urinalysis, (3) pain, or (4) systemic signs and symptoms.

Abnormal Voiding Pattern

Ninety percent of newborn infants pass urine within the first 24 hours of life, and 98% do so within 48 hours. In the first year of life, when fluid intake is high and infants' urinary concentrating ability is limited compared with older children and adults, voiding is frequent and is both diurnal and nocturnal. Beyond school age, after adequate control has been acquired, voiding is usually diurnal, is voluntary, and occurs 4 to 6 times a day. At any age, voiding should be effortless and painless, involve passage of an adequate volume of urine, and lead to complete emptying of the bladder. An abnormal voiding pattern can involve any of these parameters.

Timing

Nocturia in older children is defined as awakening at night to pass urine. Occasional nocturia can be normal, especially following copious intake of water around bedtime; this can be easily inferred if withholding of fluids at bedtime dramatically improves the condition. Otherwise, nocturia may indicate a loss of urinary concentrating ability.

Volume

The volume of urine normally passed during a single void (bladder capacity) in ounces is equal to age (years) plus 2 and plateaus by 9 years of age. Urine volume in full-term babies averages 20 mL/24 hours in the first 2 days of life, rising to 200 mL by the 10th day. Beyond the neonatal period, the total volume of urine voided in 24 hours represents roughly half of the daily fluid intake. In infants in whom intake averages 100 mL/kg/d urinary output averages 2 mL/kg/h. Age-related daily urine output values are presented in Appendix I.

A newborn can require medical attention because of a delay in the passage of urine. If both kidneys are normal in size and the bladder contains urine by percussion, delay in the passage of urine is likely normal. However, renal agenesis and obstructive uropathy should be considered. Routine prenatal ultrasound usually alerts a physician to such diagnoses.

Oligoanuria is defined in newborns as the passage of less than 0.5 mL/kg/h of urine. In neonates who are sick, oligoanuria is usually prerenal in origin and will respond to appropriate fluid administration. However, ATN, congenital renal anomalies, renal vein thrombosis, and drug-related toxicity should also be considered. A urinalysis and blood chemistry values should be obtained. In older children, oliguria is defined as a 24-hour urine output less than 300 mL/m^2; and *anuria*, less than 50 mL/m^2. This decrease in urinary flow rate can occur by 2 mechanisms. The first mechanism is the elaboration of more concentrated urine, while GFR remains normal, occurring in SIADH. The second mechanism is a decrease in renal clearance ability, which may be due to prerenal (hemodynamic), renal (parenchymal), or postrenal (obstructive) causes.

Polyuria is the passage of a larger-than-normal daily urine volume. It should not be confused with frequency of urination, in which a patient often feels the need to void but passes only a small amount of urine. If it is unclear whether a child has polyuria or frequency of urination, a 24-hour urine should be collected. Polyuria is often accompanied by polydipsia (ie, increased intake of water). Acute onset of polyuria or polydipsia suggests diabetes mellitus (a condition easily ruled out by obtaining blood and urine glucose levels) or DI. Diabetes insipidus may be central (inadequate production or release of ADH) or nephrogenic (inability to concentrate the urine in the presence of normal levels of ADH). Nephrogenic DI can be due to congenital or acquired unresponsiveness of the distal nephron to ADH and can

> ## ə➤ Pearl
>
> Oligoanuria in newborns is defined as the passage of less than 0.5 mL/kg/h of urine. In older children, oliguria is a urine output of less than 300 mL/m^2, and anuria is less than 50 mL/m^2 per 24 hours.

be an early sign of chronic renal failure owing to a variety of causes (chronic pyelonephritis, hydronephrosis, renal cystic disease, or dysplasia). Rarely, polydipsia and polyuria may be functional or psychogenic in children as part of a pattern of attention-seeking behavior.

The Act of Voiding

An infant who exhibits symptoms of urinary retention or who has difficulty initiating voiding may be suffering from a serious underlying disease. Retention in the child with neurologic deficits suggests a neurogenic bladder. In an otherwise normal male child, retention should always alert a physician to the possibility of bladder outlet obstruction (bladder neck obstruction, PUVs, urethral stricture, or severe meatal stenosis). Acute difficulty in voiding can also occur with urethritis or cystitis, in which case other signs and symptoms of inflammation are usually present. A weak urinary stream, or dribbling of urine, can be the presenting sign of an obstructive uropathy.

Dysuria, or pain on urination, is highly suggestive of UTI. It is often accompanied by frequency of urination, whereby a child often feels the urge to pass urine and typically passes only small amounts, as well as urgency (ie, the inability to voluntarily hold urine for a reasonable amount of time). Parents of a young infant might report that the child invariably screams when passing urine. The combination of dysuria, frequency, and urgency is termed the *urethral triad,* which suggests either a UTI or noninfectious urethritis due to irritation from poor hygiene or from chemical inflammation, such as can be caused by bubble baths.

Voluntary Control

Incontinence means wetting at an inappropriate time and place in a child older than 5 years. Incontinence may be continuous (associated with malformations or sphincter damage) or intermittent. Intermittent incontinence may be daytime incontinence or nocturnal incontinence, referred to as *enuresis.*[5] Incontinence may be primary (the child has never been toilet trained) or secondary (the child achieved bladder control for a time then started wetting again). Enuresis is a benign condition occurring in around 20% of children between 4 and 5 years of age, 8% at 8 years of age, and 5% at 10 years of age. Often there is a history of this trait in either parent. Daytime incontinence, especially if secondary, is more likely to indicate underlying pathology, whether infectious, anatomical, or emotional. Urinary incontinence frequently accompanies UTI in the toddler age group and can be its only manifestation of UTI in around 10% of boys. Urgency incontinence may be secondary to acute or chronic cystitis, occult neurogenic bladder, or uninhibited bladder contraction (dysfunctional void-

ing). Overflow incontinence is most often seen in patients with neurologic problems, such as myelodysplasia. Daytime incontinence is an indication for thorough urologic, neurologic, and psychosocial investigation.

Persistent dampness of the underwear in a child who is toilet trained and continent may suggest ureteral ectopia. In a girl, especially one who is overweight, wetting can also result from "vaginal reflux," whereby some urine pools in the vaginal introitus during voiding and leaks out into the underwear as the child ambulates.

Abnormal Urinalysis

Frequently, an asymptomatic abnormal finding on urinalysis is discovered in a child during a preschool screening or well-child checkup. Newborns and infants can also be referred to medical attention because of an unusual urine color or smell. Unusual-smelling urine is often the sign of an underlying metabolic disorder involving organic or amino acids. The most common are a musty urine odor, suggestive of phenylketonuria, and the characteristic sweet smell of maple syrup urine disease. Such findings warrant immediate investigation. Most of these metabolic disorders are currently found during routine neonatal screening.

Most commonly, children are referred for investigation of asymptomatic hematuria and/or proteinuria (Chapters 7 and 8). Hematuria is rare in newborns. A common complaint is pink urine, which is a benign and transient finding due to the presence of large amounts of uric acid crystals in the urine of normal newborns. Physiologic vaginal bleeding can occur in female newborns after withdrawal from the elevated levels of maternal hormones and may be confused with hematuria.

Uric acid crystals are common and normal in the urine of newborns. An increased occurrence of cases of nephrocalcinosis is found in premature infants with complicated hyaline membrane disease and bronchopulmonary dysplasia. These cases are thought to result from chronic hypercalciuria secondary to prolonged furosemide administration and are more likely to form if the infant receives a calcium supplement.

Pain

Most diseases of the urinary tract are painless. Pain most often relates to an acute process, usually inflammation or distension of a hollow viscus. Chronic hydronephrosis is not accompanied by pain. When pain is present, the examiner should inquire about its location (flank, suprapubic), possible radiation, nature (dull or colicky), and severity.

Flank pain of renal origin most commonly results from infection or inflammation of the renal parenchyma that leads to stretching of the renal capsule. When accompanied by fever, nausea, or vomiting, flank pain strongly suggests acute pyelonephritis, even in the absence of other symptoms of UTI. It can also be a prominent feature of immunoglobulin A nephropathy, where 35% to 50% of episodes of gross hematuria are accompanied by flank pain that resembles acute pyelonephritis. Flank pain can occur also in 5% of patients with APSGN. In both pyelonephritis and GN, the pain is described as persistent and dull, with little or no radiation, and is often accompanied by tenderness to percussion.

Colicky pain is usually due to the presence of a stone. Although renal stones are uncommon in children, they should be kept in mind, especially in children with a positive family history (Chapter 19). The pain in this condition is typically described as colicky, excruciatingly severe, and radiating to the groin or migrating along the course of the ureter. However, such a classic picture is rare in small children with urolithiasis, who are more likely to present with nonspecific symptoms such as nausea or vomiting and, in about 16%, generalized abdominal pain.

Abdominal, flank, or back pain is the most frequent presenting symptom of ADPKD, occurring in around 60% of patients. The pain is described as dull, nagging, or aching and occasionally colicky. Radiation to the epigastric or suprapubic area is common.

Suprapubic pain, associated with suprapubic tenderness, is highly suggestive of acute cystitis, a common condition in children, especially girls. Typically, it is accompanied by the urethral triad of dysuria, frequency, and urgency. Cystitis can be of bacterial or viral etiology and is often associated with hematuria. Suprapubic or abdominal pain in a teenage girl raises the concern of a sexually transmitted infection. Sexually transmitted infections often show pyuria on urinalysis and can be accompanied by a UTI as well.

In a child with abdominal pain, inquiry should be made for a history of recent trauma and the child examined for the presence of skin bruises. Renal or bladder injuries (hematoma or rupture) have reportedly occurred in patients with severe forms of child abuse; however, it is unusual to see injury to the urinary tract in the absence of other findings.

Systemic Signs and Symptoms

Systemic signs and symptoms of renal disease may be unrelated to the urinary tract. Thus nausea, vomiting, and failure to thrive occur with uremia, acidosis, or UTI. Metabolic acidosis is often associated with vomiting and growth retardation. The 3 most commonly encountered physical signs that strongly suggest renal pathology are edema, hypertension, and abdominal mass.

Edema can occur by 3 possible mechanisms, 2 of which directly relate to renal pathology. The first is decreased oncotic pressure of plasma owing to renal protein loss and decreased plasma protein concentration. Typical of this is nephrotic edema, which tends to be most prominent in the periorbital area, and anasarca, or generalized edema, in younger infants. Protein loss in children can also occur through the gastrointestinal tract (protein-losing enteropathy) or the skin. The second mechanism of edema is increased venous pressure resulting from volume overload, which can occur when the GFR is decreased while intake of fluids is not curtailed (edema is present in 75% of children with acute postinfectious GN). The third mechanism is increased vascular permeability owing to prematurity or an allergic reaction. Although this mechanism of edema formation does not involve the kidneys, it is noteworthy that many cases of NS in children are initially misdiagnosed as allergies. Parents might report that children have a spontaneous tendency to remove their shoes or that socks leave an imprint when taken off. Edema typically changes position and is more prominent in the periorbital area in the morning and in the dependent areas, such as lower extremities, after prolonged standing.

Hypertension is an important sign of renal disease. Essential hypertension is increasingly recognized, especially in the second decade of life, and it often accompanies obesity during the teenage years. Most hypertension in infants younger than 1 year is of vascular etiology. History of placement of umbilical lines in the neonatal period should be sought because of the incidence of thrombosis, especially if the line was left in place for a long time. Thrombosis is the most common cause of hypertension in sick newborns. Coarctation of the aorta is the other common cause; thus special attention should be paid to perfusion of the extremities, including temperature, presence of pulses, and BP. Measurement of BP in all 4 extremities may show a gradient or discrepancy that must be pursued. Congenital renal anomalies, such as cystic kidney disease, can also cause neonatal hypertension. Beyond the first year of life, severe hypertension in children is mainly due to renal vascular or parenchymal disease. Thus hypertension in a child should always prompt investigation of the kidneys (Chapter 15).

More than 50% of abdominal masses in newborns are of renal origin. Most of these masses are benign, with most representing a nonfunctioning multicystic dysplastic kidney, polycystic kidney disease, or hydronephrosis. Although tumors can be present in newborns, their incidence peaks in the toddler years. Beyond the neonatal period, approximately 55% of all children presenting with an abdominal mass have a nonsurgical condition. Of the remaining 45%, most are retroperitoneal and renal in origin. An abdominal flank mass may represent a wide variety of conditions, including enlarged kidneys (hydronephrosis, polycystic kidney disease, multicystic dysplasia), a tumor (Wilms tumor or neuroblastoma), or a renal vascular accident (renal venous thrombosis). A suprapubic mass can be a distended bladder. The incidence of malignant conditions, namely Wilms tumor and neuroblastoma, increases with age to peak at 2 to 3 years, when they become the leading cause of abdominal masses in children.

ᕍ *Pearl*

Systemic signs and symptoms of renal disease may be unrelated to the urinary tract. More than half of abdominal masses in newborns are of renal origin.

History

Family History

A history of consanguinity should be obtained if a genetic disorder is suspected, such as the infantile form of polycystic kidney disease or the Finnish type of congenital NS. Family history of neonatal death in infancy due to renal problems may suggest the infantile form of polycystic kidney disease. In a child with isolated hematuria, history of a similar finding in other family members, as well as a urinalysis on immediate family members, can help suggest the diagnosis of benign familial hematuria, and thus avoid more invasive investigation. Note, however, that not all familial hematuria is benign. Various causes of hematuria, including polycystic kidney disease, Alport syndrome, and sickle cell disease or trait, are genetically transmitted. Family history of hearing loss, with or without renal impairment, should alert a physician to the possibility of Alport syndrome, a genetically inherited condition characterized by high-frequency sensorineural hearing loss and CKD. Alport syndrome is more likely to be clinically manifested in males. Family history of CKD, dialysis, or renal transplantation raises the possibility of a genetic form of nephropathy, such as Alport syndrome or ADPKD.

Family history of renal calculi points to the possibility of a metabolic disorder underlying stone formation. Children with enuresis often have a positive family history. A family history is important in various forms of renal tubular dysfunction such as cystinosis and various genetic renal disorders (Chapter 16). Family history of hypertension should be investigated in a child with a mild elevation in BP. Vesicoureteral reflux may be present in more than one-third of asymptomatic siblings of affected children.

Perinatal History

In taking the history of a newborn with renal disease, attention should be paid to prenatal and postnatal events. Currently, most pregnant women undergo one or several prenatal ultrasounds to assess the anatomy and well-being of the developing fetus. Normal kidneys are easily visualized in utero; urine output in a fetus is high, such that a cycle of bladder filling and emptying can often be observed. Most urinary tract abnormalities are detectable at 28 to 30 weeks of gestation. Oligohydramnios is suggestive of bilateral renal agenesis, or severe bilateral renal obstruction, because urine contributes to the formation of amniotic fluid. Often a newborn exhibits physical findings of intrauterine compression such as a flattened facies and club feet. Because the presence of a normal volume of amniotic fluid is essential for adequate pulmonary development, these conditions are often associated with pulmonary hypoplasia. Polyhydramnios, on the other hand, suggests gastrointestinal tract atresia, which is commonly associated with renal and urinary tract abnormalities.

Maternal diabetes can predispose the newborn to renal vein thrombosis that can present in the neonatal period with hematuria, abdominal mass, and renal insufficiency. Maternal drug intake could predispose a newborn to a variety of congenital renal anomalies and can also affect fetal renal function in the absence of renal parenchymal pathology. Intake of angiotensin-converting enzyme inhibitor by the mother, for example, can lead to oligoanuria in a newborn. Infusion of oxytocin to the mother during the course of labor together with administering a large amount of hypotonic fluids places a newborn at risk for significant hyponatremia and fluid overload because the effects of oxytocin overlap with ADH.

𝕒 Pearl

Physicians taking the history of a newborn with renal disease should pay attention to prenatal and postnatal events.

During delivery, the placenta and umbilical cord should be carefully examined. The presence of amnion nodosum should alert an examiner to the possible occurrence of renal agenesis or severe obstructive uropathy. Single umbilical artery is associated with genitourinary anomalies in 27% of cases. Obviously, a history of maternal hemorrhage, fetal distress, or neonatal depression can predispose a baby to ATN.

Patient History

Growth

Growth retardation and failure to thrive are common findings in children with CKD, chronic UTI, DI in the infant, and RTA.

Congenital Anomalies

Various surface anomalies suggest the presence of concomitant congenital renal anomalies. Malformations of the external ears, the presence of preauricular pits (usually with proteinuria), or the presence of supernumerary nipples should alert the physician to the possible presence of renal malformations. The absence or severe laxity of abdominal musculature in a boy suggests the prune-belly syndrome, which in its complete form consists of the triad of bilateral cryptorchidism, absent abdominal muscles, and complex malformations of the upper urinary tract.

Anomalies of other organ systems are associated with renal abnormalities and will be considered later under each system. Several genetic syndromes are associated with renal and urologic anomalies, and imaging studies of the urinary tract should be performed as part of the initial investigation (Chapter16 and Appendix IV). Various congenital anomalies including aniridia, hemihypertrophy, and ambiguous genitalia are associated with the occurrence of Wilms tumor.

Congenital heart disease, particularly ventricular septal defect, is associated with a higher incidence of renal anomalies than in the general population. The incidence of urologic anomalies in patients with cardiac defects is sufficiently high to warrant performing a renal ultrasound and visualizing the kidneys in the course of cardiac catheterization at the time when the contrast is concentrated and excreted by the kidneys. Obviously, any cardiac problem leading to a reduction in cardiac output can lead to a reduction in GFR. In addition, congestive heart failure presenting in a child with no previous cardiac problems should prompt a study of the urine sediment in search of RBC casts because fluid overload is a common presentation in patients with APSGN.

The respiratory tract is rarely involved in children with renal disease. However, it should be noted that tachypnea or dyspnea can be signs of congestive heart failure. In addition, pulmonary pathology such as pneumonia or assisted ventilation can predispose to SIADH.

The incidence of genitourinary anomalies is higher in children with gastrointestinal anomalies, such as imperforate anus and esophageal or rectal atresia. The level of the rectal atresia correlates with the number of anomalies seen, with a greater number existing in patients with high atresia. The incidence increases in children with tracheoesophageal fistulae.

Anorexia, nausea, and vomiting can be nonspecific symptoms of renal disease, such as uremia, urolithiasis, or RTA. Diarrhea is a prominent symptom of UTI in younger infants. Severe fluid deficits due to increased fluid losses or poor intake can predispose to prerenal impairment in glomerular filtration. Chronic constipation can predispose a child to UTIs; chronic retention of stools is also often associated with holding of the urine, which can lead to dysfunctional voiding.

Hypospadias, hydrocele, undescended testes, and other genital abnormalities are common and easily detected conditions. Because association with underlying upper urinary tract abnormalities is not usually higher than in the general population, it remains controversial whether these findings should prompt imaging of the upper urinary tract. It is generally agreed that children with coronal hypospadias do not need imaging, whereas children with perineal hypospadias do. Severe epispadias can be accompanied by exstrophy of the bladder and occur more commonly in boys. Ambiguous genitalia, along with abnormal gonadal differentiation, nephropathy, and Wilms tumor, constitute Denys-Drash syndrome. Patients with ambiguous genitalia and nephropathy should be followed closely for the possible development of Wilms tumor. Note the age at which and the ease with which toilet training was achieved. Resistive toilet training (which involves conflict between parent and child) can lead to a child voluntarily withholding stool and urine, which may lead to chronic constipation, UTIs, and dysfunctional voiding.

Patients with congenital kyphosis or scoliosis have a reported higher incidence of genitourinary anomalies than the general population. Skeletal malformations, such as bowed legs, can be consequent to RTA, renal hypophosphatemic rickets, or renal osteodystrophy associated with chronic renal failure. Orthopedic manipulation and traction have been reported to trigger hypertension.

≈ Pearl

Anomalies of other organ systems, especially cardiovascular and gastrointestinal, are associated with renal and urinary tract abnormalities.

Meningomyelocele with agenesis of the sacral segments predisposes a patient to a neurogenic bladder, with consequent urinary retention and infection. A patient with hydrocephalus and shunt is at risk for shunt nephritis, usually concomitant with an active shunt infection. History of headaches can be a sign of hypertension. Any central nervous system pathology, including meningitis or intracranial tumor, can result in SIADH.

Infection
Parents should be questioned for a history of recurrent UTIs or unexplained fevers. Such history is of extreme importance in children with decreased renal function because most pyelonephritic scars occur at an early age and can lead to loss of functional renal mass. In addition, children with recurrent UTIs should be suspected of having an associated anomaly, such as obstruction, vesicoureteral reflux, urinary stasis, or renal stone. History of recent or ongoing infection outside the urinary tract should be elicited because renal disease such as acute GN may be associated with streptococcal pharyngitis or impetigo, shunt nephritis associated with infection of a ventriculoatrial or peritoneal shunt, and the GN of subacute bacterial endocarditis.

Psychosocial History
Evaluation of family dynamics is of primary importance in enuresis and suspected psychogenic DI. Children should be asked about the tendency to hold their urine and about availability, accessibility, and use of bathrooms at school.

Dietary History
Dietary intake is important in the evaluation of a child with polyuria or polydipsia. Excessive intake of foods generating a large osmolar load (such as milk or peanut butter) can lead to these symptoms in small infants because their urine-concentrating ability is limited. These signs will abate with dietary adjustments. On the other hand, children with genuine DI will often spontaneously curtail their intake of protein and favor high-carbohydrate foods. History of anorexia and decreased intake, also associated with spontaneous avoidance of protein foods, characterizes a child with CKD. A dietary review to determine daily sodium intake is important in a child with hypertension.

Drug Intake
Various drugs are nephrotoxic, producing a decrease in GFR. The most commonly used of these are loop diuretics, such as furosemide, and the aminoglycoside antibiotics. In patients suspected of having aminoglycoside nephrotoxicity, a review of the drug levels obtained during the course

of therapy is essential because nephrotoxicity is often related to elevated trough levels. Loop diuretics and aminoglycosides can decrease GFR with no detectable decrease in urine output (high-output renal failure). Semi-synthetic penicillins, such as methicillin, are notorious for causing interstitial nephritis, manifesting primarily as hematuria and decreased GFR. Such patients show other symptoms suggesting a drug reaction, such as fever, skin rash, or eosinophilia.

Keep in mind that although renal prostaglandins play a minor role in determining renal function in normal children and adults, they are of major importance in preserving renal function in newborns and in conditions associated with renal hypoperfusion. Thus prostaglandin inhibitors, such as aspirin or nonsteroidal anti-inflammatory drugs, can lead to an acute decrease in GFR in newborns (eg, when given to close a patent ductus arteriosus) and in older children with preexisting renal dysfunction.

Intake of drugs leading to renal dysfunction should be considered in the evaluation of a child undergoing treatment for a malignancy. Chemotherapy given to a child with a large tumor mass can lead to hyperuricemia and consequent acute obstructive uric acid nephropathy with renal failure. Vincristine is known to cause SIADH. Amphotericin B, used for the treatment of various systemic fungal infections, often leads to hypokalemia and a dose-dependent decrease in GFR.

Physical Examination

General Appearance

Potter syndrome is the name initially used to describe bilateral renal agenesis. It consists of typical facies with flattened midportion of the face, wide-set eyes, beaked nose, low-set ears, and a prominent fold originating at the inner canthus of the eye, often with clubbing of the feet and pulmonary hypoplasia (Figure 18-1). Height and weight should be measured and plotted on appropriate growth charts; failure to thrive or growth retardation can be a clue to renal disease, whereas obesity is often accompanied by high BP. Assessment of hydration status is obviously important; dehydration in a child with azotemia would suggest prerenal etiology. Edema should be noted because it may indicate hypoproteinemia or fluid overload. Congenital anomalies, such as hemihypertrophy and ambiguous genitalia, should be noted.

Vital Signs

Fever in younger children can be the only sign of UTI. About 7% of female infants with unexplained fever may have a UTI. Blood pressure measurement should be an integral part of a complete physical examination, even in infants and younger children, and should be interpreted in relation to age and sex by comparing to normal values (Chapter 15). Hypertension is defined as the average systolic and/or diastolic BP equal to or greater than the 95th percentile for age and sex on at least 3 separate occasions. It is important to use the appropriate cuff in measuring BP. A small cuff will result in overestimation of the BP, whereas too large a cuff will underestimate it. Using the wrong size cuff is a very common cause of alarming BP readings in pediatrics.

The use of a Dinamap monitor, an oscillometric device, has gained popularity in clinics and hospitals because of its ease of use, especially with small, uncooperative children. Although this method is fairly reliable for general screening and monitoring, values outside the normal range should be confirmed by the auscultatory method. If an elevated reading is obtained, BP should be measured in the 4 extremities because aortic coarctation is a very common cause of hypertension in younger children.

Tachycardia as a sign of congestive heart failure should be noted in evaluating an azotemic child because prerenal failure can occur as a result of low cardiac output. An increased respiratory rate can suggest metabolic acidosis with respiratory compensation through hyperventilation.

Skin

Patients with CKD may have pallor due to anemia or a yellowish discoloration of their skin. Various other skin changes or rashes can accompany renal disease. Alopecia, lanugo hair, or a malar rash in a child being investigated for hematuria or proteinuria suggests SLE. A palpable purpuric rash localized over the buttocks or lower extremities is typical of anaphylactoid (Henoch-Schönlein) purpura, as is localized edema over the scalp, face, scrotum, or extremities. Adenoma sebaceum in a butterfly distribution around the nose is a common finding in tuberous sclerosis, a condition often accompanied by renal tumors. Neurofibromas or café-au-lait spots (Von Recklinghausen disease) in a hypertensive child raise the suspicion of vascular hypertension and pheochromocytoma, which is rare in the pediatric age group.

Eyes

Aniridia, or absence of the iris of the eye, may be associated with Wilms tumor. Eye abnormalities primarily involving the lens, such as cataracts, can be observed in older patients with Alport syndrome, as well as in patients with the Lowe oculocerebrorenal syndrome (Fanconi syndrome with mental retardation and ocular abnormalities). Slit-lamp examination of the eye is mandatory in a child with Fanconi syndrome to look for corneal or retinal deposition of cystine crystals that are diagnostic of cystinosis. Fundoscopic examination, looking for hypertensive changes, helps differentiate acute from chronic hypertension. Hypertensive changes are classified into 4 grades: grade I—increased arteriolar light reflex; grade II—arteriovenous nicking; grade III—cotton wool exudates and flame-shaped hemorrhages; and grade IV—papilledema. Grades I and II suggest chronic hypertension, whereas III and IV usually accompany acute increases in arterial pressure; papilledema is seen in malignant hypertension.

Heart and Lungs

Patients with congenital heart disease, particularly ventricular septal defect, are associated with a higher incidence of renal anomalies than the general population. The presence of a hemic murmur can suggest anemia, a frequent finding in CKD. Careful cardiac examination should be performed, especially in a child with hypertension. A murmur best heard at the second or third intercostal space along the sternal edge and radiating to the back or a soft systolic murmur of collateral flow heard around the left scapular area suggests aortic coarctation, a common cause of hypertension in younger children. Femoral pulses should be palpated. In a child with hypertension, cardiomegaly, signs of congestive heart failure due to increased afterload, or cardiac arrhythmias should be sought. Decreased cardiac output can be the cause of prerenal failure. In a child with azotemia, signs of congestive heart failure should be noted, including accessory heart sounds, a gallop rhythm, or venous congestion (prominent neck veins, hepatomegaly, or peripheral edema).

Lungs should be examined for the presence of rales that suggest congestive heart failure due either to a primary cardiac problem or to fluid overload. Signs of pleural effusion (decrease in breath sounds and dullness to percussion around the base of the lung) can often be detected in edematous patients with NS.

Abdomen

The widespread use of prenatal ultrasonography should not obviate careful palpation of the abdomen for an abdominal mass. In newborns, a patent urachus can be suspected from passage of urine from the umbilicus; it is easily ligated surgically. The abdomen should be examined for absence or laxity of the abdominal muscles (prune-belly). Presence of meningomyelocele or anal atresia should be noted. Large abdominal masses can obviously manifest as abdominal distension with an increased abdominal girth.

The location of an abdominal mass, as well as its surface characteristics, can help determine its etiology. Upper abdominal masses most likely arise from the kidneys, adrenal glands, liver, or spleen. In older children, polycystic kidneys can sometimes be palpated as bilateral flank masses. It is often mentioned that the mass of hydronephrosis is smooth and cystic, whereas that of a Wilms tumor is smooth and firm and that of neuroblastoma is nodular. A pelvic mass in a boy suggests an enlarged bladder with outlet obstruction, whereas in a girl it is more likely to be a hydrocolpos.

The abdomen should be examined for ascites. Bulging flanks with dullness to percussion, while the periumbilical area remains tympanic, suggest the presence of ascites. A fluid wave is obtained with difficulty in children. Shifting dullness may be easily demonstrated. A small amount of fluid is difficult to detect by physical examination, and ultrasonography of the abdomen may be necessary. In a child with nephrotic ascites, the abdominal girth should be measured. This is best done with the child standing and always at a fixed distance from a landmark such as the umbilicus.

Flank tenderness should be elicited on both sides by gently tapping the costovertebral angle with a closed fist. Auscultation of the abdomen is likely to be unrevealing in a child with renal disease. However, in the presence of hypertension, a flank bruit should be sought by listening over the flank with the bell of the stethoscope in a quiet environment. The presence of hypertension suggests renovascular etiology of the hypertension.

The suprapubic area should be examined. Exstrophy of the bladder is obvious. The bladder is not palpable in a normal child. A palpable bladder with a thickened wall suggests hypertrophy owing to an anatomical obstruction, such as PUVs, or increased bladder work as can occur with severe reflux. Suprapubic tenderness is often present in a child with cystitis. Bladder fullness can be assessed by percussion. Urinary retention in a child with a neurologic problem (cerebral palsy or meningomyelocele) can predispose to UTI.

Extremities

The extremities should be examined for pitting edema, most apparent over the tibia and median malleolus. In a bedridden patient, edema is more easily noticed in the presacral area. Arthritis suggests a connective tissue disease such as SLE and is a component of Henoch-Schönlein purpura, the most common vasculitis of childhood. Skeletal abnormalities, such as bowing of the legs, can be a sign of renal osteodystrophy in children with CKD and also commonly occur in children with RTA or hypophosphatemic rickets.

Genitalia

Examination of the external genitalia is an important part of the evaluation of a child with abnormal urinary findings such as hematuria or pyuria. The urethral meatus should be examined for ulcerations, erosions, or prolapse that would explain the presence of RBCs in the urine. A normal meatus in a boy is a 2- to 3-mm slit. Adhesions can lead to meatal stenosis, with dysuria or genital discomfort. It should be noted whether a boy is circumcised or not because uncircumcised boys have a much higher incidence of UTIs than those who are circumcised. Poor hygiene, especially in uncircumcised boys, or vulvovaginitis in girls, can lead to the urethral triad and to the presence of white cells or squamous cells in the urine. Signs of sexual abuse should also be sought.

The child's underwear should be examined. Wet underwear in a child who is toilet trained can be a sign of urinary urgency due to a UTI or suggest vaginal reflux. Encopresis could also explain the occurrence of UTI in a child with an otherwise normal urinary tract. Cryptorchidism, hypospadias, or the presence of ambiguous genitalia should be noted.

Voiding

Physical examination of an infant or child with a reported voiding abnormality should include, if possible, actual observation of voiding. This is particularly important in boys because of a higher incidence of bladder outlet obstructive lesions. Children with PUVs will strain to urinate and exhibit a weak stream or dribbling. On the other hand, a child with meatal stenosis will have a strong but very thin stream. A child who is able to void a sizable amount of urine soon after emptying the bladder should be suspected of retention.

Rectal Examination

Rectal examination can be useful to evaluate an abdominal mass. It is also important to assess the rectal sphincter in a child with new onset of incontinence. Eliciting the bulbocavernosus reflex (squeezing the glans and observing rectal sphincter contraction) is indicated when a neurologic deficit is suspected.

Neurologic Examination

Audiometry should be performed when a child with unexplained hematuria or decreased renal function is suspected of having Alport syndrome. High-frequency sensorineural loss is the typical finding in this condition; hearing impairment is often not noted clinically because it does not involve speech range. Sensorineural hearing loss can also result from the use of 2 common classes of nephrotoxic drugs, namely loop diuretics and aminoglycoside antibiotics. Various cranial nerve palsies, including facial (VII) and ocular (III) nerve palsies, can result from severe hypertension.

References

1. Avner ED, Harmon WE, Niaudet P. *Pediatric Nephrology.* 5th ed. Baltimore, MD: Lippincott Williams and Wilkins; 2003
2. Barakat AY, ed. *Renal Disease in Children: Clinical Evaluation and Diagnosis.* New York, NY: Springer-Verlag; 1990
3. Belman AB, King LR, Kramer SA. *Clinical Pediatric Urology.* 4th ed. London, UK: M Dunitz; 2002
4. Kaplan BS, Meyers KEC. *Pediatric Nephrology and Urology.* St Louis, MO: Mosby; 2004
5. Neveus T. The new International Children's Continence Society's terminology for the paediatric lower urinary tract—why it has been set up and why we should use it. *Pediatr Nephrol.* 2008;23:1931–1932

Chapter 3

Examination of the Urine

Agnes B. Fogo and Amin J. Barakat

Abbreviations

ATN	Acute tubular necrosis
DNP	Dinitrophenylhydrazine
GN	Glomerulonephritis
HCO_3^-	Bicarbonate
hpf	High-power field
K	Potassium
Na	Sodium
NS	Nephrotic syndrome
Posm	Plasma osmolality
RBC	Red blood cell
RTA	Renal tubular acidosis
sg	Specific gravity
SLE	Systemic lupus erythematosus
TS	Total solid
Uosm	Urine osmolality
UTI	Urinary tract infection
WBC	White blood cell

Introduction

A carefully performed urinalysis using physical, chemical, and microscopic examination offers important information regarding the kidney.[1-9] The results of any urinalysis depend on proper collection, preservation, and careful examination. Numerous specific tests are also available for specific diagnoses

ℰ❧ Pearl

A carefully performed urinalysis using physical, chemical, and microscopic examination offers important information regarding the kidney.

when indicated by initial routine screening tests. Urinalysis is an easy and informative tool to the practicing physician. Primary care physicians should be comfortable performing and interpreting urinalyses.

Specimen Collection and Preservation

The urine should be collected in a clean, dry container. First morning voided specimens yield the most concentrated urine and are more likely to show formed elements and allow detection of bacteria because of overnight incubation in the bladder. Preservation methods are necessary if the urine is not tested within 1 hour of collection. Adequate preservation for 24 hours without interference with routine dipstick tests may be achieved by refrigeration or the use of chemicals. No available method is adequate for prolonged preservation of RBCs.

Urine culture requires a "clean-catch" midstream specimen collected into a sterile, covered container. The area around the urethral meatus should be cleaned with an antiseptic solution in a front-to-back fashion in females and with the foreskin retracted in uncircumcised males. The first few milliliters of the voided specimen are voided outside before the clean-catch sample is collected. For infants and small children, special plastic bags with adhesive may be used. The entire perineal area covered by the bag is cleaned, avoiding fecal contamination. The bag should be checked every 15 minutes to ensure a clean urine collection. One-third of infants will produce a urine specimen within the first hour. Suprapubic needle aspiration is an alternative method that should be performed by experienced physicians and only if necessary (Chapter 6).

For routine urinalysis, about 10 mL of urine is needed, although a much smaller sample (2.5 mL) is sufficient to perform a multiple reagent strip, copper reducing test, and sg. A timed urine collection, usually 24 hours, may be necessary for quantitative determination of various substances. To start the collection, the bladder is emptied, discarding the initial urine voided. The time is noted, and all urine for the next 24 hours is collected. The normal 24-hour volume increases from 15 to 60 mL in the term newborn to 250 to 450 mL at 2 months of age, to an adult range of 700 to 1,500 mL by 8 years of age. Adequacy of a 24-hour collection may be assessed by measuring the amount of creatinine excreted and comparing it to ranges for age and body weight (usually 8–20 mg/kg/d). For accurate results, the sample must be complete and the container should be refrigerated during the collection period. Special precautions are necessary for some collections, such as vanillylmandelic acid, calcium, citrate, oxalate steroids, and others. The most commonly used procedures for collection should be verified with the reference laboratory used because methods may vary.

ॐ *Pearl*

A first morning voided specimen is more likely to show formed elements and bacteria. Urine culture requires a clean-catch midstream specimen.

Quality Control and Instrumentation

Quality control involves all aspects of specimen handling and ensures accurate results. Specimen identification is the most likely area for errors. It is imperative that the container (not the lid) be properly labeled and that identification of the sample is maintained throughout transportation, specimen preparation, and testing until the results are correctly recorded. Known positive and negative controls should be run routinely in the laboratory to ensure that test procedures and reagents give correct results. Corrective action should be taken if results do not fall within the known and expected range. Urine must be at room temperature during testing, and the color change must be read at the right time interval. Any excess of urine must be properly drained off because "run-over" (reagent buffers from one area of the strip seeping over to another) may give false results.

Instruments in the clinical laboratory should be checked regularly to ensure proper performance. Reagent strips must be stored in a cool, dry place and should not be refrigerated. A loose cap on the container may result in deterioration of the reagents and cause false-positive or false-negative results. Reagent strips are usually read by automation. The TS refractometer used to measure the sg should be calibrated periodically. Automated urine cell analyzers are available.

ॐ *Pearl*

Instruments in the clinical laboratory should be checked regularly, and controls should be run routinely.

Physical Examination

Gross examination of the urine provides important information. Normal urine is clear, transparent, and yellow in color due to the presence of the pigment urochrome and urobilin, a breakdown product of hemoglobin. The appearance may be altered by the presence of cellular or other material. Substances that change urine color and appearance are presented in Table 3-1.

The odor of urine reflects its components, although it is seldom diagnostic. Freshly voided normal urine has an aromatic odor due to volatile acids. On standing, a characteristic ammonia odor results from degradation of urea. In some diseases, urine does have an unusual characteristic odor. The urine of diabetics has a fruity odor due to acetone. Foul or putrid odor is indicative of infection. Maple syrup disease derives its name from the characteristic scent of the urine. Other metabolic diseases with an abnormal odor include phenylketonuria (musty) and hypermethioninemia (fishy).

ও Pearl

Change in appearance or color of urine may indicate disease.

Any persistent unusual odor of urine in infants should alert the physician to the possibility of a metabolic disorder, and appropriate screening tests should be done (see following sections).

Specific Gravity

The sg of urine reflects the relative proportion of solutes in a given volume of urine. Urea, creatinine, chlorides, sulfates, phosphates, and bicarbonates compose 70% to 90% of the sg; the remainder reflects the presence of various organic compounds. Specific gravity may range from 1.003 to 1.030, but it usually remains between 1.010 and 1.025. An sg of 1.023 or more in any random urine specimen indicates normal concentrating ability. Water diuresis can decrease urine sg to 1.001. Abnormally low values may be a result of intrinsic renal loss of concentrating ability, central or nephrogenic diabetes insipidus, or polydipsia. The most common causes of an increase in sg are dehydration, elevated urinary protein and glucose, and the presence of preservatives or contrast media. Specific gravity may also help in differentiating prerenal failure (elevated sg and urine Na^+ <20 mEq/L) from ATN (sg <1.012, and elevated urine Na^+ up to 60 mEq/L).

Table 3-1. Urine Appearance	
Appearance	**Cause**
Clear, colorless, or pale yellow	Dilute—increased fluid intake, diabetes mellitus, or diabetes insipidus
Turbid or cloudy	Amorphous phosphates or carbonates with alkaline pH, urates (pinkish), cells, bacteria, yeast, spermatozoa, mucin, x-ray media, fecal contamination
Milky	Fat (nephrosis), chyle (lymphatic obstruction), pus
Yellow-orange to yellow-brown	Concentrated, urobilin, bilirubin, pyridium, nitrofurantoin, dilantin, acriflavine (green fluorescence)
Red to red-brown	Hemoglobin, RBC, myoglobin, porphyrin, beet ingestion, aniline dyes (candy), rifampin, theophylline, iodine
Brown-black	Phenothiazines, methyldopa, metronidazole, phenols
Brown-black to brown-purple on standing	Porphyrins, melanins, homogentisic acid (alkaptonuria)
Red-pink	Phenolsulfonphthalein, bromsulphalein, rhubarb
Blue-green	*Pseudomonas*, methylene blue, amitriptyline, methocarbamol, chlorophyll pigment (mouthwash), riboflavin
Yellow-green	Bilirubin, biliverdin

Abbreviation: RBC, red blood cell.

Multistix 10 SG reagent strip (Miles Laboratories, Elkhart, IN) is the most convenient way to measure urine sg. The color of the strip changes with the ion concentration in the specimen, and the changes are empirically correlated to sg levels and given as increments of 0.005 between 1.000 and 1.030. Elevated glucose, urea, or nonionic contrast dyes will not influence the result, whereas increased protein (which may be ionic) may cause elevated sg. Alkaline or highly buffered urine may give falsely low readings. Correction by adding 0.005 to the sg if urine pH is higher than 6.5 is therefore recommended.

Specific gravity may be measured also by a urinometer, which measures sg based on buoyancy, and the TS refractometer. The latter is a handheld instrument that measures the refractive index of a solution, which is directly proportional to the sg. The TS meter has the further advantage of requiring only one drop of urine, but it has to be calibrated daily with distilled water and adjusted if necessary to give an sg of 1.000. Both instruments will show an increased sg in the presence of increased glucose, protein, or contrast media. The sg increases by 0.003 for each 1 g protein/100 mL, 0.004 for each 1 g glucose/100 mL, and 0.001 for each 0.15 g NaCl/100 mL. The newest advance in sg measurement, the falling drop direct method, is currently available in some automated urinalysis instruments.

Although both sg and osmolality reflect solute concentration, the latter is a measure of the number of particles in a solution and is not affected by the weight of the solutes. Osmolality thus reflects the concentrating ability of the renal tubules. Osmolality is measured by freezing point depression or by vapor pressure depression; 1 osm of any solute added to 1 kg water lowers the freezing point of water by 1.86°C. The normal range in a newborn is 15 to 585 mOsm/kg, with a mean of 240 mOsm/kg. Regular diet and kidney maturation increase the normal range in children to 300 to 800 mOsm/kg. Neonates normally have some concentrating ability and are able to increase osmolality to a mean of 950 mOsm/kg after 12 to 14 hours of fluid deprivation. By 2 years of age, the concentrating ability after dehydration approaches the adult range (1,200 mOsm/kg). Osmolality of less than 800 mOsm/kg after water deprivation indicates a loss of concentrating ability. With advanced renal disease, Uosm approaches that of plasma and the glomerular filtrate (285 mOsm/kg), indicating complete loss of diluting or concentrating ability of the renal tubule. In prerenal failure, Uosm remains greater than Posm, whereas in ATN they become similar.

> ## ◈ Pearl
>
> Specific gravity of 1.023 or more in any random urine specimen indicates normal concentrating ability. In prerenal failure, Uosm remains higher than Posm; in ATN, they become similar.

Chemical Examination

Routine chemical screening assays of urine are often done by reagent strip testing. These consist of a plastic strip with multiple pads, each impregnated with specific reagents, indicators, and buffers. The reagent portion is immersed into the fresh, well-mixed urine specimen and immediately removed. The excess urine is removed by running the edge of the strip against the container rim, and the color change of the strip is compared under adequate light at the appropriate reading time with the standard color chart provided by the manufacturer. The Clinitek Atlas automated urine chemistry analyzer is a fully automated spectrophotometer that reads these colorimetric reactions on the reagent strips. It also reads sg by an optic refractive method. Proper storage and handling of reagent strips with appropriate quality control is imperative. Some substances that color urine (azo dye–containing drugs, pyridium, nitrofurantoin) may interfere with or mask the proper reagent strip color reactions. Confirmatory or more specific tests may be performed by separate chemical assays. The characteristics of reagent strips used in urinalysis are presented in Table 3-2.

pH

Normal urine pH varies from 4.5 to 8.5; however, urine is normally slightly acidic due to acid production from normal metabolism. Urine pH is usually determined by a strip indicator sensitive to pH changes. Strips detect pH reliably from 5.0 to 8.5. More precise measurements, when indicated, such as in suspected cases of RTA, may be done on a freshly voided specimen using a pH meter with a glass electrode.

The kidney normally excretes 50 to 100 mEq of hydrogen daily as titratable acid and ammonium. Transient acidity may occur after eating cranberries or after high protein intake. Persistent increase in urinary acidity may be present with respiratory or metabolic acidosis, fever, phenylketonuria, alkaptonuria, methanol intoxication, renal tuberculosis, severe diarrhea, starvation, or uremia.

Alkaline urine is seen if a urine sample has been allowed to stand for a prolonged time interval, thus allowing the escape of carbon dioxide and conversion of urea to ammonia. Postprandially, urine is normally alkaline. Diets high in citrate (oranges), infection with urea-splitting organisms, respiratory or metabolic alkalosis, hyperaldosteronism, Cushing syndrome, and RTA also cause alkaline urine.

Protein

Urine contains small amounts of protein, normally 100 mg/m^2/24 hours. In children, two-thirds of the physiologic urine protein consists of albumin and one-third represents a mixture of Tamm-Horsfall protein and globulin. This ratio is reversed in adults. Tamm-Horsfall protein, a large glycoprotein, may be present normally at a concentration of 2 to 2.5 mg/dL.

Protein may be detected by reagent strips that use buffered tetrabromophenol blue (N-Multistix, Miles Laboratories) or tetrachlorophenoltetrabromo-sulfophthalein (Chemstrip, Boehringer, Ingelheim, Germany)

Table 3-2. Characteristics of Reagent Strips Used in Urinalysis

Test	Chemstrip	Multistix	False-Positive Results	False-Negative Results
pH	5–9	5–8.5 visual 5–9.0 pH meter	None	None
Protein	6 mg/dL (albumin)	15–30 mg/dL (albumin)	Highly alkaline urine,[b] phenazo-pyridine,[a] antiseptics, and urine detergents[a,b]	Low levels of proteins other than albumin, very dilute urine, pH <4.5[a,b]
Glucose	40 mg/dL	75–125 mg/dL	Peroxide, oxidizing cleaning agents	Decreased sensitivity: high sg,[a,b] ketones >40 mg/dL[b]
Ketones	9 mg/dL (acetoacetic acid) 70 mg/dL (acetone)	5–10 mg/dL (acetoacetic acid)	Phenylketones, phenolphthalein, levodopa metabolites (red reaction vs violet for ketones), highly pigmented urines, sulfhydryl-containing compounds,[a,b] high sg[b]	
Blood	0.03 mg/dL hemo-globin, 5 RBC/hpf	0.015–0.062 mg/dL hemo-globin, 5–20 RBC/hpf	Myoglobin, bacterial peroxidases, oxidizing cleaning agents, men-strual contamination[a,b]	Decreased sensitivity: high protein, ascorbic acid, high sg[b]
Bilirubin	0.5 mg/dL	0.4–0.8 mg/dL	Pyridium, indican, other sub-stances that color urine red, chlorpromazine?[a,b]	Ascorbic acid >25 mg/dL, light exposure[a,b], decreased sensitivity: high nitrite[a]

Abbreviations: RBC, red blood cell; hpf, high-power field; WBC, white blood cell; sg, specific gravity.

[a]Chemstrip test used.

[b]Multistix test used.

		Table 3-2. Characteristics of Reagent Strips Used in Urinalysis, continued		
Test	**Chemstrip**	**Multistix**	**False-Positive Results**	**False-Negative Results**
Urobilinogen	0.4 mg/dL	0.2 mg/dL	Phenazopyridine,[a] Ehrlich reagent interfering substances (sulfon-amides, p-aminobenzoic acid)	Decreased sensitivity: formalin >200 mg/dL, light exposure[a,b]; nitrite >5 mg/dL [a]
Nitrite	0.05 mg/dL	0.06–0.1 mg/dL	Substances coloring urine red[a,b]	Decreased sensitivity: high sg, short bladder incubation, ascorbic acid >25 mg/dL[a,b]
Leukocytes	92.7% sensitivity correlates with >105 bacteria/mL	5–15 WBC/hpf correlates with >105 colonies/mL	Oxidizing cleaning agents, nitro-furantoin[b]	Cephalocin, gentamicin, albumin >500 mg/dL[a]; decreased sensitivity: glucose >3 g/dL, high sg, tetracycline, high-concentration oxalic acid[b]; cephalexin[a,b]

Abbreviations: RBC, red blood cell; hpf, high-power field; WBC, white blood cell; sg, specific gravity.

[a]Chemstrip test used.

[b]Multistix test used.

indicators. At a constant pH, the binding of the protein to the reagent results in changing colors from yellow to green-blue with increasing protein concentrations (from 30 to >1,000 mg/dL). The reagent strips are much more sensitive to albumin than globulins, hemoglobin, or Bence-Jones protein (see Table 3-2). High-performance liquid chromatography may be indicated as a sensitive and specific test to detect significant albuminuria early in high-risk patients (ie, those with kidney disease, hypertension, or diabetes). Qualitative testing for protein may also be obtained by precipitation methods, by heating, or by adding sulfosalicylic acid. The latter method is more sensitive, detecting as low as 5 to 10 mg/dL of all urine proteins, including albumin, globulins, glycoproteins, and Bence-Jones protein.

Quantitative protein determination on a timed (24-hour) collection is done by precipitation methods, heat and acetic acid precipitation being the most sensitive and detecting protein levels as low as 2 to 3 mg/dL. False-positive acid precipitation may occur with some radiographic contrast media. A semiquantitative method is the urine protein/creatinine ratio (Chapter 8).

Marked proteinuria (>4 g/1.73 m^2/d) may be seen in amyloidosis, severe GN, SLE, malignant nephrosclerosis, or severe renal venous congestion such as renal vein thrombosis. Moderate proteinuria (0.5–4 g/1.73 m^2/d) may be seen in most renal diseases, including any of the types listed earlier, diabetic nephropathy, preeclampsia, interstitial diseases, or lower urinary tract disease. Mild proteinuria (<0.5 g/1.73 m^2/d) may be present in chronic GN, tubular diseases, polycystic kidney disease, or nephrosclerosis without malignant hypertension. Proteinuria is nephrotic when it is greater than 40 mg/m^2/h or 50 mg/kg/d.

Postural or orthostatic proteinuria is a benign condition occurring only when a child is in the upright position. Nonrenal conditions such as strenuous exercise, fever, emotional stress, cold or heat exposure, or congestive heart failure may all be associated with functional proteinuria (Chapter 8).

ᕱ❧ Pearl

A semiquantitative method of measuring protein in the urine is the urine protein/creatinine ratio.

Glucose and Reducing Substances

Reducing substances in urine are normally very low (<100 mg/dL); most are contributed by glucose. The amount of glucosuria depends on the blood glucose level and the amount of tubular reabsorption. The normal renal threshold for glucose is 160 to 180 mg/dL, although some patients may have a benign congenitally lowered renal glucose threshold.

Screening tests for sugars in the urine employ either glucose oxidase, which is specific for glucose, or copper reduction tests, which react with any reducing substance. The glucose oxidase test becomes less sensitive as the urine sg increases. When indicated, the specific nonglucose sugar in the urine may be identified by paper chromatography.

The commonly used multiple reagent strips N-Multistix and Chemstrip both use glucose oxidase and detect 75 to 100 mg/dL and 40 mg/dL, respectively. Moderately high ketones (40 mg/dL) may decrease sensitivity for trace glucose levels with N-Multistix. Significant glucosuria is usually an indication of diabetes mellitus. Other possible causes of hyperglycemia and glucosuria, such as some endocrinopathies, glycogen storage diseases, thiazide diuretics, or steroid administration, should be considered. Postprandially, glucose in blood and urine may be transiently elevated. Glucosuria without hyperglycemia is seen in some tubular defects, such as Fanconi syndrome, cystinosis, and lead poisoning.

Spillover of carbohydrate in the urine occurs in disorders of carbohydrate metabolism (galactosuria, lactosuria, fructosuria, pentosuria) or may be physiologic due to increased ingestion of the sugar. The most significant in children is galactose resulting from an inborn error of metabolism (galactose-1-phosphate uridyl transferase deficiency). Lactose may be seen in patients with lactase deficiency. Lactosuria is common in premature infants and newborns until 3 to 4 days of age, when the gastrointestinal flora is established. Pentosuria may rarely occur because of an inborn error of metabolism, but it is more commonly a result of ingestion of large amounts of cherries or plums.

Ketones

The ketone bodies acetoacetic acid, β-hydroxybutyric acid, and acetone are intermediates of fatty acid metabolism with normal proportions of 20%, 78%, and 2%, respectively. Small amounts (2–4 mg/dL) are normally present in the blood, with increases seen after the renal excretory capacity has been overcome.

Screening tests use the sodium nitroprusside or nitroferricyanide reaction to acetoacetic acid as an indicator of the presence of ketone bodies. Sensitivity is 5 to 10 mg/dL. Normal urine levels are up to 2 mg/dL of acetoacetic acid and 20 mg total ketones. Ketosis may develop in any conditions associated with abnormal or decreased carbohydrate metabolism such as diabetes mellitus, low carbohydrate intake as in prolonged vomiting or starvation, low carbohydrate levels relative to increased metabolic demands seen in severe prolonged exercise, or glycogen storage disease.

Blood

Red blood cells in the urine may originate from any site of the urinary tract from glomerulus to urethra. Bleeding may be microscopic or gross. Hematuria may be seen in numerous diseases (Chapter 7). When hematuria is renal in origin, proteinuria and casts are also often seen.

The normal range of RBC excretion in the urine is wide. Quantitative studies indicate normal ranges of 240,000 RBCs or less per 12 hours, with lower levels for females. In most laboratories, by standard methods, these values correspond to 1 RBC per 2 to 3 hpf, or approximately 500 RBC/mL; however, up to 3 RBC/hpf may be considered normal. The detection of blood is based on the lysis of the RBC and the peroxide-like activity of the released hemoglobin. Intact RBCs produce a speckled pattern, in contrast to the smooth color change seen with hemoglobin (see later discussion). When sg is 1.004 or less, RBCs will be almost completely lysed within 2 hours. In acid urine (pH <6), some lysis also occurs. Therefore, RBCs may not be detected on microscopic examination under these conditions, although the hemoglobin dipstick test will detect the hemoglobin released from lysis. None of the preservative reagents adequately preserve blood over a 24-hour period. Interference with the dipstick test is presented in Table 3-2.

✏ Pearl

Red blood cells in urine may originate from any site of the urinary tract. Renal hematuria is usually accompanied by proteinuria and RBC casts.

Hemoglobin and Myoglobin

Hemoglobinuria, like hematuria, produces red discoloration of the urine and gives a positive dipstick test for blood. Chemical and microscopic examinations on a freshly voided specimen are necessary to differentiate the two. Hemoglobinuria without hematuria is the result of excess free hemoglobin in the blood and is seen with hemolytic anemia; transfusion reactions; paroxysmal nocturnal hematuria; paroxysmal cold hemoglobinuria; severe infectious diseases; after severe burns; renal infarcts; poisoning with snake venoms, mushrooms, or strong acids, and strenuous exercise and with some prosthetic heart valves.

Myoglobin is derived from skeletal muscle and is a small, easily filtered molecule that is seen in the urine following muscular damage such as that caused by trauma, convulsions, prolonged severe exercise, heatstroke, electric shock injury, myocardial infarction, and other injuries. Acute kidney injury may result from high levels due to renal tubular cell toxicity. Both hemoglobin and myoglobin are detected by their peroxidase-like activity. The Multistix and Chemstrip reagent pads cause lysis of intact RBCs when they touch the reagent area. The result is that free hemoglobin or myoglobin gives a uniform green color, whereas the lysis of intact RBCs on the reagent pad causes a green spot or speckled reaction. The sensitivity ranges are 0.015 to 0.016 mg/dL of free hemoglobin or 5 to 20 RBC/hpf (see Table 3-2). Myoglobin can be differentiated from hemoglobin, although both produce clear red urine, because the plasma remains colorless with increased myoglobin in contrast to the red-pink plasma seen with hemoglobinemia. Additional tests, such as elevated serum creatine phosphokinase levels to detect muscle injury, electrophoresis, or ammonium sulphate tests (precipitates hemoglobin but not myoglobin), may also aid in the differentiation.

Bilirubin

Bilirubin is formed from hemoglobin breakdown and becomes water soluble when conjugated in the liver to glucuronide. Most bilirubin is excreted in the bile and enters the enterohepatic circulation. Intestinal bacteria further break bilirubin down to urobilinogen, a portion of which is reabsorbed. Small amounts of bilirubin and urobilinogen are normally excreted in the urine. Elevated urine bilirubin is seen with liver parenchymal disease.

Normal random urines may show trace positive reactions, and clinical correlation is necessary to interpret this finding. Substances that interfere with these tests are presented in Table 3-2.

Bacteria

Chemical testing for microorganisms is based on the presence of nitrite formed by bacterial reduction of the nitrates normally present in urine. Neither bacteria nor nitrite is present in normal clean-catch urine samples. Testing should be done on a first-morning void because urine must be incubated with the bacteria for at least 4 hours to allow nitrite formation. The sensitivity of this chemical test in an early morning specimen is about 90%.

࣌ *Pearl*

A positive nitrite test indicates the presence of significant bacteria, while a negative test does not rule out UTI.

A positive test indicates the presence of significant bacteria, whereas a negative test does not rule out UTI. False-negatives may be due to a short bladder incubation time or because the bacteria lack the reductase enzyme to produce nitrite. False-positive results may occur due to interference from agents that color the urine red. Occasionally, further reduction of nitrite to nonreacting nitrogen may occur. Rarely, a patient's diet, and thus the patient's urine, may be void of nitrate. Due to these factors, the degree to which the test is positive does not correlate with the degree of bacteria in the urine. With either Chemstrip or Multistix reagent strips, high levels of ascorbic acid (>25 mg/dL) decrease the sensitivity or may cause false-negative results with small amounts of nitrite.

Screening for WBCs using the presence of leukocyte esterase in these cells is also available. Leukocytes in the urine are most commonly due to infection, although they may be seen with various other conditions presented later in this chapter. The test detects the leukocyte esterase from intact and lysed WBCs. Sensitivity is 5 to 15 WBC/hpf for Multistix, which correlates well with 10^5 bacteria/mL or greater. The Chemstrip reagent has greater than 97% sensitivity for detection of significant bacteria. Test sensitivity is decreased with high sg, as well as elevated glucose, oxalic acid, albumin, and certain antibiotics (see Table 3-2).

Electrolytes

Measurement of electrolytes in the urine is performed by flame photometry without interference by other substances. Electrolyte values in the urine normally vary widely in response to diet and fluid intake. Sodium excretion is useful for volume status assessment and evaluation of acute kidney injury. Decreased urine Na^{+2} (<10–15 mEq/L) is most commonly seen with effective volume depletion. In acute kidney injury due to ATN, Na^{+2} is usually greater than 20 mEq/L, whereas in prerenal failure urine Na^{+2} is usually less than 20 mEq/L. Urinary Na^{+2} is also used to calculate the fractional excretion of Na^{+2}, the

> **Pearl**
>
> Urinary Na^{+2} is usually less than 20 mEq/L in prerenal failure and greater than 20 meq/L in ATN.

most accurate renal failure index. Chloride excretion parallels that of Na^{+2}, and thus urine chloride usually adds little information to that given by urine Na^{+2}. However, in cases of hypovolemia with metabolic alkalosis because some excess HCO_3^- is excreted as $NaHCO_3$, the resulting elevated urinary Na^{+2} concentration does not reflect the volume status. In this instance, urine chloride remains low and thus provides useful information.

Urine K^+ excretion reflects dietary intake. With K^+ depletion due to extrarenal losses or to diuretic use, excretion may fall to very low levels. Higher levels associated with hypokalemia suggest the presence of renal K^+ wasting. In renal failure, the ability to excrete K^+ is impaired. Thus urine K^+ is inappropriately low, and hyperkalemia ensues. Urine Na^{+2}/K^+ ratio may be of diagnostic value (see Appendix I).

Other Studies

Inborn Errors of Metabolism

When an inborn error of metabolism is suspected, specific diagnostic tests are performed. After routine urinalysis, a reducing substance test (eg, copper reduction test) or Clinitest (on fresh urine) will detect metabolic defects associated with increased carbohydrate excretion. If the glucose oxidase test is negative, the specific abnormal carbohydrates or reducing substances may be identified by specific enzymatic reactions, gas chromatography, or thin-layer chromatography.

The mucopolysaccharidoses are a specific group of diseases of carbohydrate metabolism owing to deficiency of one or more lysosomal enzymes. There is a resulting increase in urinary excretion of mucopolysaccharides and abnormalities due to accumulation within tissues. Screening on random or 24-hour urine samples is performed by precipitation, electrophoresis, or thin-layer chromatography tests. The mucopolysaccharidoses strip test is based on the metachromatic reaction of a basic dye with the anionic mucopolysaccharides. The toluidine blue test is based on the same reaction. False-positive results occur with heparin and numerous other substances.

The DNP test detects elevated ketoacids, which are seen in numerous conditions; among them are phenylketonuria, maple syrup urine disease, and tyrosinosis. Comparison with routine urinalysis is necessary because ketones also will give a positive result. Therefore, a positive DNP test is common in a neonate who normally excretes increased ketones. The cyanide nitroprusside test detects sulfhydryl-containing amino acids and thus is used to screen for cystinuria and homocystinuria. Dilute or highly acid urine may produce a false-negative reaction. The nitrosonaphthol test detects tyrosine and its metabolites. False-positive reactions may occur with gastrointestinal disease with bacterial overgrowth, resulting in increased p-hydroxyphenyl acetic acid. Specific tests are available to identify the elevated amino acids and other compounds.

The normal range of total urinary amino acids in children from 2½ to 12 years of age is 3.3 to 6.2 mg/kg/h, and in infants it is 3.8 to 6.5 mg/kg/h. If increased levels are detected by thin-layer chromatography, individual amino acids can be identified by specific reaction or separation techniques. Several spot screening tests are also available.

Disorders of purine or pyrimidine metabolism (such as Lesch-Nyhan, xanthinuria, orotic aciduria, and gout) are characterized by hyperuricemia and excess urates in the urine. An infant with these diseases may thus present with a red or pinkish-tinged diaper owing to excess urates. Examination of the urine identifies many of these abnormal crystals. Specific enzyme defects may be identified in some of these diseases.

Disorders of porphyrin metabolism may be detected by screening for urinary porphobilinogen. The urine may be deep red, turning darker with light exposure. Other screening tests detect other urinary porphyrins (coproporphyrin, uroporphyrin, protoporphyrin) by their red fluorescence under ultraviolet light after extraction. Specific quantification may then be done. Normal daily levels are 70 to 250 mg (coproporphyrin), 10 to 30 mg (uroporphyrin), 2 mg (porphobilinogen), and 1 to 7 mg (aminolevulinic acid).

Miscellaneous

Urine creatinine levels are used to assess renal clearance and adequacy of timed urine collections. The Jaffe reaction measures noncreatinine chromogens in the plasma that are not present in the urine. This offsets the overestimation of creatinine clearance caused by the low tubular secretion of creatinine. Thus the calculated creatinine clearance approximates the true glomerular filtration rate (Chapter 4).

Microscopic Examination

The urinary sediment may normally contain some elements from the kidney and urinary tract, such as crystals, low numbers of epithelial cells, RBCs, WBCs, and hyaline casts (Figure 3-1). Significant information can be

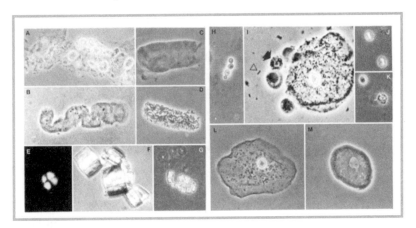

Figure 3-1.
Microscopic urinalysis (all by phase microscopy except E, which is polarized; magnification in parenthesis). **A.** Cellular cast (×200). **B.** Waxy cast (×200). **C.** Hyaline cast (×200). **D.** Coarse granular cast (×200). **E.** Talc-"Maltese cross" appearance (×500). **F.** Uric acid crystals (×500). **G.** Calcium oxalate crystals (×500). **H.** Yeast (×500). **I.** Large squamous epithelial cell with adjacent darkly granular polymorphonuclear leukocytes (arrow) and small, rod-shaped bacteria (triangle). **J.** Normal red blood cells (RBCs) (×500). **K.** Dysmorphic RBCs (×500). **L.** Renal epithelial cell (×500). **M.** Renal tubular cell (×500). RBC indicates red blood cell. (Reprinted with permission from Barakat AY. *Renal Disease in Children: Clinical Evaluation and Diagnosis.* New York, NY: Springer-Verlag; 1990:47–48.)

obtained from careful preparation and examination of the urinary sediment. The fresh or properly preserved sample should be thoroughly mixed prior to centrifugation. Ten milliliters is centrifuged at 400 rpm for 5 minutes. The supernatant is decanted, leaving a standard, uniform urine volume of 0.5 or 1.0 mL. If a stain is used, it should be added before the specimen is gently resuspended. One drop of the resuspended sediment is placed on a clean, labeled glass slide, covered with a 22 × 22 mm cover slip (avoiding air bubbles), and immediately examined. The entire slide must initially be examined at low power with special attention to the edges where formed elements tend to cluster. Findings are quantified over at least 10 low-power fields. High-power examination (40×) of 20 fields should be done and the urine elements counted. With conventional bright field microscopy, there is little contrast between urine and casts because of their similar refractive index. Optic contrast can be increased by a combination of shutting down the iris diaphragm, lowering the condenser, and decreasing the light source brightness. Staining of the sediment may also help visualization and identification of formed elements. Phase contrast microscopy amplifies phase differences and translates these into intensity differences that can be recognized by the human eye. Thus excellent visualization of all elements of the sediment is possible without staining.

⅔ Pearl

Excellent visualization of all elements of the urine sediment is possible without staining.

Various stains may be used, although the Sternheimer-Malbin stain is the most frequently used for WBCs, epithelial cells, and casts. Eosin stains RBCs but not yeast. Prussian blue stains hemosiderin, and the Papanicolaou stain is superior for identification and study of nucleated cells.

Cells

Normal urine contains epithelial cells, WBCs, and RBCs with a wide range of normal numbers. Based on laborious quantitative studies (Addis count) of urine collections from healthy patients, normal ranges for excretion over 24 hours are up to 130,000 RBCs; 650,000 WBCs and epithelial cells; and 2,000 hyaline casts.

Red blood cells are biconcave, anucleate cells measuring 6 to 7 μm in diameter. Normally, the urine may show up to 3 RBC/hpf. The morphology of the RBCs by phase microscopy or a simple Wright stain may indicate the source of bleeding. Dysmorphic RBCs with irregular membranes, distortion, and cell-to-cell variation indicate a glomerular origin of the RBCs, whereas RBCs with normal morphology suggest nonglomerular origin (Chapter 7). Crenated RBCs seen in hypotonic urine are symmetrical and show less variability than dysmorphic cells. A careful search for RBC casts is imperative because their presence is diagnostic of glomerular hematuria.

The presence of increased WBCs in urine is referred to as *pyuria* or *leukocyturia*. Polymorphonuclear leukocytes (pus cells) are larger than RBCs. They are round, have a characteristic multilobed nucleus, and measure 12 to 15 μm in diameter. The upper limit of normal WBC excretion is 5 WBC/hpf, although most clean-catch specimens have less than 1 WBC/hpf. More than 10 WBC/mm^3 on clean, midstream uncentrifuged urine using a counting chamber is considered abnormal. Pyuria may originate from any part of the urinary tract. Although the most common cause of pyuria is UTI, the absence of pyuria, particularly in preschool children, does not rule it out. Sterile pyuria may arise from various conditions including dehydration, fever, trauma from instrumentation, foreign body or calculus, chemical inflammation, gastrointestinal and respiratory infection, urogenital abnormalities, RTA, and GN. Pyuria persisting after infection has cleared should suggest urinary tract obstruction or congenital abnormality. Persistent pyuria requires adequate workup including cultures for anaerobes and tuberculosis, renal ultrasound, voiding cystourethrogram, and cystoscopy.

Renal tubular cells measure 15 to 24 μm in diameter and frequently have eccentric nuclei. Increased numbers (>15/hpf) are indicative of renal tubular damage such as ATN, papillary tip necrosis, or graft rejection. However, slightly increased numbers are normally seen in newborns. Renal tubular cells that have degenerated or are filled with lipid show a maltese cross formation under polarized light. These cells are called *oval fat bodies* and are characteristically seen in patients with the NS.

Bacteria, yeast, parasites, and ova may be present in the urine. Bacteria are very small rod-shaped or round cocci. The presence of any number of bacteria in a noncentrifuged clean-catch urine sample correlates well with more than 10^5 colonies/mL and suggests a UTI. Culture defines the specific organism and its sensitivity to antibiotics. Yeasts are 3 to 5 μm (smaller than RBCs); they do not lyse with acetic acid and do not stain with eosin.

🪸 Pearl

Normal urine may show up to 3 RBC/hpf. Sterile pyuria may be seen in patients with dehydration, fever, calculus, gastrointestinal and respiratory infection, and urogenital abnormalities

Mycelial branching forms or budding yeast may be present, the most common of which are the *Candida* species. Ova and parasites such as *Enterobius vermicularis* are most often due to fecal contamination.

Casts

Casts originate in the renal tubules and have a matrix composed of the Tamm-Horsfall mucoprotein. They are tubular in shape with rounded or blunted ends depending on the site of formation. They may be curved, straight, or convoluted. The absence of dark edges serves to differentiate them from fibers; artifacts that may appear castlike. Cast formation is increased with acid urine and low urine flow. Casts are classified based on their structure and components as hyaline, cellular, and mixed casts. Elements are added to the mucoprotein matrix before it is passed in the urine, thus the cast gives important information on processes occurring within the kidney at the site of formation.

The morphology of a cast is also dependent on how long it has been retained before passage, with a generally accepted progression from cellular to coarsely granular to finely granular to waxy. The cast diameter is dependent on the site and conditions of formation. Casts are usually uniform in diameter; being narrower in children than in adults. Narrow casts may indicate swollen tubular epithelium, which has reduced the tubular lumen size. Broad casts, often measuring more than 150 μm in diameter, may be seen with any type of casts but are most commonly waxy. They are usually of greater prognostic importance because they originate in collecting or abnormally dilated tubules and are the result of urinary stasis in the lower portion of the duct. Broad casts are formed when entire groups of nephrons have decreased functional capacity, and they are often described as renal failure casts.

Hyaline casts are the most commonly found and least diagnostic of the casts. They are colorless, homogeneous, and transparent. They are formed by precipitation of protein in the tubular lumen and may have additional elements, cells, and debris. A few hyaline casts are found in normal urine, and increased amounts are frequently present following physical exercise, diuretics, dehydration, and many types of renal disease. These casts have a refractile index similar to urine and therefore are more difficult to detect with bright field microscopy. Phase microscopy greatly enhances the ease of identification. Hyaline casts dissolve in water and in an alkaline medium and hence may not be seen in advanced renal failure where the urine is dilute and alkaline.

Cellular casts may contain epithelial or blood cells. Epithelial casts are formed by conglutination of desquamated cells from the epithelial lining of the tubule. Red blood cell casts are always pathologic and usually indicate glomerular bleeding. They may be present in any form of GN, renal infarction, renal vein thrombosis, or renal trauma. They appear as yellow-to-brown cylinders with variable numbers of RBCs identified. Degeneration and cell lysis produce a more homogeneous yellow-brown cast. White blood cell casts indicate renal origin of leukocytes and are indicative of pyelonephritis, interstitial nephritis, SLE, or other inflammatory diseases. They appear refractile and granular; the multilobed nucleus of the polymorphonuclear leukocyte is discernible unless the cast is too degenerated. Differentiation from epithelial cell casts may then be difficult. Occasional epithelial cells are expected within a cast owing to normal cell turnover. However, large numbers of these cells in a cast indicate tubular damage. Epithelial cell casts are often present with RBC and WBC casts in cases of GN or pyelonephritis. Staining, particularly with the Papanicolaou stain, facilitates differentiation between WBC and epithelial casts, accentuating the epithelial cell's single, round central nucleus.

With time, cellular casts begin to disintegrate, forming coarsely granular, finely granular, and finally waxy casts. Waxy casts are yellow tanned, dense, and homogeneous and differ from hyaline casts in that they have a high refractive index. The progress of this cellular degeneration is slow, and the presence of waxy casts is indicative of oliguria or anuria. Fatty degeneration of tubular epithelial cells produces fatty casts. These contain large amounts of fat globules and may be seen in NS. They appear transparent with highly refractile fat droplets showing maltese cross formation under polarized light.

ॐ *Pearl*

Hyaline casts are the most commonly found and least diagnostic of the casts. Red blood cell casts are diagnostic of glomerular hematuria.

Mixed casts may contain the preceding elements in combination. Their significance is determined by the dominant component so that a hyaline granular red cell cast has the same significance as a red cell cast.

Crystals

Urine that has been allowed to stand for a time may show precipitation of many crystals, very few of which are of clinical significance. The type of crystals formed is dependent on the pH of the urine. Normal crystals seen in acid urine are uric acid, amorphous urates, calcium oxalate or, less commonly, calcium sulfate or hippuric acid.

Crystals that are always abnormal and appear in acid to neutral urine are cystine, leucine, tyrosine, cholesterol, and those resulting from radiographic dye or antibiotics such as sulfonamides. Cystine is typically hexagonal and occurs with cystinosis or cystinuria. Leucine has regular concentric striations and is seen in maple syrup urine disease or severe liver disease. Tyrosine appears like sheaves of fine, highly refractile needles and is seen with inborn errors of tyrosine metabolism or severe liver disease. Cholesterol consists of flat plates with notched corners and is indicative of nephritis, NS, or lymphatic obstruction. Sulfonamides produce brown or clear sheaves of needles; radiographic dyes produce variable-sized needles singly or in sheaves. The sg of the urine is usually very high with these dyes (>1.050).

In alkaline urine, one may normally see calcium phosphate, calcium carbonate, or ammonium biurate. Uric acid characteristically forms a rhombic prism, diamond- or rosette-shaped, showing numerous interference colors under polarized light. These are increased with greater cell turnover, especially with leukemia therapy, or in gout. Calcium oxalate is envelope- or dumbbell-shaped and is pathologically increased with ethylene glycol intake, diabetes mellitus, liver disease, or Crohn disease of the small bowel; after small bowel resection; and also in hyperoxaluria, a rare hereditary disease. There may also be increases in chronic renal disease or with ingestion of large amounts of vitamin C. Amorphous urates, calcium sulphate, and hippuric acid have no diagnostic

≈ Pearl

Normal crystals appearing in acid urine are uric acid, amorphous urates, and calcium oxalate. Abnormal crystals include cystine, leucine, and tyrosine.

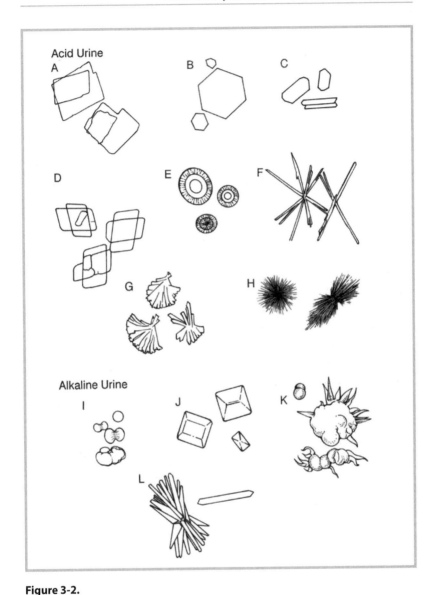

Figure 3-2.
Crystals seen in acid or alkaline urine (drawn at magnification 150–200). **A.** Cholesterol. **B.** Cystine. **C.** Hippuric acid. **D.** Hypaque. **E.** Leucine. **F.** Renografin. **G.** Sulfonamides. **H.** Tyrosine. **I.** Calcium carbonate. **J.** Triple phosphate. **K.** Ammonium biurate. **L.** Calcium phosphate. (Reprinted with permission from Barakat AY, *Renal Disease in Children: Clinical Evaluation and Diagnosis.* New York, NY: Springer-Verlag; 1990:53.)

significance. Triple phosphate (ammonium magnesium phosphate) appears as prisms, often coffin lid–shaped, and may be implicated in urinary calculus formation. Other potentially stone-forming crystals include calcium phosphate. Amorphous phosphates and thorn-apple-like ammonium biurate crystals are of no diagnostic significance. Differentiation of specific crystals may thus be determined based on presence in alkaline, neutral, or acid urine and specific solubility and heat precipitation tests. Most important, the presence of numerous commonly seen nondiagnostic crystals should not obscure examination of the rest of the sediment for important diagnostic clues to renal disease. The characteristic appearance of commonly seen crystals is illustrated in Figure 3-2.

References

1. Foot CL, Fraser JF. Uroscopic rainbow: modern matula medicine. *Postgrad Med J.* 2006;82:126–129

2. Tsai JJ, Yeun JY, Kumar VA, Don BR. Comparison and interpretation of urinalysis performed by a nephrologist versus a hospital-based clinical laboratory. *Am J Kidney Dis.* 2005;46:820–829

3. Simerville JA, Maxted WC, Pahira JJ. Urinalysis: a comprehensive review. *Am Fam Physician.* 2005;71:1153–1162

4. Fuller CE, Threatte GA, Henry JB. Basic examination of urine. In: Henry JB, ed. *Clinical Diagnosis and Management by Laboratory Methods.* 20th ed. Philadelphia, PA: WB Saunders; 2001:367–402

5. Free HM, ed. *Modern Urine Chemistry: Application of Urine Chemistry and Microscopic Examination in Health and Disease.* Elkhart, IN: Miles Laboratories; 1987

6. Boeckx RL. Urine drug screening by gas chromatography-mass spectrometry: application to a pediatric environment. *Clin Lab Med.* 1987;7:401–414

7. Sheets C, Lyman JL. Urinalysis. *Emerg Med Clin North Am.* 1986;4:263–280

8. Free AH, Free HM. Urinalysis: its proper role in the physician's office. *Clin Lab Med.* 1986;6:253–266

9. Graff L. *A Handbook of Routine Urinalysis.* Philadelphia, PA: JB Lippincott; 1983

Chapter 4

The Role of the Clinical Laboratory in the Diagnosis of Renal Disease

Tarak Srivastava, Uttam Garg, and Uri S. Alon

Abbreviations

AG	Anion gap
BUN	Blood urea nitrogen
CKD	Chronic kidney disease
CV	Coefficient of variance
EDTA	Ethylenediaminetetraacetic acid
ESRD	End-stage renal disease
GFR	Glomerular filtration rate
HDL	High-density lipoprotein
K/DOQI	Kidney Disease Outcomes Quality Initiative
LDH	Lactate dehydrogenase
LDL	Low-density lipoprotein
LH	Luteinizing hormone
PTH	Parathyroid hormone
RTA	Renal tubular acidosis
SD	Standard deviation
TP	Tubular phosphate
TSH	Thyroid-stimulating hormone

Introduction

Clinical laboratory medicine plays a key role in the diagnosis and management of renal disease because most noninfectious kidney diseases have minimal symptoms and signs until late in their clinical course. The monitoring of therapy and disease progression relies heavily on laboratory assessments. It is important to obtain an optimal sample for a valid laboratory result, which can be challenging in children, especially in premature infants and neonates. Although venipuncture is practical and even preferred, finger and heel sticks are commonly used for blood collection in small children. Avoid the temptation to squeeze or milk the puncture site because it leads to hemolysis and dilution with interstitial fluid and, subsequently, an inaccurate result. If blood is to be drawn for electrolytes, pH, carbon dioxide partial pressure, or lactic acid, it is preferable not to use a tourniquet and to avoid hand clenching. In general, for chemistry analyses, the most commonly used and preferred anticoagulant is heparin, although EDTA and sodium citrate are also used. Tubes for blood collection should be filled with the prescribed minimum volume to avoid spurious results from inappropriate anticoagulant-to-specimen ratio. The more recent chemistry analyzers need significantly less blood volume (3–20 µL) compared with the older analyzers (0.1–1 mL) for each

Pearl

An optimal sample collection is crucial for valid and informative results.

analysis and can use either serum or plasma. Plasma is a preferred sample because it speeds up the turnaround time. It eliminates the need to wait for the sample to clot and also produces much less hemolysis, which commonly interferes with many chemistry tests. Urine can be collected either as a spot random or as a timed (6-, 12-, or 24-hour) sample. For spot random urine, first-morning urine is preferred because it has less variability. It is important to note the time correctly in shorter-timed collection periods to avoid an error. In contrast to adults, for safety reasons, timed urine collections in children are done in sample jugs without adding the additives. Urine should be refrigerated and brought to the laboratory as soon as possible after the collection has been completed. The appropriate additives to the urine are added in the laboratory; for example, hydrochloric acid is added for the catecholamine assay, and boric acid is added to a urine sample for oxalate and citrate assays. A specimen may be rejected by the laboratory if the child is not properly prepared (fasting vs nonfasting) or if the specimen is unlabeled or improperly labeled, is improperly collected, is improperly preserved, or has an inadequate volume.

Reference Range

The terms *normal values* or *normal ranges* are misnomers and should actually be referred to as *reference ranges*. Reference range generally refers to the middle 95% of the values obtained from healthy individuals. The common variables that affect reference ranges include age, sex, ethnicity, pregnancy, and normal physiologic fluctuations such as circadian rhythms or seasonal variations. The magnitude of the effect of circadian rhythm should not be underestimated because, for instance, urinary potassium excretion can vary 5-fold during a 24-hour period in contrast to only 7% variation in serum potassium concentration.[1] Establishing appropriate reference ranges in children is a big challenge. Although not uncommon in routine practice, it is not appropriate to use adult reference ranges for children because these may vary significantly. Pay special attention to reference range in the laboratory report to prevent misinterpretation. For example, (1) alkaline phosphatase values change significantly with age in concert with rapid skeletal growth during infancy and puberty, and an adult reference range would not be appropriate; (2) the reference range for LDH can vary 2-fold to 4-fold among laboratories depending on the analytic methods used, which can lead to discrepancy when laboratory results are compared without paying attention to the reference ranges; and (3) it is also important to keep in mind the units used by the laboratory, especially when interpreting results in patients who are referred from another country.[2]

Other variables that are equally important in interpreting test results in certain clinical settings are hydration status, lean body mass, posture, diet, exercise, other concomitant test results, concurrent medications, and collection and handling of the specimen.[3] This is especially true when interpreting the results of certain hormones such as renin, aldosterone, PTH, and vitamin D because these test results in isolation may have no value. Although for most analytes the reference ranges are based on chronologic age, it may be important to consider physiologic age based on pubertal stage or bone age, especially in cases of sex hormones. The reference range for common analytes is presented in Appendix I.

✦ Pearl

Analytic and biologic variables must be accounted for when interpreting reported laboratory results.

Basic Statistics in Clinical Laboratory Medicine

Reference range for a particular test generally refers to the middle 95% of values obtained from a reference healthy population. This means that for any given test, the results of 5% of healthy individuals will fall outside (2.5%

above and 2.5% below) this limit. When multiple tests are done on a healthy individual, the probability that all test results will fall within the reference ranges decreases. For example, the probability that a healthy person will have 2 different test results within the reference range is $0.95 \times 0.95 = 0.9025$, or 90.25%. For 5, 10, and 20 tests, the probability that all test results will be within reference ranges is 77.4%, 59.9%, and 35.8%, respectively. In other words, the higher the number of tests conducted, the greater the probability that one or more of the test results will fall outside the reference range in an individual. Establishment of good reference ranges requires samples from a large number of healthy individuals, which is particularly challenging in children. The pediatric reference ranges are often derived using smaller numbers of individuals and extrapolation from adult values.[1-3] Therefore, the probability that a test result will fall outside the reference range is even higher for children.

In addition to physiologic variations, the test results are also affected by analytic variations. All laboratory assays have inherent errors, which are generally divided into random and systematic errors. A random error or imprecision of a test can move in either a negative or positive direction without any prediction. This imprecision is generally expressed as SD or CV, a normalized measure of dispersion of a probability distribution defined as the ratio of SD to the mean and expressed as percentage. A small CV implies good precision, whereas a large CV implies poor precision. For example, when the laboratory reports a CV (or random error) of 5% for serum creatinine and accepts results within ±2 SD, it denotes that for a sample with serum creatinine of 1 mg/dL, the laboratory may report the result anywhere from 0.90 to 1.10 mg/dL on repeated measurements from the same sample. The systematic error denotes the bias of a result compared with another method, most often a reference method. In other words, a systematic error refers to how close a reported test result is to the true value (ie, accuracy, of the result). For example, when creatinine is measured by a kinetic Jaffe method and is compared with the gold standard gas chromatography-isotope dilution mass spectrometry, the systematic error has been reported as large as 0.23 mg/dL.[4]

In addition to understanding of concepts of reference range and assay variability in clinical laboratory medicine, it is important to understand the performance of a test result in identifying a particular disease or abnormality. Neither accuracy nor analytic precision addresses the clinical utility of a test. To understand it, several common statistical descriptors, such as sensitivity, specificity, and predictive values, are used to discriminate individuals who are healthy from those who are diseased. Sensitivity of a test refers to the frequency of a positive test result in the presence of a particular disease (ie, positivity in disease), and the specificity of a test refers to the frequency of a negative test result in persons who do not have the disease (ie, negativity in health). A test with a high sensitivity will identify almost all patients with the disease. The larger the number of false-negative tests, the less sensitive the test. A common mnemonic used to remember this is SNout (in a test with a high sensitivity, a negative result effectively rules out the diagnosis). On the other hand, a test with a high specificity will identify almost all patients without the disease. The larger the number of false-positive tests, the less specific the test. A common mnemonic to remember this is SpPin (in a test with high specificity, a positive result effectively rules in the diagnosis). Calculation of sensitivity and specificity of a test requires categorization of individuals as healthy or diseased by some other means (Table 4-1). Sensitivity and specificity of a particular test move in opposite directions (ie, with increasing sensitivity of a test, there will be a decrease in specificity, and vice versa).

In an ideal test, both sensitivity and specificity will approach 100%. However, in reality either by performance of the test or selection of a par-

Table 4-1. Statistics Commonly Used in Interpretation of a Laboratory Test in a Disease Condition

For example, a rapid respiratory syncytial virus (RSV) antigen detection assay in children with confirmed presence or absence of RSV by viral culture. An example of an assay kit is shown.

		Disease		Total
		Present	Absent	
Diagnostic test	Positive	90 (TP)	10 (FP)	100
	Negative	5 (FN)	95 (TN)	100
Total		95	105	200

Sensitivity = TP/(TP + FN) = 95%
Specificity = TN/(FP + TN) = 90%
Positive predictive value = TP/(TP + FP) = 90%
Negative predictive value = TN/(FN + TN) = 95%
Efficiency = (TP + TN)/(TP + TN + FN + FP) = 92.5%

Abbreviations: FN, false negative; FP, false positive; TN, true negative; TP, true positive.

ticular cutoff, a test will be high in either sensitivity or specificity. Sensitivity of a test should be high when missing an individual with a disease has a high impact on the outcome. For example, screening tests for human immunodeficiency virus and phenylketonuria should have high sensitivity. Confirmation tests for these diseases should have high specificity. On the other hand, specificity of a test should be high when a false-positive but not a false-negative result has more implication on the final outcome (ie, tests for drug abuse for legal purposes).

Another statistical descriptor that is commonly used to assess the diagnostic value of a test is predictive value. Positive and negative predictive value of a test refers to true positive and true negative rates, respectively. In contrast to sensitivity and specificity, which are inherent properties of a test and are independent of prevalence of a particular disease, predictive values take into account the prevalence of the disease. When the prevalence of a given disease changes from high to low, given the same sensitivity and specificity of a test, its positive predictive value decreases markedly as the false-positive rate becomes disproportionately high.

᠅ Pearl

The higher the number of tests conducted in an individual, the greater the probability that one or more of the test results will fall outside its reference range.

Another test characteristic is efficiency, which takes into account the ability of a test to correctly identify both true positives and true negatives. It is defined as percent of correct results (ie, true results divided by all results). In addition to the standard sensitivity, specificity, and predictive values described earlier, other statistical terms that are also used are *odds ratio, positive likelihood ratio, negative likelihood ratio, prevalence,* and *pretest odds* and *posttest odds* to better understand the interpretation and use of laboratory tests in the clinical setting.[5]

Effects of Renal Disease on Laboratory Values

The kidney plays an important role in the homeostasis of fluid and electrolytes, acid-base balance, and mineral metabolism and has specific endocrine functions. Thus the presence of renal disease will have an impact on laboratory results, which can be both specific and nonspecific. Some of the clinically relevant changes in laboratory values subsequent to renal dysfunction that need to be considered during laboratory interpretation are discussed later in this chapter.

Lipid Profile

In CKD, there is abnormal lipid metabolism leading to hypertriglyceridemia and decreased HDL. The K/DOQI guidelines recommend that all children, as well as adults with CKD, should be evaluated for dyslipidemia.[6] One should take into account that many laboratories use the Friedewald formula to calculate LDL cholesterol:

$$\text{LDL cholesterol (mg/dL)} = \text{total cholesterol} - [\text{HDL cholesterol} + (\text{triglycerides}/5)]$$

The Friedewald formula was developed from healthy control subjects.[7] Concerns have been raised about the use of the Friedewald formula in patients with ESRD, given the accumulation of intermediate-density lipoproteins.[8] The formula has a poor correlation with the reference method in ESRD when the serum triglycerides are higher than 400 mg/dL.[9] Therefore, LDL cholesterol should be measured by either the new direct methods or by the reference method of ultracentrifugation when serum triglycerides are higher than 400 mg/dL in children with ESRD.[8,9]

Hormone Evaluation

The kidney normally plays an important role in the metabolism, secretion, degradation, and excretion of a number of hormones, their associated receptors, and binding proteins. This leads to either increased or decreased hormone levels, disturbed activation of prohormones, altered bioactivity, altered hormone binding to carrier proteins, and/or altered tissue sensitivity at the receptor and postreceptor levels.[10] Abnormalities detected in the thyroid hormone axis are characterized by low total and free thyroxine T_4 and T_3, with normal TSH, normal or decreased thyroid hormone-binding globulin, and normal or decreased TSH-releasing hormone tests; this is similar to sick euthyroid syndrome seen in other chronic diseases. A normal or low reverse T_3 in patients with CKD helps differentiate it from the sick euthyroid state of other chronic diseases in which the reverse T_3 is elevated. The abnormalities detected in the somatotropic hormone axis in children with renal dysfunction consist of growth hormone insensitivity, which is manifested by normal or elevated levels of growth hormone, normal or decreased levels of total insulin-like growth factor-1, and decreased growth hormone receptor activity. The abnormalities detected in the gonadotropic hormone axis in advanced renal dysfunction are characterized as a compensated state of hypergonadotropic hypogonadism manifested by normal or elevated levels of the gonadotropic hormones, follicle-stimulating hormone, and LH and the loss of the LH pulsatile pattern.[10]

Drugs and Toxins

In children with renal dysfunction, certain drugs (such as cimetidine, trimethoprim, ciprofloxacin, and flucytosine) lead to an elevation in serum creatinine but not BUN because they interfere with the tubular secretion of creatinine.[11] On the other hand, drugs such as angiotensin-converting enzyme inhibitors, nonsteroidal anti-inflammatory drugs, cyclosporine, and tacrolimus will cause elevation in serum creatinine because of their direct effect on renal hemodynamics.

Solute Excretion in Urine

Urine creatinine is commonly used as the denominator for measurement of various solute excretion rates expressed as solute/creatinine ratio (eg, calcium, protein, citrate, and catecholamines). It is important to remember that these values can be applied only to children with normal muscle mass and not to individuals with poor muscle mass because of their decreased urine creatinine excretion. The urinary excretion of creatinine is dependent on age and muscle mass; thus the urinary ratio may appear to be much higher in infants and toddlers due to low urine creatinine excretion compared with a school-aged child. In addition, urinary creatinine may be spuriously high in malnourished children and spuriously low in very muscular adolescents. Urine osmolality can be used instead of urine creatinine in these special clinical situations.[12] Many tubular assessments done in routine clinical practice for RTA or diabetes insipidus have the built-in assumption that the renal function is normal; hence these laboratory assessments are not valid when done in the setting of renal dysfunction.

Serum Chemistry Levels

The levels of a few laboratory analytes are out of the reference range in the presence of renal dysfunction, as discussed earlier under Hormone Evaluation. Similarly, the serum levels of amylase and lipase can be up to 2 to

3 times the upper limit of the reference range in children with ESRD, which can lead to misdiagnosis of acute pancreatitis. Also, serum levels of creatinine kinase LDH, and gamma-glutamyl transpeptidase can be elevated, and serum levels of aspartate aminotransferase and alanine aminotransferase decreased in subjects on hemodialysis in the absence of pathology.[13] Laboratory values of oxalate in urine and serum are dependent on the degree of renal dysfunction. In the early stages of primary hyperoxaluria, urine oxalate is more informative for diagnosis, whereas in the late stages of the disease, with moderate to severe renal dysfunction, serum oxalate is of more diagnostic help.

❧ Pearl

One must be cognizant of changes in laboratory results without the presence of co-morbid diseases in children with CKD.

Specific Individual Analytes

Creatinine

Creatine is synthesized primarily in the liver and then transported to the muscle. The rate of conversion of creatine to creatinine is relatively constant at 1.6% to 1.7% of the total daily pool.[14] Total body content of creatine is relatively constant and is proportional to muscle mass. Muscle mass is the single most important determinant of the amount of creatinine produced every 24 hours. Dietary intake of creatinine does not affect the creatinine in any meaningful way, although it can transiently affect serum concentration and urine excretion of creatinine.[15] Because the conversion of creatine to creatinine is relatively constant and creatinine is freely filtered through the glomerulus without reabsorption by the tubule, the major determinant of serum creatinine levels besides muscle mass is renal function. Most autoanalyzers in use today measure serum creatinine by a modified Jaffe kinetic rate color reaction. The picric acid Jaffe reaction has been well-recognized over the years to overestimate serum creatinine concentration in healthy individuals by 20% to 30% (but not in urine) because of the presence of noncreatinine chromogens compared with a more precise and accurate measurement of serum creatinine by high-performance liquid chromatography and mass spectrometry.

The literature has many formulas to estimate GFR based on the principle that creatinine excretion is constant and equal to creatinine production, which in turn is proportional to muscle mass and can be estimated from an individual's age, sex, height, and weight. The assumptions in estimated GFR calculations are that (1) serum creatinine has attained its steady-state value (the equation is not helpful in acute renal failure where serum creatinine is rapidly changing) and (2) creatinine is predominantly filtered at the glomerulus with nonconsequential secretion or reabsorption by the tubule (which is not true in moderate to severe renal failure). The Schwartz equation is used most commonly in clinical practice in children, and the estimated GFR for different ages and sex using this equation is shown in Table 4-2.[16-18] The observation that many of the complications of CKD can be prevented or delayed through early detection and treatment prompted the K/DOQI work group to develop a formal staging system for stratification of CKD based on the level of kidney function, independent of the primary renal diagnosis[19] (Table 14-1). One must remember that the equation to estimate GFR using the Schwartz equation was developed using the kinetic Jaffe assay. The enzymatic assay for creatinine is not affected by noncreatinine chromogen like the Jaffe method, thus giving a lower value for serum creatinine. There is risk of overestimating GFR when using the Schwartz equation if serum creatinine is measured using newer assays.

Blood Urea Nitrogen

Although results are expressed as urea nitrogen, particularly in the United States, it is urea that is measured in clinical laboratories, and it is serum or plasma and not whole blood that is used for the measurement. The factor for converting mass units of urea nitrogen to mass units of urea is 2.14.

Urea is the end product of protein metabolism in the liver. It is filtered by the renal glomeruli, partially reabsorbed by the renal tubules, and excreted in the urine. The reabsorption of urea makes it a poor measure of GFR. Many factors, such as increased protein intake, increased endogenous protein catabolism, congestive heart failure, use of diuretics, hyperalimentation, ketoacidosis, intestinal bleeding, dehydration, infection, and many medications, can increase plasma urea concentration.

In clinical practice, urea helps in differentiating prerenal from renal azotemia. In children with severe renal failure (predialysis), GFR is esti-

Table 4-2. Normal GFR in Children and Young Adults Using the Schwartz Equation[a]		
Schwartz Equation	Age (Sex)	Mean GFR ± SD (mL/min/1.73 m²)
GFR = 0.33 × (length/S_{Cr}) in preterm		
GFR = 0.45 × (length/S_{Cr}) in term	1 wk (males and females)	40.6 ± 14.8
GFR = 0.45 × (length/S_{Cr}) in 2–8 wk	2–8 wk (males and females) >8 wk (males and females)	65.8 ± 24.8 95.7 ± 21.7
GFR = 0.55 × (length/S_{Cr}) in 2–12 y	2–12 y (males and females)	133.0 ± 27.0
GFR = 0.70 × (length/S_{Cr}) in 13–21 y boys	13–21 y (males)	140.0 ± 30.0
GFR = 0.55 × (length/S_{Cr}) in 13–21 y girls	13–21 y (females)	126.0 ± 22.0

Abbreviations: GFR, glomerular filtration rate; SD, standard deviation.
[a]GFR is expressed in mL/min/1.73 m²; length in cm; and S_{Cr} (serum creatinine) in mg/dL.

mated using an arithmetic mean of urea clearance and creatinine clearance, and urea is used to assess the adequacy of peritoneal dialysis and hemodialysis. In special situations (such as drug interference with the creatinine assay and in children who are severely hyperbilirubinemic and undergoing hemofiltration), in which creatinine results can be misleading, urea can be helpful.[20] Urea at a GFR of less than 75% of normal has a specificity and sensitivity of 91% and 67%, respectively, whereas for creatinine, these values are 96% and 69%, respectively. Although urea measurement has its limitations, it is commonly used to assess renal function in conjunction with creatinine.[21]

Electrolytes-Anion Gap

Sodium, with its accompanying anions, contributes to most of the extracellular osmolality. Essentially all dietary sodium taken in is excreted through the kidneys. Following glomerular ultrafiltration, 60% to 70% of sodium is reabsorbed in the proximal tubules and 25% to 30% in the ascending loop of Henle. A small fraction of sodium (10%–15%) is presented to the distal tubule, where it is tightly regulated by the renin-angiotensin-aldosterone system to maintain sodium balance. In the past, sodium measurement was done by flame photometry, which has been almost completely replaced by ion-specific electrodes for sodium assay. Depending on the analyzer, the sodium in a sample can be determined without dilution (direct potentiometry) or with dilution (indirect potentiometry) by an ion-specific electrode. When sodium is measured by flame photometry or indirect potentiometry, pseudohyponatremia due to hyperlipidemia (or, less often, by hyperproteinemia) can occur. This is due to the electrolyte exclusion effect (ie, other molecules replacing water in relation to sodium). This phenomenon of pseudohyponatremia is not seen with direct potentiometry. The clinical observation of hyponatremia or hypernatremia is invariably a result of conditions associated with water excess or water loss rather than the rare situations of poor intake or salt poisoning. Clinical history, physical examination, and review of drugs with simultaneous measurement of serum and urine for electrolytes, creatinine, and osmolality can help one to tease out the pathophysiologic disturbance in serum sodium, which can then be confirmed by appropriate tests (Chapter 11).

Potassium is the major intracellular cation. Potassium, like sodium, is filtered through the glomeruli and is almost completely reabsorbed in the proximal tubules and ascending loop of Henle. The net excretion of potassium in urine is by secretion into the luminal fluid under the influence of aldosterone and rate of tubular flow in the distal tubule. Ion-specific electrodes are almost exclusively used for measurement of potassium. Various factors can artificially increase serum potassium level. The common causes of artificially increased potassium include hemolysis due to sample shaking, delay in sample processing, and grossly elevated leukocyte count. Serum is more affected than plasma. Therefore, use of plasma for potassium measurement is recommended. In addition to severe metabolic acidosis, the common cause of pathologic elevation of serum potassium is decreased urinary excretion of potassium by the kidneys in acute kidney injury and CKD. A disturbance in serum potassium in children with normal renal function requires additional evaluation. Clinical history, physical examination, review of drugs, assessment of growth, blood pressure, acid-base status, and simultaneous measurement of serum and urine for electrolytes, creatinine and osmolality, serum renin, and aldosterone can help narrow down the differential diagnosis for abnormal serum potassium, which can then be confirmed by appropriate tests (Chapter 11).

Serum contains a large number of solutes: the 4 ions with highest plasma concentrations (Na^+, K^+, Cl^-, HCO_3^-) are routinely measured and are used for calculation of AG. The sum of cations (sodium and potassium) normally exceeds the sum of measured anions (chloride and bicarbonate); the unmeasured anions are represented by $AG = (Na^+ + K^+) - (Cl^- + HCO_3^-)$. The AG is commonly used in the interpretation of acid-base disturbances (Chapter 12). Causes of metabolic acidosis with normal and high AG are presented in Table 12-3. Occasionally the AG is abnormally small or even has a negative value. If laboratory error is eliminated, the small AG is most likely the result of reduced concentration of the normal unmeasured anion, albumin. Consequently, in the face of severe hypoalbuminemia, which may mask high AG acidosis, the AG must be corrected using the equation developed by Figge et al[22]:

$$\text{Albumin-corrected AG} = AG + 2.5 \, (4.4 - \text{albumin in g/dL})$$

Less common causes of a reduced or negative AG are pseudohyperchloremia (an artifactual increase in plasma chloride), sometimes due to bromism or hyperlipidemia; or an increased concentration of cations (such as positively charged globulins in patients with multiple myeloma or those on lithium therapy).

Calcium-Phosphorous-PTH-Vitamin D

Plasma calcium mainly exists in 3 forms: approximately 47% protein bound, approximately 43% ionized (the biologically active form), and approximately 10% complexed to other anions. Most of the main laboratory chemistry analyzers measure total calcium, whereas blood gas analyzers measure ionized calcium. When collecting a blood sample for calcium measurement, it is important to collect serum or plasma in a heparin tube because sodium citrate, EDTA, and potassium oxalate-containing tubes will give erroneous calcium results. Also, it is important to pay attention to the units in the laboratory report because most US clinical laboratories report total serum calcium in milligrams per deciliter and ionized calcium in millimoles per liter.

Phosphate is another major ion whose metabolism is significantly affected by the kidneys. If possible, TP/GFR must be measured when evaluating a child with a mineral disorder because it provides more biologic information than an isolated serum phosphate value.[23] Most of the total body phosphate is in the bones and striated muscle, and only approximately 1% is in the plasma. The commonly used methods of phosphate measurement in clinical laboratories are either dye binding or enzymatic assays.

Parathyroid hormone secretion by the parathyroid gland is tightly regulated by the level of serum-ionized calcium through the calcium sensing receptor and is also affected by serum phosphorous, magnesium, and $1,25(OH)_2$-vitamin D concentrations. Vitamin D has many metabolites that circulate in the serum. The clinical laboratory commonly measures $25(OH)$-vitamin D and $1,25(OH)_2$-vitamin D. The initial metabolite formed following hydroxylation of vitamin D in the liver is $25(OH)$-vitamin D, which is then subsequently hydroxylated in the kidneys to $1,25(OH)_2$-vitamin D. At times, the report will have the additional information of $25(OH)$-vitamin D_2 (plant source of vitamin D, ergocalciferol) and $25(OH)$-vitamin D_3 (endogenous vitamin D, cholecalciferol). D_2 and D_3 are not different metabolically or functionally at the cellular level.

In the homeostasis of calcium and phosphorous metabolism there is an interplay between 3 organs—the gastrointestinal tract, bone, and kidneys—which is further orchestrated by hormones, such as $1, 25(OH)_2$-D, PTH, calcitonin, fibroblast growth factor-23, and so on. Often a primary defect in one organ induces compensatory mechanisms in the remaining 2 organs, like an increased absorption of calcium in the gut secondary to a primary renal loss. Thus, in evaluation of a disorder affecting the calcium and/or phosphate metabolism, it is necessary to have simultaneous measurement of serum calcium (total and ionized), phosphorous, alkaline phosphatase, creatinine, PTH, and vitamin D metabolites with urine calcium, phosphorus, and creatinine, combined with appropriate radiologic studies. For instance, normal serum PTH in the face of low serum ionized calcium and normal skeletal survey indicates hypoparathyroidism, even though serum PTH is normal.

Proteinuria-Microalbuminuria

Normally children lose a small amount of protein (<4 mg/m^2/h) in the urine. Under normal circumstances proteins smaller in size than albumin are filtered at the glomerulus. These small proteins are then reabsorbed and metabolized in the proximal renal tubule. A minute amount of albumin always comes through in the glomerular ultrafiltrate and is metabolized in the tubules like the other proteins. In addition, the renal tubules and uro-epithelium of the pelvis, ureter, bladder, and urethra secrete proteins into the urine. The net protein in the urine is the result of protein in the glomerular ultrafiltrate that is not reabsorbed by the renal tubules and those proteins that are secreted into the urine. Thus in different kidney diseases the amount and nature of the protein in the urine will differ. In glomerular diseases, the increased proteinuria is the result of increased glomerular permeability and is associated with large amounts of protein, with the presence of high-molecular-weight proteins such as albumin and immunoglobulin G, known as glomerular proteinuria. In diseases like multiple myeloma and light- and heavy-chain diseases, there is an "overflow proteinuria" from increased amounts of freely filtered low-molecular-weight proteins (such as Bence Jones protein), which were not completely reabsorbed by the tubules. In tubulointerstitial kidney disease, there is failure of the renal tubules to reabsorb the normally filtered low-molecular-weight proteins (such as α1-microglobulin, ß2-microglobulin, and retinol binding protein), which is termed *tubular proteinuria.* These low-molecular-weight proteins are measured in the clinical laboratory either by urinary electrophoresis or by specific immunoassay for individual low-molecular-weight proteins, whereas total protein is measured using standard dye methods (Chapter 8).

Routine urinalysis done with a urine dipstick is able to detect abnormal proteinuria (predominantly albumin) (Chapter 3). Under normal circumstances there is a small amount of albumin in the urine that cannot be detected by the routine urine dipstick method. This proteinuria has been termed *microalbuminuria.* This, however, is a misnomer because it is not the name of a substance but instead refers to abnormal amounts of albumin in the urine before the subject develops overt proteinuria. Microalbuminuria is measured in the laboratory by immunoassay on both random spot urine samples and in 24-hour urine samples. The normal excretion rate for urinary albumin is less than 30 mg/g creatinine in random spot urine and less than 20 µg/min in a timed urine collection. The clinical importance of this abnormal but low amount of urinary albumin is that it correlates with progression of CKD. Studies have shown that decreasing the amount of urinary albumin (microalbuminuria) excretion in diabetic adults with therapy delays the progression of CKD.[24] Data in the literature are also suggestive of a beneficial effect in patients with nondiabetic CKD. Although not many large-scale studies have been conducted in children, these observations have been extrapolated to children from adults.

Interpretation of Laboratory Data

The purpose of clinical laboratory testing is to assist physicians in determining the diagnosis and to monitor treatment and disease progression. By knowing several basic concepts of clinical laboratory medicine, limitations of a test, and related basic statistical analyses, a clinician can better understand when and how to use these laboratory tests in renal diseases. Three aspects must be considered during interpretation of every test result: (1) analytic issues that go into reporting a test result, (2) statistical issues that need to be considered for a given test and, finally, (3) the clinical setting in which the test results need to be interpreted.

For a given laboratory test, there can be issues related to analytic errors that are assessed by random error (or CV) and systematic error (or bias). The assay result can vary owing to the nature of the instrument and for the same instrument between laboratories. The same analyte can be reported by central laboratories using different methods that are usually not known to the physician. For example, serum creatinine can be performed by a modified kinetic Jaffe reaction or by an enzymatic assay. This can lead to misinterpretation of results when a child is transferred from an outlying primary care facility to a tertiary center. The term *normal values,* as discussed previously, is a misnomer and they should actually be referred to as *reference ranges.* Due to the statistical way a reference range is created, even a healthy individual might have a few abnormal test results. One must be cognizant that no test is perfect or has 100% sensitivity or specificity. The sensitivity and specificity of a test do not change, whereas the predictive values of a test do change based on the prevalence of a disease in the population being tested. If the prevalence of a given disease is rare, then for the same given sensitivity and specificity of a test, its positive predictive value will decrease markedly because the false-positive rate will be disproportionately high for a rare true-positive result. This should be considered, for example, when a nasal aspirate test is ordered for influenza before the onset of an influenza season because the test will give many false-positive results and will need virology confirmation, whereas it can be taken as a true positive in the middle of the influenza season without the need for virology confirmation.

A laboratory test result should always be interpreted in the overall clinical and biochemical setting. For example, total serum calcium below the reported reference range would still be appropriate in children with hypoalbuminemia. On the other hand, normal total serum calcium may be clinically inappropriately high in children on dialysis who are hyperphosphatemic. The previous discussion of the role of hypoalbuminemia in AG assessment alluded to the fact that in the setting of hypoalbuminemia, a normal AG reported by the laboratory could in reality indicate high AG acidosis. Certain laboratory results cannot be interpreted in isolation without additional laboratory tests, imaging studies, and clinical data. For example, a PTH level is fully informative only in the setting in which serum calcium, creatinine, albumin, phosphorous, vitamin D levels (and at times magnesium), and urine calcium and TP/GFR are known, as well as the clinical condition in which the test was conducted (CKD, ESRD, nephrolithiasis, rickets, etc).

> ### ❧ Pearl
>
> One must consider the analytic issues of the laboratory, the sensitivity and specificity of a test in the setting of disease prevalence, and the clinical setting in which the test was requested when interpreting a laboratory report.

Thus a basic knowledge of clinical laboratory medicine is helpful in ordering and interpreting test results. This is especially important due to the complexity of renal physiology and pathophysiology and often the need to obtain information about several variables to allow the support of a clinical diagnosis. When confronting unacceptable test results, clinicians should consult with their colleagues in the laboratory for better clarification of the potential reasons for the discrepancy.

References

1. Oxley DK, Garg U, Olsowka ES. Maximizing the information from laboratory test—the Ulysses syndrome. In: Jacobs DS, Demott WR, Oxley DK, eds. *Laboratory Test Handbook.* 5th ed. Hudson, OH: Lexi-Comp, Inc.; 2001:15–33

2. Srivastava T, Garg U, Chan YR, Alon US. Essentials of laboratory medicine for the nephrology clinician. *Pediatr Nephrol.* 2007;22:170–182

3. Olsowka ES, Garg U. Specimen collection and point of care testing. In: Jacobs DS, DeMott WR, Oxley DK, eds. *Laboratory Test Handbook.* 5th ed. Hudson, OH: Lexi-Comp, Inc.; 2001:35–39

4. Myers GL, Miller WG, Coresh J, et al. Recommendations for improving serum creatinine measurement: a report from the Laboratory Working Group of the National Kidney Disease Education Program. *Clin Chem.* 2006;52:5–18

5. Sackett DL, Straus SE, Richardson WS, Rosenberg W, Haynes RB. Diagnosis and screening. In: Sackett DL, Straus SE, Richardson WS, Rosenberg W, Haynes RB, eds. *Evidence-Based Medicine—How to Practice and Teach EBM.* 2nd ed. New York, NY: Churchill Livingstone; 2000:67–94

6. National Kidney Foundation K/DOQI clinical practice guidelines for managing dyslipidemias in chronic kidney disease. *Am J Kidney Dis.* 2003;41(suppl 3):S1–S92

7. Friedewald WT, Levy RI, Fredrickson DS. Estimation of the concentration of low-density lipoprotein cholesterol in plasma, without use of the preparative ultracentrifuge. *Clin Chem.* 1972;18:499–502

8. Senti M, Pedro-Botet J, Nogues X, Rubies-Prat J. Influence of intermediate-density lipoproteins on the accuracy of the Friedewald formula. *Clin Chem.* 1991;37:1394–1397

9. Nauck M, Kramer-Guth A, Bartens W, Marz W, Wieland H, Wanner C. Is the determination of LDL cholesterol according to Friedewald accurate in CAPD and HD patients? *Clin Nephrol.* 1996;46:319–325

10. Srivastava T, Warady BA. Overview of the management of chronic kidney disease in children. 2006; UpToDate Online version 14.3

11. Andreev E, Koopman M, Arisz L. A rise in plasma creatinine that is not a sign of renal failure: which drugs can be responsible? *J Intern Med.* 1999;246:247–252

12. Richmond W, Colgan G, Simon S, Stuart-Hilgenfeld M, Wilson N, Alon US. Random urine calcium/osmolality in the assessment of calciuria in children with decreased muscle mass. *Clin Nephrol.* 2005;64:264–270

13. Vaziri ND, Kim I. Serum enzyme levels. In: Daugirdas JT, Ing TS, eds. *Handbook of Dialysis.* 2nd ed. Boston, MA: Little Brown and Company; 1994:416–421

14. Heymsfield SB, Arteaga C, McManus C, Smith J, Moffitt S. Measurement of muscle mass in humans: validity of the 24-hour urinary creatinine method. *Am J Clin Nutr.* 1983;37:478–494

15. Crim MC, Calloway DH, Margen S. Creatine metabolism in men: urinary creatine and creatinine excretions with creatine feeding. *J Nutr.* 1975;105:428–438

16. Schwartz GJ, Haycock GB, Edelmann CM Jr, Spitzer A. A simple estimate of glomerular filtration rate in children derived from body length and plasma creatinine. *Pediatrics.* 1976;58:259–263

17. Schwartz GJ, Feld LG, Langford DJ. A simple estimate of glomerular filtration rate in full-term infants during the first year of life. *J Pediatr.* 1984;104:849–854

18. Schwartz GJ, Gauthier B. A simple estimate of glomerular filtration rate in adolescent boys. *J Pediatr.* 1985;106:522–526

19. National Kidney Foundation K/DOQI clinical practice guidelines for chronic kidney disease: evaluation, classification and stratification. *Am J Kidney Dis.* 2002;39(suppl 1):S1–S266

20. Chadha V, Garg U, Warady BA, Alon US. Sieving coefficient inaccuracies during hemo-diafiltration in patients with hyperbilirubinemia. *Pediatr Nephrol.* 2000;15:33–35

21. Rodgerson DO. Renal function. In: Howanitz JH, Howanitz PJ, eds. *Laboratory Medicine: Test Selection and Interpretation.* New York, NY: Churchill Livingstone; 1991:41–65

22. Figge J, Jabor A, Kazda A, Fencl V. Anion gap and hypoalbuminemia. *Crit Care Med.* 1998;26:1807–1810

23. Alon U, Hellerstein S. Assessment and interpretation of the tubular threshold for phosphate in infants and children. *Pediatr Nephrol.* 1994;8:250–251

24. Strippoli GF, Craig MC, Schena FP, Craig JC. Role of blood pressure targets and specific antihypertensive agents used to prevent diabetic nephropathy and delay its progression. *J Am Soc Nephrol.* 2006;17(4 suppl 2):S153–S155

Chapter 5

Imaging of the Kidney and Urinary Tract

S. Sedberry-Ross and H. Gil Rushton

Abbreviations

AAP	American Academy of Pediatrics
ACE	Angiotensin-converting enzyme
ADPKD	Autosomal dominant polycystic kidney disease
AP	Anterior-posterior
CT	Computed tomography
DMSA	Dimercaptosuccinic acid
DTPA	Diethylene triamine penta-acetic acid
eBC	Estimated bladder capacity
ERPF	Estimated renal plasma flow
GFR	Glomerular filtration rate
IVP	Intravenous pyelography
KUB	Abdominal plain film of kidney, ureter, and bladder
MAG3	Mercaptoacetyl triglycine
MCDK	Multicystic dysplastic kidney
MIBG	Metaiodobenzylguanidine
MRA	Magnetic resonance angiography
MRI	Magnetic resonance imaging
PUV	Posterior urethral valve
RCC	Renal cell carcinoma
RMS	Rhabdomyosarcoma
RNC	Radionuclide cystography
RPD	Renal pelvic diameter
Tc-99m	Technetium 99
UPJ	Ureteropelvic junction
UTI	Urinary tract infection
UVJ	Ureterovesical junction
VCUG	Voiding cystourethrogram
VUR	Vesicoureteral reflux

Introduction

Radiologic imaging of the genitourinary tract in pediatric patients has continued to evolve during the past decade. Prenatal imaging has become routine and allows early detection of many genitourinary anomalies. Ultrasound, VCUG, and nuclear scintigraphy with Tc-99m-DMSA and Tc-99m-MAG3 diuretic renal scans are critical in the evaluation and diagnosis of disease and often play a key role in deciding between observational management and intervention. Spiral CT and gadolinium-enhanced MRI have significantly improved and often play an important role in evaluation and diagnosis. Imaging of the genitourinary tract in pediatric patients is fundamental to the management and treatment of many genitourinary abnormalities. This chapter provides a review of available imaging modalities and offers a guide to imaging of specific urinary tract abnormalities and illnesses in children.

Imaging Modalities

Abdominal Plain Film of Kidney, Ureter, Bladder

The KUB provides limited but useful information. Evaluation of bowel gas or colonic stool content can be useful in documenting constipation in children with voiding disorders, many of whom have a more generalized elimination dysfunction. Radiopaque stones in the kidney, ureter, or bladder may be noted. One important use in pediatric urology patients is evaluation for skeletal or spinal abnormalities that may be associated with genitourinary pathology.

Intravenous Pyelogram

Intravenous pyelography is a contrast study that begins with a scout film, followed by a film over the kidneys after an intravenous contrast is administered. Tomographic images of the kidneys are then obtained. Prone films allow optimal visualization of the renal collecting system and are obtained after 10 to 20 minutes if there is concern for obstruction.[1]

The role of IVP in pediatric urology has largely been replaced by sonography and nuclear scintigraphy. In neonates, immature kidneys are unable to concentrate the intravenous contrast, further limiting its usefulness. In older children, it can be used to evaluate the ureters if other studies fail to provide adequate information. A single-shot excretory urogram is often obtained in unstable trauma patients undergoing emergent laparotomies. Approximately 32% of patients may avoid unnecessary renal exploration if the imaging technique is done properly.[2]

Ultrasound

Ultrasonography, which uses high-frequency sound waves to image anatomic structures, is one of the most important and widely used imaging modalities in pediatrics. It is a painless, noninvasive technique that allows visualization of organs in real time without exposure to ionizing radiation or nephrotoxic contrast agents. Other advantages include availability, flexibility, and accurate anatomical structural detail. However, ultrasound provides no functional information, and retroperitoneal structures can be difficult to evaluate. Body habitus and bowel gas may interfere with the examination.[3] Furthermore, the quality of the ultrasound is operator-dependent, and clarity can vary depending on skill and experience.

The mainstay of ultrasound imaging is a real-time, 2-dimensional, grayscale display. With this technique, variations in the amplitudes of the echoes arising from tissues, such as renal parenchyma, are displayed as varied shades of gray on a monitor. Tissues such as fat have high-signal intensities and appear white on the monitor. These structures are described as hyperechoic. For example, peripelvic fat adjacent to the normal renal pelvis appears as whitish tissue in the central portion of the kidney (Figure 5-1). In contrast, if there is no internal echo, such as when imaging urine in the bladder or a hydronephrotic renal pelvis, the structure appears black and is described as anechoic (Figure 5-2). A structure is described as hypoechoic if its signal is less intense, and therefore less echoic, than a surrounding structure. If echogenicities are the same, they are described as isoechoic.

Color Doppler ultrasound is an important tool in the evaluation of blood flow. The Doppler effect is a change in the frequency of a wave as it is reflected from a moving object. It measures the velocity of a moving object and determines the flow direction. Color Doppler ultrasound provides an estimate of the average velocity of flow within a vessel and color codes the information. The flow direction is assigned the color red or blue, indicat-

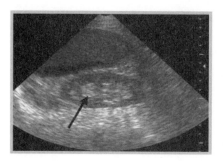

Figure 5-1.
Ultrasound of a normal kidney. Hyperechoic peripelvic fat adjacent to the normal renal pelvis appears as whitish tissue in the central portion of the kidney as indicated by the arrow.

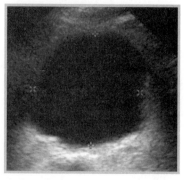

Figure 5-2.
Normal bladder ultrasound. Ultrasound of a normal bladder filled with urine appears black and is described as anechoic.

ing flow toward or away from the transducer, respectively. The color-coded vascular information is then superimposed on a grayscale image.[4]

Power (energy) Doppler sonography, a modification of standard color Doppler ultrasonography, is more sensitive in depicting slow flow in smaller and deeper vessels (intrarenal arteries) than color Doppler.[5] It is also valuable in ultrasonography of an acute scrotum because of its increased sensitivity to low-flow states, which would indicate testicular torsion. In contrast to color Doppler, power Doppler ultrasonography does not provide any information relative to velocity or the direction of blood flow.[4]

ஃ Pearl

Ultrasound is one of the most important imaging modalities in pediatrics. It is painless and non-invasive and it allows visualization of organs without exposure to ionizing radiation or nephrotoxic contrast agents.

Three- and 4-dimensional ultrasonography, which is currently available in sophisticated areas of radiology such as high-risk perinatology centers, offers increased accuracy and improved appreciation of anatomical relationships. However, these techniques require highly trained skilled technologists and a complex and expensive computational infrastructure.

Prenatal Ultrasound

Approximately 50% of the 4 million pregnant women in the United States are scanned annually to evaluate for fetal anomalies.[6] Overall sensitivity of the prenatal ultrasound varies. Levi[7] compiled data from 36 studies and more than 900,000 fetuses and concluded that the overall sensitivity for the detection of fetal abnormalities was 40.4% (range 13.3%–82.4%). Sensitivity for detection of genitourinary anomalies, which account for approximately 20% of all abnormalities identified, is somewhat higher.[7]

By 16 to 17 weeks of gestation, the kidneys and bladder can be identified in 90% of fetuses.[8] Prenatal ultrasound imaging includes longitudinal and transverse views of the kidneys and bladder.[9] The kidneys can be seen as hypoechoic paraspinal structures with an echogenic renal pelvis. Kidney size is measured to ensure appropriate growth for gestational age (Figure 5-3). Kidneys are examined for any abnormal cystic or solid structures or for evidence of hydronephrosis. The fetal bladder is evaluated for any abnormalities, such as ureteroceles or bladder diverticulum. Bladder distension may be noted and can indicate obstruction. Bladder filling can be noted as early as 14 to 15 weeks.[8] Abnormal shape of the urinary bladder can be an indication of cloacal abnormalities, and absence of the bladder on serial

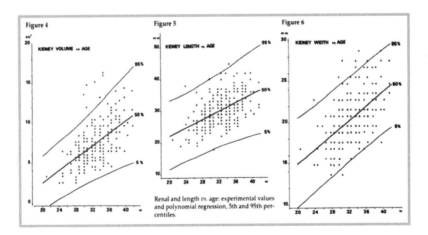

Figure 5-3.
Renal length versus age: experimental values and polynomial regression, 5th and 9th percentiles. (Reprinted with permission from Jeanty P, Dramaix-Wilmet M, Elkhazen N, Hubinont C, van Regemorter N. Measurements of fetal kidney growth on ultrasound. *Radiology.* 1982;144[1]:159–162.)

scans may indicate bladder exstrophy. The volume of amniotic fluid should always be assessed.

The most common abnormality detected on prenatal ultrasound is hydronephrosis, the severity of which can vary. To provide prognostic criteria for this variability, a grading system was developed by the Society for Fetal Urology (Figure 5-4). Measurements of the prenatal RPD have also been shown to correlate with the significance of postnatal clinical outcome.

ᴥ Pearl

The most common abnormality detected on prenatal ultrasound is hydronephrosis.

Grignon et al[10] found that 94% of patients with an RPD greater than 20 mm had significant clinical manifestations that required long-term follow-up or

Grade of Hydroephrosis	Renal Pelvis	Renal Parenchymal Thickness
Grade 0	No dilatation	Normal
Grade I	Mild dilatation	Normal
Grade II	Moderate dilatation but limited to renal pelvis	Normal
Grade III	marked dilatation, renal pelvis is dilated and calyces dialted	Normal
Grade IV	Severe pelcicalyceal dilatation	Thinned

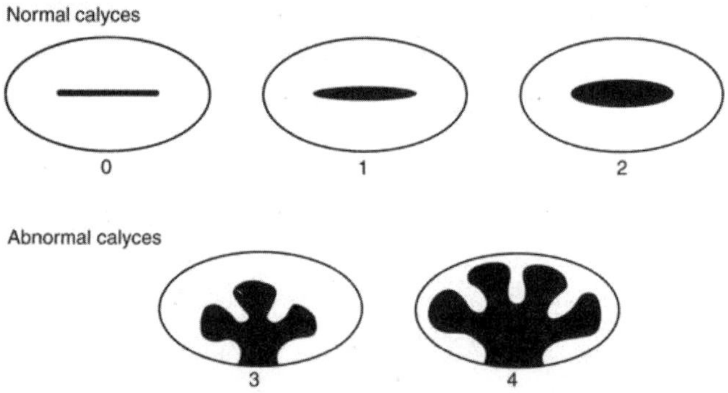

Figure 5-4.
The Society of Fetal Urology grading system for antenatally detected hydronephrosis (Reprinted with permission from Belarmino JM, Kogan BA. Management of neonatal hydroephrosis. *Early Hom Dev.* 2006; 82:9–14.)

surgery. In this study, 50% of patients with an RPD 10 to 15 mm in size had a significant abnormality, and only 3% of those with an RPD less than 10 mm needed long-term intervention. Renal pelvic diameter has been found to correlate with diagnosis in some cases. Mild hydronephrosis (5–9 mm) is often the result of VUR, whereas more severe hydronephrosis (>15 mm) is associated with UPJ obstruction.

Prenatal Hydronephrosis

In the face of fetal hydronephrosis, the goal is term delivery (also see Chapter 17). Fetuses with unilateral hydronephrosis and a normal contralateral kidney have adequate renal reserve, so postnatal growth and development should be normal. These children should be evaluated after birth. In cases of bilateral dilation of the urinary tract, pulmonary development is unlikely to be compromised as long as amniotic fluid levels remain normal on serial ultrasounds. In these instances, prenatal observation with term delivery and early postnatal evaluation is encouraged (Figure 5-5).

In fetuses with bilateral hydronephrosis associated with oligohydramnios, management depends on estimated fetal renal function and gestational age of the fetus. Fetal ultrasound and fetal urine chemistry compositions (Table 17-1) allow classification into good and poorly functioning groups. Fetuses with good renal function parameters that develop oligohydramnios after 32 weeks of gestational age are usually best managed by prenatal corticosteroids and preterm delivery. If oligohydramnios develops between 20 and 32 weeks of gestational age and fetal renal function parameters are good, prenatal intervention may be considered.[8] Before 20 weeks, severe oligohydramnios associated with renal abnormalities is incompatible with survival. Options for interventions are beyond the scope of this chapter. However, it is important to have accurate communication between the perinatologist, obstetrician, pediatric urologist, pediatric nephrologist, neonatologist, and pediatrician so that optimal management plans can be made.

Voiding Cystourethrogram

Voiding cystourethrogram is a contrast study that should include assessment of the spine and pelvis; masses or opaque calculi; bladder capacity, contour, and emptying capability; the presence and grade of reflux; and urethral appearance.[11] Following a preliminary plain film of the abdomen, a urethral catheter or feeding tube is passed into the bladder. Contrast medium is instilled,

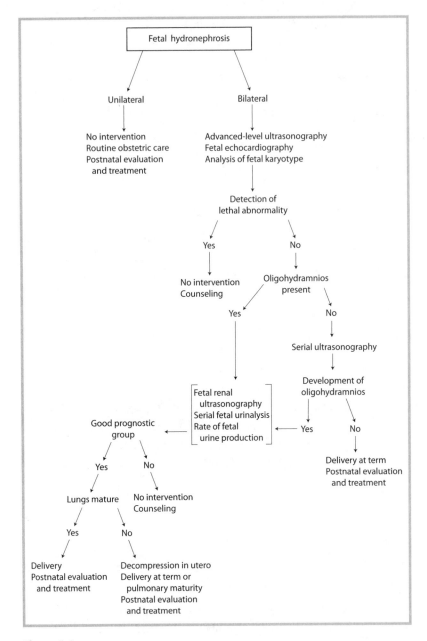

Figure 5-5.

Algorithm for management of fetal hydronephrosis. (Reprinted with permission from Gloor JM. Management of prenatally detected fetal hydronephrosis. *Mayo Clin Proc.* 1995;70(2):145–152.)

and the bladder filled to capacity. Fluoroscopic monitoring is performed during filling and voiding. Although fluoroscopic exposure is kept at a minimum, there is an inevitable radiation dose to the gonads, particularly the ovaries.[1]

During contrast instillation, filling defects, if present, are seen as darker areas surrounded by white contrast. The filling phase is important in identifying abnormalities such as ureteroceles because these may collapse as the bladder fills. Once the bladder is at full capacity, anteroposterior images and steep oblique images centered on the UVJ are obtained. This decreases radiation exposure to the gonads and enhances the detection of VUR and other abnormalities such as bladder diverticula.[12]

Imaging during voiding is important because 20% of VUR may be missed if these images are not obtained.[11] Voided volume is measured and allows the technician to determine actual bladder capacity and compare this volume with eBC[1]:

$$eBC = age\ (yrs) + 2 \times 30$$

Maximum filling volumes less than the estimated capacity often are clinically insignificant but may indicate a neuropathic bladder, an infected bladder, or an error on the part of the technician. Larger than expected filling volumes may reflect infrequent voiding or could indicate dysfunctional voiding that requires further urologic evaluation.

The VCUG is also important for evaluation of the urethra. Urethral disease is rare in girls, but an anteroposterior image of the urethra should be obtained.[11] Images of the male urethra during voiding are important to evaluate for PUVs or other urethral pathology such as a stricture. In boys, the entire urethra must be imaged because disease can occur anywhere from the bladder base to the urethral meatus.

At the conclusion of voiding, each renal fossa should be imaged. These images may demonstrate reflux that

ᕮᐤ *Pearl*

Voiding cystourethrogram is an important contrast study that assesses presence and grade of reflux; urethral appearance; masses or opaque calculi; and bladder capacity, contour, and emptying capability.

is not appreciated during fluoroscopy. In children with high-grade reflux, delayed abdominal imaging performed 15 minutes after voiding can help differentiate simple reflux from reflux associated with possible obstruction at the UPJ or UVJ.[12]

Nuclear Medicine

Radionuclide Cystography

Radionuclide cystography is an ideal imaging study for patients requiring repeat or longitudinal follow-up studies and/or for sibling screening for VUR.[1] It is also preferred by many for postoperative follow-up imaging after antireflux procedures. A dose of 0.5 mCi of Tc-99m-pertechnetate in iso-

Pearl

Radionuclide cystography is a low-dose radiation imaging study ideal for patients requiring follow-up or postoperative studies and/or sibling screening for VUR.

tonic saline is instilled in the bladder through a catheter. Continued observation under the gamma camera provides a detailed cystogram. This increases the sensitivity of the study without an increase in ionizing radiation. Unfortunately, an accurate grade of VUR cannot be determined. However, bladder capacity at the point of reflux can be determined, there is less gonadal radiation ($4–5 \times 10{-}5$ Gy), and the study is more sensitive than VCUG.[1] These qualities make this study ideal for following patients with known VUR.

Technetium 99m-Mercaptoacetyl Triglycine

Tc-99m-MAG3 diuretic renal scan is a nuclear medicine study used to evaluate both renal function and drainage of the renal collecting system. Tc-99m-MAG3 is a radionuclide that is excreted predominantly by renal tubular secretion. The active secretion of Tc-99m-MAG3, independent of GFR, makes it the agent of choice for imaging patients with suspected urinary obstruction.[12]

Patients are hydrated intravenously, and a urinary catheter is inserted into the bladder to keep it empty during the study. Images of the kidneys and bladder are obtained for approximately 20 to 40 minutes after injection of the radioisotope, and radiotracer counts are then plotted on a time graph creating a 3-phase curve.[12] If hydronephrosis and delayed spontaneous drainage of the isotope from the upper collecting system is observed, a diuretic (usually furosemide 1 mg/kg; max 40 mg) is administered intravenously, and additional images are obtained for another 15 to 20 minutes to evaluate drainage from the dilated collecting system.

The first phase of the curve is characterized by a rapid rise in radioisotope counts reflecting perfusion to the kidneys. The second phase increases more gradually, reflecting renal clearance of the radiotracer. Renal function is evaluated after 2 to 3 minutes following injection, which is the point in the second phase when activity is proportional to ERPF in each kidney.[12] The curve normally peaks after 2 to 5 minutes, which initiates the third phase and in turn demonstrates a gradual decline in radiotracer indicating excretion.[12] Counts in the bladder will increase as the kidneys drain. If retention of isotope is seen within a dilated renal pelvis or ureter, a

⮞ Pearl

Tc-99m-MAG3 diuretic renal scan is a nuclear medicine study used to evaluate hydronephrosis by assessing both renal function and drainage of the renal collecting system.

diuretic is given to stimulate urine output so as to further evaluate drainage of the upper collecting system. A nonobstructive renogram excludes clinically significant obstruction (Figure 5-6). When obstruction is present, the third phase of the renogram will be flattened depending on the sever-

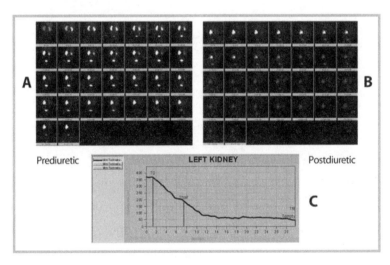

Prediuretic   LEFT KIDNEY   Postdiuretic

Figure 5-6.
Mercaptoacetyl triglycine diuretic renal scan: nonobstructive hydronephrosis. Note prompt uptake of radiotracer by the left and right kidney. **A.** Prediuretic images reveal prompt excretion of radiotracer by the right system with retained radiotracer in the left system. **B.** In postdiuretic images the left kidney is cleared of radiotracer. **C.** This is also demonstrated by the downward slope of the drainage curve and a normal T1/2 (time to half maximum counts) of <15 minutes.

ity of obstruction (Figure 5-7). As obstruction becomes more severe, renal function is depressed and uptake of the radiotracer is reduced, thus altering the second phase of the renogram curve. If diuretics are administered, a nonobstructed system will respond with abrupt clearance of the radiotracer, whereas an obstructed system will retain radiotracer in the collecting system. In some cases, the system cannot tolerate the increased flow and will become distended.[12] Sources of potential false-positive renograms are dehydration, poor renal function, and massive dilation of the collecting system with urinary stasis.

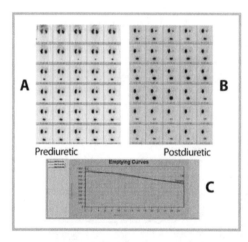

Prediuretic   Postdiuretic

Figure 5-7.
Mercaptoacetyl triglycine diuretic renal scan: obstructive hydronephrosis. Note prompt uptake of radiotracer by the left and right kidney. **A.** Prediuretic images reveal prompt excretion of radiotracer by the right system with retained radiotracer in the left system. **B.** In postdiuretic images the left kidney continues to retain the radiotracer. **C.** This is also demonstrated by the very slow downward slope of the drainage curve compared with a steep downward slope in the nonobstructed system.

Dimercaptosuccinic Acid

Tc-99m-DMSA is a chelating agent that is taken up and fixed in the renal cortex, specifically the proximal convoluted tubules. There is little accumulation of the agent in the renal papilla and medulla, and there is minimal excretion. This reflects renal cortical activity without focusing on the collecting system[4,12] (Figure 5-8).

ॐ Pearl

Tc-99m-DMSA scan is used to identify acute pyelonephritis, renal cortical scarring, some congenital anomalies of the kidneys, and renal trauma.

Tc-99m-DMSA is used to identify acute pyelonephritis, renal cortical scarring, and some congenital anomalies of the kidneys, such as ectopic kidneys. It provides differential function of renal units and can indicate a nonfunctioning moiety like MCDK or nonfunctioning polar moieties in a duplex renal system.

Tc-99m-DMSA is the imaging modality of choice in diagnosing acute pyelonephritis, which shows decreased accumulation of the radiotracer in the infected area. This is due to ischemia, inflammatory edema, and decreased cellular enzyme function that is necessary for the tubules to bind the agent.[4] These areas are not associated with volume loss but are areas of photon deficiency with preservation of the normal renal contour (Figure 5-9). These defects may resolve over time or may result in renal scarring, especially in infants younger than 1 year. Renal scars are diagnosed when there are areas of photopenia associated with renal cortical volume loss. Consequently, the reniform shape of the kidney is distorted as a result of scarred areas (Figure 5-10).

Dimercaptosuccinic acid scan is also useful in follow-up of patients with renal trauma to evaluate renal differential function and to provide information concerning the severity of the damage. This information is important in recommending long-term follow-up for sequelae such as hypertension.[13]

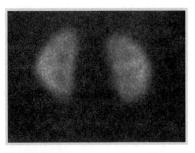

Figure 5-8.
Normal dimercaptosuccinic acid with uptake of radiotracer equal throughout the renal parenchyma. Note the smooth, even edges of the kidney with normal renal contour.

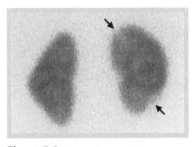

Figure 5-9.
Dimercaptosuccinic acid (DMSA): acute pyelonephritis. Acute inflammation prevents normal radiotracer DMSA uptake and creates areas of photopenia as indicated by the arrows. However, the normal renal contour is preserved.

?➤ *Pearl*

Diethylene triamine penta-acetic acid is the imaging modality of choice to measure GFR.

Diethelyne Triamine Penta-acetic Acid

Tc-99m-DTPA is a chelating agent that is removed almost entirely by glomerular filtration. Therefore, it is the imaging modality of choice to measure GFR. Imaging with Tc-99m-DTPA provides information about renal perfusion early in the study, and delayed images provide information about renal function and the collecting system. A disadvantage of using DTPA is a variable degree of plasma protein binding (1%–10%), which can underestimate GFR.[12]

Glucoheptonate

Tc-99m glucoheptonate is an organic anion that is rapidly removed from the kidney via glomerular filtration and tubular secretion. Because of its rapid clearance, it can to be used to find ERPF. The major disadvantages of using hippuran are the radioisotopes used to label it, which give higher radiation doses. Also, the photon is poorly imaged by conventional gamma cameras. These factors, and its high expense, limit its use at most major pediatric medical centers.[12]

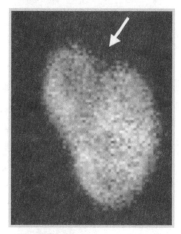

Figure 5-10.
Dimercaptosuccinic acid: renal scarring. Renal scarring results in contraction of the normal renal contour, as indicated by the arrow.

Computed Tomography

The spiral CT and electron beam CT have improved the ability to image the kidneys, including the collecting system and renal vasculature. Computed tomographic imaging is based on the attenuation of x-ray photons as they pass through patient tissues. A computer then mathematically reconstructs a cross-sectional image of the body from measurements of x-ray transmission through thin slices of body tissue.[14]

Noncontrast CT images are used to evaluate stone disease and detect renal parenchymal calcifications. Precontrast attenuation measurements of renal masses and evaluation of hemorrhagic events can be determined.[15] The arterial phase images at 25 seconds and can evaluate vascular abnormalities, such as arteriovenous malformations, and can provide detail of vascular anatomy. The corticomedullary phase, obtained at 30 to 70 seconds post–contrast injection, may offer better characterization of renal masses. The nephrographic phase, obtained at 90 to 180 seconds, is important in the evaluation of renal parenchyma for neoplasms and inflammatory disease and can evaluate renal veins for possible tumor thrombus when there is a renal neoplasm. Delayed images obtained at 3 to 5 minutes after contrast is excreted into the collecting system can demonstrate filling defects in the collecting system and image the ureters. Images at 20 minutes will evaluate the bladder. Because of the paucity of fat in the neonate, CT examination is limited except to evaluate retroperitoneal or abdominal masses.[4] However, it can be an important imaging modality in older children. In a stable trauma patient, CT imaging is the imaging modality of choice based on its accuracy and ability to diagnose urologic and nonurologic abdominal and pelvic injuries. A renal protocol CT scan consisting of a noncontrast phase followed by contrast and delayed phases allows for evaluation of the renal vasculature, parenchyma, and collecting system, respectively. Computed tomography can better characterize tumors of the genitourinary system that are initially diagnosed with ultrasound. In these cases, CT is indicated to establish the presence of function in the contralateral kidney, to evaluate for bilateral disease, and to stage the tumor.

☙ Pearl

Computed tomography is the gold standard for diagnosing renal calculi and evaluating a trauma patient and the extent of disease in patients with neoplasms.

Although CT is a valuable imaging modality, there are risks and disadvantages associated with its use. Intravenous contrast media are excreted by way of the kidney through glomerular filtration. These agents are nephrotoxic and can induce acute impairment of renal function after exposure. In addition, patients with asthma and severe allergies are at increased risk of subsequent reaction to contrast agent injection. Furthermore, most young children require sedation for the study. Perhaps the most important consideration in the pediatric patient is ionizing radiation exposure. Therefore, CT scanning of children should be reserved for situations in which ultrasonography, nuclear medicine, and MRI cannot provide the needed information.

Magnetic Resonance Imaging

Magnetic resonance imaging is a multiplanar diagnostic imaging modality that acquires images based on proton density, T1 and T2 relaxation flow, magnetic susceptibility, and diffusion.[4] The addition of faster imaging times and gadolinium, a nonnephrotoxic contrast agent that has virtually no side effects, has made MRI an attractive imaging technique in the pediatric population.

Currently MRI is reserved for the evaluation of more complex cases. Magnetic resonance imaging can provide details of the genitourinary system in the fetus.[16] It is excellent for assessing tissue characteristics and determining relationships with surrounding structures. It also provides excellent anatomical detail of the upper collecting system, making it useful in the evaluation of duplex systems associated with ectopic ureters. Magnetic resonance imaging is also valuable in the diagnosis of intrarenal and perirenal masses, metastatic evaluation of other tumors, and evaluation of pelvic structures including the ovaries and uterus.[4]

ẻ❧ Pearl

Magnetic resonance imaging is valuable in the diagnosis of renal and perirenal masses, evaluation of pelvic structures, and metastases.

Although MRI is an important imaging modality, it does have significant limitations. Children usually need sedation for MRI. In addition, MRI is expensive, and with the exception of a few academic institutions, most pediatric hospitals do not have access to the up-to-date units needed to fully evaluate the urinary tract of a pediatric patient.

Imaging of Genitourinary Tract

Urinary Tract Infection

Imaging recommendations for children with their first culture-documented UTI vary from institution to institution (Chapter 6). Ultrasound may be performed to evaluate for evidence of obstruction, particularly in children who did not have prenatal ultrasound imaging after 30 to 32 weeks of gestation.[17] Cystography (contrast or isotope) is used to evaluate for VUR, ureteroceles, or PUV in boys. Renal cortical scans using Tc-99m-DMSA are used to detect acute pyelonephritis and/or renal scarring (see Figures 5-9 and 5-10).

According to the AAP, all children younger than 2 years diagnosed with their first UTI should be evaluated with a renal and bladder ultrasound to screen for hydronephrosis or evidence of obstruction.[18] The AAP also recommends a VCUG or RNC in children 2 months to 2 years of age with their first UTI.[19]

Imaging evaluation in all children younger than 5 years and in older girls with febrile or recurrent infections is recommended.[19] In older boys with a first episode of acute cystitis, a sonogram (if negative) is sufficient. However, if evidence is found of hydronephrosis or bladder wall thickening, a VCUG should be performed to evaluate the urethra and to evaluate for VUR.[19] In girls with a normal sonogram evaluation, isotope cystography can be performed to evaluate for VUR and to avoid radiation to the gonads. Although these practices are currently in place, it should be noted that there is only fair evidence to support these recommendations (see Chapter 6 and Figures 5-11 and 6-1). Tc-99m-DMSA scintigraphy is the study of choice for confirming the diagnosis of acute pyelonephritis in children.[20]

Ultrasonography, followed by VCUG or isotope cystogram, followed by a possible Tc-99m-DMSA scintigraphy is the most common sequence for evaluation of children with febrile UTIs, but recent studies have questioned this approach. Because Tc-99m-DMSA can identify children with acute pyelonephritis who are at risk for renal scarring, independent of the presence or absence of VUR, an alternative approach in children with a culture-documented UTI and a normal prenatal ultrasound is to initially obtain a Tc-99m-DMSA scintigraphy study. If lesions are noted, further evaluation with a VCUG is recommended. Hanssan et al[21] found that performing the Tc-99m-DMSA first may prevent unnecessary VCUGs in 48.5% of children.

Contrast CT may be used to evaluate for pyelonephritis and is very sensitive for detection of perirenal or intrarenal abscesses. However, because there is considerable radiation exposure with CT, a Tc-99m-DMSA should be the first-line study to evaluate children for acute pyelonephritis. Magnetic resonance imaging can obtain the information normally obtained by nuclear scan, ultrasound, and VCUG in a single study without exposing children to ionizing radiation.[22] However, widespread use of this imaging modality in children with UTIs is currently limited because of cost, lack of availability, and the need for sedation.

⅌ Pearl

Ultrasound, followed by VCUG or RNC and possibly Tc-99m-DMSA scintigraphy, is the most common sequence for evaluation of children with febrile UTI.

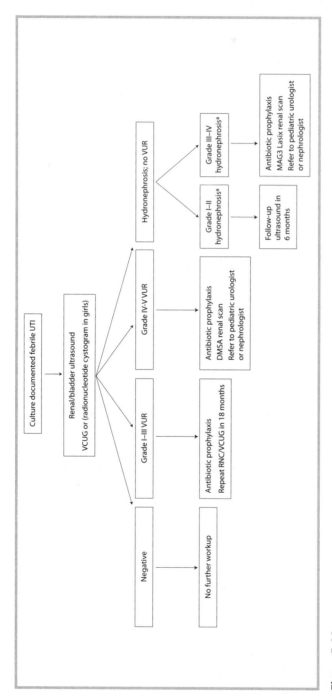

Figure 5-11.

Standard workup for culture-documented febrile UTI. DMSA indicates dimercaptosuccinic acid; RNC, radionuclide cystography; VCUG, voiding cystoure-throgram; VUR, vesicoureteral reflux.

[a]Any UTI under age 5 years.

Febrile or recurrent UTI in older girls.

Older boys with febrile UTI or abnormal sonogram.

Hydronephrosis

The causes of prenatal and postnatal hydronephrosis are multiple (Table 5-1). In the era of the prenatal ultrasound, an incidental radiologic diagnosis of hydronephrosis is common. These ultrasound findings often dictate decisions for further workup with the goal of accurately diagnosing pathology without subjecting a large number of healthy children to invasive investigations. In newborns with abnormal findings on prenatal ultrasound, the increased risk of urinary infection merits initiation of antibiotic prophylaxis until urologic diagnosis has been established.

Postnatal imaging recommendations in patients with a normal postnatal ultrasound who had demonstrated prenatal hydronephrosis are controversial. In cases of persistent postnatal hydronephrosis or newly diagnosed hydronephrosis, the etiology of the hydronephrosis is obstructive, refluxing, or nonobstructive. As discussed earlier, the diameter of the renal pelvis can give some indication of the etiology and help direct the initial evaluation. Hydronephrosis is often graded as mild, moderate, or severe. The Society for Fetal Urology grading system uses 4 grades to describe the severity of hydronephrosis on ultrasound (see Figure 5-4).

Studies have reported that routine VCUG in the evaluation of newborns with a prenatal diagnosis of hydronephrosis can result in the detection of VUR in 10% to 40% of cases.[23,24] However, in these studies most of the patients had persistent postnatal dilation of the upper collecting system. At

Table 5-1. Differential Diagnosis of Hydroenphrosis[a]		
Renal Pelvis	**Renal Pelvis and Ureter**	**Renal Pelvis, Ureter, Bladder and Possibly Urethra**
UPJ obstruction	VUR (high grade)	PUV
VUR	Megaureter obstructive nonobstructive	Neurogenic bladder
MCDK	Duplex collecting system in association with ectopic ureter, uretercrocele or lower pole VUR	Prolapsing ureterocele

Abbreviations: MCDK, multicystic dysplastic kidney; PUV, posterior urethral valve; UPJ, ureteropelvic junction; VUR, vesicoureteral reflux.

[a]Hydronephrosis can be limited to the renal pelvis or may be associated with dilation or abnormalities of other areas of the collecting system. A differential diagnosis can be considered depending on the area involved.

our institution, we no longer recommend routine VCUG if the postnatal ultrasound is normal. However, if the postnatal sonogram was performed in the first week of life, we do repeat the sonogram at 3 to 4 months of age to avoid missing hydronephrosis that may have been underestimated during a period of perinatal dehydration (Chapter 17).

Vesicoureteral reflux is graded according to the International Reflux Study in Children (Figure 5-12). Vesicoureteral reflux is associated with 2 important sequelae: pyelonephritis and renal scarring. Therefore, it is important that children remain on antibiotic prophylaxis if a diagnosis of VUR is confirmed. Vesicoureteral reflux spontaneously resolves or improves in most patients, depending on the grade of reflux. Spontaneous resolution of VUR diagnosed after a UTI occurs in about 90% of patients with grade I; 80% with grade II; 50% with grade III; and 10% with grade IV; with virtually no resolution of grade V on long-term follow-up.[25] However, recent studies focusing on newborns with high-grade VUR detected prenatally have shown much higher resolution rates, even with grade V VUR. Spontaneous resolution of reflux usually occurs within the first few years of life, after which the rate of reflux resolution remains constant throughout childhood at 10% to 15% per year.[26] Follow-up recommendations include RNC at 12- to 18-month intervals and continuation of antibiotics until resolution of the reflux or until the child is toilet trained.[1] In cases of persisting VUR, breakthrough UTIs, or noncompliance with medical management, children should be evaluated by a pediatric urologist. A VUR management algorithm is presented in Figure 18-5.

Hydronephrosis may be secondary to obstruction. Obstruction of the urinary tract is most often associated with significant dilation of the AP diameter of the renal pelvis, which is defined as greater than 15 mm, or hydronephrosis with associated dilation of the calices.[1] Significant hydronephrosis in the absence of hydroureter and a normal bladder is most often due to UPJ obstruction or MCDK. Ureteropelvic junction obstruction is the most common cause, accounting for 48% of all dilated collecting systems.[3] Currently, with the use of prenatal screening, most cases of UPJ obstruction are diagnosed prenatally; however, presentation in older children may occur with bouts of episodic abdominal or flank pain and vomiting (Dietl crisis), UTI, or hematuria after minor trauma.[1]

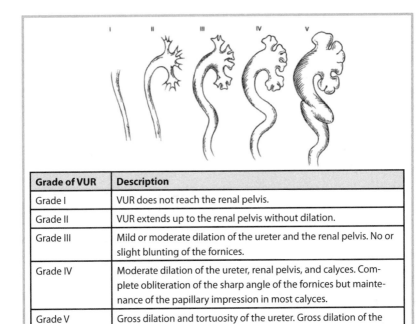

Grade of VUR	Description
Grade I	VUR does not reach the renal pelvis.
Grade II	VUR extends up to the renal pelvis without dilation.
Grade III	Mild or moderate dilation of the ureter and the renal pelvis. No or slight blunting of the fornices.
Grade IV	Moderate dilation of the ureter, renal pelvis, and calyces. Complete obliteration of the sharp angle of the fornices but maintenance of the papillary impression in most calyces.
Grade V	Gross dilation and tortuosity of the ureter. Gross dilation of the renal pelvis and calyces. The papillary impressions are not visible in most calyces.

Figure 5-12.
The International Reflux Grading System. VUR indicates vesicoureteral reflux. (Reprinted with permission from Fernbach SK, Feinstein KA, Schmidt, MB. Pediatric voiding cystourethrography: a pictorial guide. *Radiographics.* 2000;20:155.)

Ureteropelvic Junction Obstruction

In UPJ obstruction, the calyces and renal pelvis are dilated to varying degrees (Chapter 18). Renal parenchyma may be thinned and may appear more echogenic. In the most severe cases, small cysts may be present, indicating a degree of dysplasia. Although usually detected by ultrasound, a 99mTc-MAG3 diuretic renal scan is the imaging modality of choice for a suspected UPJ. This provides quantitative assessment of differential renal function of the hydronephrotic kidney relative to the contralateral renal unit. It also provides semiquantitative assessment of drainage from the dilated collecting system.

When UPJ obstruction is diagnosed in an infant, 2 options are available: expectant surveillance or operative intervention. Surveillance has been initially recommended in newborns with prenatally detected hydronephrosis if the AP diameter of the renal pelvis is less than 30 mm and/or differential function is greater than 40%. Even in the presence of severe UPJ obstruction, spontaneous resolution is possible. Spontaneous resolution or improvement was reported in 78% of 31 kidneys with moderate or severe hydronephrosis and a differential function of greater than 35%. However, careful long-term follow-up is necessary because more than 30% of UPJ obstruction cases may require pyeloplasty.[27] Follow-up includes serial 99mTc-MAG-3 diuretic renal scans at 6- to 12-month intervals, depending on the degree of obstruction, to assess drainage and function.

Indications for surgical intervention in patients with prenatally detected hydronephrosis include increasing dilation on follow-up studies, poor initial or deteriorating differential renal function (<35%–40%), worsening drainage over time, or persistent obstruction with stable function but no evidence of improvement after 4 to 5 years of observation.[1] When the AP diameter is greater than 30 mm, 60% to 100% of these units will eventually lose function.[28] Surgical intervention is usually necessary in these children, as well as when function is less than 40% at initial evaluation.[1] In contrast to prenatal hydronephrosis, older children with UPJ obstruction usually present with symptoms of abdominal/flank pain, infection, or hematuria. Because spontaneous improvement is unlikely in this age group, early surgical intervention is usually indicated without a period of surveillance.

> **꽃 Pearl**
>
> Tc-99m-MAG3 diuretic renal scan is the imaging modality of choice for a suspected UPJ obstruction.

Renovascular Hypertension

Hypertension occurs in approximately 1% to 3% of children.[3] However, recent studies indicate that the incidence may be increasing. Renal disorders are one of the most common etiologies of hypertension in the pediatric population and should be considered in children diagnosed with high blood pressure (Chapter 15). Infants and children younger than 10 years who are diagnosed with hypertension and older children with severe hypertension require advanced laboratory and imaging evaluation. Renal ultrasound with Doppler imaging is often the initial imaging modality.[4]

Renal scintigraphy in conjunction with an ACE inhibitor, most often captopril, is a reliable study in the evaluation of renovascular hypertension and renal artery stenosis. This study is not useful in neonates because glomerular function rate is low. Normally, imaging with a Tc-99m-MAG3 or Tc-99m-DTPA after administration of an ACE inhibitor will reveal equal uptake and drainage of the radiotracer. If the renal artery diameter is decreased by 50%, the test will reveal decreased uptake by the involved kidney. If abnormalities are noted, it is important to next perform renal scintigraphy without the presence of an ACE inhibitor. If the repeat study without an ACE inhibitor is normal, renovascular disease is highly suspected. Overall, the sensitivity of captopril renography appears to be approximately 90% to 93% and the specificity approximately 93% to 98%.[3]

Renal angiography remains the gold standard for evaluation of renal artery disease.[3] Magnetic resonance angiography is quickly becoming a popular alternative to the conventional renal angiogram because it is noninvasive. It uses gadolinium, a noniodinated contrast material, and produces no ionizing radiation. However, imaging of distal arteries is often inferior, sedation is required in younger children, and MRA is contraindicated in cases of magnetic implants.

Renal Cystic Disease

Multicystic dysplastic kidney has characteristic sonographic findings including communication between dilated calices and the renal pelvis, the presence of walls between cysts, larger cysts located in the periphery of the kidney, and the absence of identifiable renal parenchyma (Figure 18-3). In neonates with prenatally suspected MCDK, an ultrasound can be obtained prior to discharge from the nursery because, unlike hydronephrosis, hydration status plays no part in the accurate diagnosis.

Contralateral reflux has been reported in up to 28% of children with MCDK, leading some physicians to recommend routine VCUG in the evaluation of these patients.[1] Contralateral UPJ obstruction is also a common concomitant urologic anomaly, and other ureteral anomalies may occur. Merrot et al[29] found a 15% incidence of ipsilateral genital abnormalities, indicating the need for careful physical examination of these children. Confirmation that the dilated moiety is indeed a nonfunctioning MCDK is usually necessary. A Tc-99m-MAG3 scan is recommended because it will provide information concerning function of the suspected MCDK and drainage of the contralateral system if hydronephrosis is present.

The management of MCDK is no longer controversial. Initial surveillance includes ultrasound every 6 months for the first year of life. If MCDK is stable in size or shows evidence of involution, no further follow-up imaging or treatment is necessary. Yearly blood pressure monitoring is also recommended because hypertension may rarely occur in these patients. The risk of malignant degeneration is remote. Nephrectomy is rarely indicated for MCDK (Chapter 18).

Autosomal recessive polycystic kidney disease is easily diagnosed by ultrasonography (Figure 16-1). The kidneys are markedly enlarged bilaterally, but usually maintain their uniform shape. The ectatic dilated renal tubules give the kidneys a homogeneous hyperechoic appearance.[9] Autosomal dominant polycystic kidney disease is the third most common systemic hereditary condition, accounting for approximately 10% of patients undergoing dialysis.[30] Although ADPKD is usually a disease of adults, about 2% to 5% of patients manifest an early clinical course and may die perinatally.[31] Ultrasound is very sensitive and has become the primary mode of diagnosis. Ultrasound screening for ADPKD in children with a positive family history usually begins between the ages of 10 to 15 years. Ultrasound reveals multiple renal cysts of varying sizes located in the parenchyma of both kidneys (Figure 16-2). Earlier in the course of the disease the cysts are fewer in number and good corticomedullary differentiation may be appreciated.[9] Over time, the cysts enlarge and may compress or distort the renal parenchyma. The false-negative rate of screening by ultrasound is approximately 14% in patients younger than 30 years because macroscopic cysts may not actually develop until later in life.[32]

Simple cysts are rare but may be present in children. Much like in adults, on ultrasound simple cysts are round or ovoid with sharply defined, smooth walls. Internally they are fluid filled and thus anechoic.[32] Simple cysts are benign and do not require long-term follow-up. However, it is reasonable to obtain a follow-up sonogram after 1 year to make certain that new cysts have not developed and to monitor for any significant increase in the size of the cyst. Multiple cysts are often seen in patients with ADPKD, tuberous sclerosis, or von Hipple Landau syndrome. Juvenile nephronophthisis and medullary renal cystic disease are causes

ᘓ❧ Pearl

Ultrasound is the primary imaging mode used in the diagnosis of renal cystic disease.

of progressive renal insufficiency in children. Ultrasound findings include small to normal in size, hyperechoic kidneys that have small (0.1–1.0 cm) cysts in the medulla and at the corticomedullary junction.[3] In these patients, careful follow-up is key. Yearly sonography and serum creatinine to evaluate progression of the disease and to look for solid tumors are necessary. Computed tomography or MRI may be used to further evaluate suspicious or solid-appearing lesions. Multilocular cystic nephromas are lesions described sonographically as multiple cystic lesions that do not communicate and contain highly echogenic septations with sonolucent loculi.[3] These lesions may be associated with foci of Wilms tumor and have been considered premalignant. Children with these lesions should be referred to a pediatric urologist for surgical evaluation.

Solid Renal and Adrenal Masses

Solid masses in a pediatric patient are often found by ultrasound, by a parent, or incidentally by a primary care physician during a routine physical examination. Flank or abdominal pain, gross hematuria, and hypertension are clinical indicators of a possible renal mass.

Malignancies of the kidney represent 6.3% of cancer diagnosed among children younger than 15 years and 0.6% in children between the ages of 15 and 19 years.[33,34] Initially, plain radiographs and ultrasonography are routinely obtained for patients who have any suspicious mass. Contrast CT or MRI provides additional details on tumor consistency, extent of local disease, and distant organ involvement. Radiologic findings vary among different tumor types. Subtle differences may give some indication of the diagnosis; however, precise diagnosis cannot be obtained on the basis of preoperative imaging studies, and confirmatory histologic evaluation is necessary.

Pearl

Masses are diagnosed by plain radiographs and ultrasonography. Computed tomography with contrast or MRI provides additional details.

Renal Tumors

Computed tomography scan of the abdomen is the standard diagnostic modality for Wilms tumor. Examination of the renal vein and inferior vena cava is necessary to exclude extension of tumor, which occurs in approximately 4% of children.[3] Magnetic resonance imaging is superior to CT and ultrasonography in evaluating intravascular involvement. Computed tomography of the chest is also required to look for pulmonary nodules.[3]

Suspected clear cell sarcoma, rhabdoid tumors of the kidney, and congenital mesoblastic nephroma (the most common renal tumor in infants <6 months) may be studied with ultrasonography, CT, or MRI. Clear cell sarcomas of the kidney are associated with both bone and brain metastasis. Thus both skeletal surveys and bone scans are recommended after a histologic diagnosis is confirmed. Rhabdoid tumors are aggressive tumors that may be associated with primary brain tumors, so MRI or CT evaluation of the brain is important. Congenital mesoblastic nephroma cannot be distinguished radiologically from other tumors. However, ultrasound may show concentric rings, and CT may demonstrate splaying of the calyces instead of parenchymal displacement. Angiomyolipomas are benign lesions, but they can cause substantial morbidity when greater than 4 cm in size because these have an increased risk of hemorrhage. Annual ultrasounds are indicated to assess size and to evaluate for rare cases of RCC that may develop, particularly in children with tuberous sclerosis. Magnetic resonance imaging is an alternative imaging modality if ultrasonography is limited, as in the case of obesity. Renal lymphoma may manifest as a solitary lesion or as multiple lesions. Computed tomography imaging of lymphomatous renal masses often demonstrate homogeneous attenuation, unlike primary renal tumors, which are most often heterogeneous. On ultrasound, lesions are usually hypoechoic, reflecting tissue homogeneity. Renal cell carcinoma accounts for 1.4% of renal tumors in patients younger than 4 years, 15.2% between the ages of 5 and 9, and 52.6% between 10 and 15 years, with a peak incidence at age 11.[35,36] In children, RCC most commonly presents with pain, hematuria, or a flank mass. Ultrasound reveals a solid mass. Contrast-enhanced CT will reveal an enhancing renal mass.

Adrenal Tumors

Neuroblastoma is one of the most common solid tumors of early childhood. Imaging is important for both diagnosis and treatment planning. In children with neuroblastoma, plain radiographs may demonstrate a calcified abdominal or posterior mediastinal mass.[3] Ultrasound demonstrates a solid mass that is typically a mixed heterogenous echo pattern. Computed tomography scan reveals a large perirenal mass with calcification characteristic of neuroblastoma. Magnetic resonance imaging is useful in patients in whom there is a suspicion of spinal canal involvement. The radiolabeled iodine ^{131}I-MIBG scan is highly specific and sensitive for evaluating the extent of disease, bone involvement, and recurrence of disease after completion of therapy.[3] The complementary use of Tc-99m-methylene diphosphate bone scans can virtually eliminate any false-negative MIBG results.[3] However, only histologic evaluation of tissue can confirm the diagnosis.

Adrenocortical carcinoma and pheochromocytoma are rare tumors of childhood. Adrenocortical carcinoma may present with Cushing syndrome, whereas pheochromocytoma often presents with symptoms associated with catecholamine excess, such as hypertension. Adrenocortical carcinomas are most often evaluated with ultrasound or CT. Pheochromocytoma limited to the adrenal gland may be evaluated by ultrasound. However, ultrasound is less sensitive in the detection of tumors outside of the adrenal gland. The MIBG scan is an alternative imaging modality for locating multifocal pheochromocytoma. Jalil et al [37] found an overall sensitivity of 89% for CT, 98% for MRI, and 81% for ^{131}I-MIBG, indicating that MRI is the better imaging modality for pheochromocytoma. These tumors are hyperintense ("light-bulb sign") on T2-weighted imaging, making even small pheochromocytomas easy to diagnose.

Adrenal hemorrhage is somewhat uncommon and is most often diagnosed with ultrasound prenatally.[38] Adrenal hemorrhage may be followed with serial ultrasounds every 3 to 6 months to ensure resolution.

Renal Ectopia and Agenesis, Horseshoe Kidney

Renal ectopia occurs when the kidney does not lie in its normal location (Figure 18-2). Ultrasound is usually the initial imaging study. Ultrasound can readily identify most cases of fusion anomalies and ectopy of the kidney. The Tc-99m-DMSA renal cortical scan is the method of choice for assessing the size, location, and relative function of the ectopic renal parenchyma. Rarely, a small dysplastic ectopic kidney may be associated with an ectopic ureter. These small ectopic kidneys are frequently missed on ultrasound but detected on the Tc-99m-DMSA renal scan or MRI.

Bilateral renal agenesis is incompatible with life (Chapter 18). Unilateral renal agenesis is a relatively common urologic anomaly occurring in 1:1,000 autopsies and in 1:1,500 prenatal ultrasound studies.[39,40] This anomaly is usually discovered incidentally on prenatal ultrasound or during evaluation for

UTI or congenital abnormalities. Ultrasound will reveal an empty renal fossa and no evidence of the kidney in known ectopic positions. Tc-99m-DMSA or Tc-99m-MAG3 can provide anatomical and functional confirmation in a single study. Computed tomography and MRI also may be used to confirm the diagnosis of unilateral renal agenesis. Voiding cystourethrogram should be considered to evaluate the contralateral kidney because VUR occurs in up to 37% of these patients.

Horseshoe kidney is fusion of only the caudal aspect of the kidney (also see Chapter 18). This anomaly is suspected when both kidneys are located lower than normal with evidence of malrotation. In the horseshoe kidney, the isthmus connecting the 2 kidneys can often be visualized with a Tc-99m-DMSA or Tc-99m-MAG3 renal scan.[9] Horseshoe kidneys are associated with an increased incidence of UPJ obstruction. If hydronephrosis is detected, a Tc-99m-MAG3 renal scan is recommended to determine both function and drainage of the system.

Urolithiasis

Urolithiasis in the pediatric population is relatively uncommon (Chapter 19). Several radiologic studies are available to diagnose kidney stones, including KUB, IVP, ultrasound, and CT. Magnetic resonance imaging is insensitive in the detection of calcifications. Plain abdominal radiography only detects radiopaque stones and has a low sensitivity (62%) and specificity (67%) for the diagnosis of urolithiasis[41] (Figure 19-1). For many years, the gold standard for diagnosing urolithiasis was an IVP. However, IVP has been replaced by ultrasound and CT scans. Ultrasonography avoids radiation exposure and hence can be repeated frequently. However, a recent study by Palmer[9] reported a poor detection rate of 59% in children when ultrasound was used as the initial diagnostic test. Ultrasound may detect larger stones, but small calculi or those located in the ureter may be missed. When identified, calculi appear as echogenic foci with posterior shadowing. If the stone is obstructing, hydronephrosis or hydroureter may be seen (Figure 19-2).

Computed tomography scan, which is often the initial study in children presenting with abdominal pain, is highly accurate in the diagnosis of urolithiasis (89%–100%). When urolithiasis is suspected, it is important to obtain a noncontrast CT because intravenous contrast can mask the presence of a stone. The calculus is seen as high-attenuation focus (Figure 5-13).

If the stone is obstructing, hydronephrosis will be present. If located in the ureter, dilation proximal to the stone and edema of the ureteral wall with periureteral stranding may be seen.

Although noncontrast, narrow spiral CT is the most sensitive study for urolithiasis, there is significant radiation exposure to pediatric patients.[42] Therefore, evaluation by CT should be limited to those patients with a nondiagnostic ultrasound who continue to have symptoms suspicious for nephrolithiasis. Plain radiographs, if a stone is radiopaque, or ultrasound may be used to evaluate stone movement once a diagnosis is established.

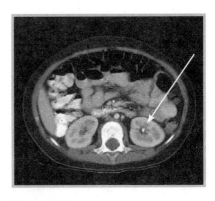

Figure 5-13.
Renal calculi appear as a high-attenuation focus as indicated by the arrow.

❧ Pearl

Ultrasound and noncontrast spiral CT are the most valuable imaging studies in the diagnosis of urolithiasis. Due to radiation exposure, CT evaluation should be limited to those patients with a nondiagnostic ultrasound and continued symptoms.

Ureteral Abnormalities

Megaureter

By far, the most common cause of hydroureter is VUR, most commonly seen in grades IV and V reflux. However, ureteral dilation not associated with VUR can occur. A ureter greater than 7 mm in diameter is referred to as *megaureter* and can be refluxing, as with high-grade VUR (obstructed or nonobstructed).[9]

In pediatric patients, ultrasound is often the initial study in the diagnosis of a megaureter. Longitudinal and transverse sonographic images of the bladder are highly sensitive in detecting distal ureteral dilation. A VCUG should be obtained to evaluate for VUR and to evaluate the bladder and urethra in search of other causes for the dilation, such as ureterocele, PUV, ectopic ureter, or neurogenic bladder.[1] If the VCUG fails to provide a diagnosis, a Tc-99m-MAG3 diuretic renal scan is obtained to evaluate for obstruction.[9]

Fifty-two percent to 72% of children with nonobstructing, nonrefluxing (primary) megaureter have resolution of the hydroureteronephrosis.[43,44] Therefore, expectant management is reasonable in affected children who have good differential renal function (>40%) on initial Tc-99m-MAG3 renal scans. Imaging should include yearly ultrasound and/or Tc-99m-MAG3 diuretic renal scans depending on the severity of the hydroureteronephrosis.

Duplex collecting systems are relatively common. Prenatal ultrasonography has resulted in an increased detection of duplex systems. On ultrasound, a simple duplication is demonstrated by a larger-than-normal kidney with 2 central hyperechoic foci separated by a band of normal echogenic renal parenchyma. There is no evidence of hydronephrosis or hydroureter in these cases, and the bladder is normal.[9] In cases of simple duplication, no additional imaging studies are indicated because these normal variants are not associated with an increased risk of infection.

Dilation of the fetal urinary tract is associated with complex renal duplication in 4.7% of cases.[45] More complex cases occur in the presence of ureteroceles, ectopic ureters, UPJ obstruction, or VUR. Ultrasound may reveal variable degrees of hydronephrosis of the upper pole and/or lower pole moiety. Dilation of the upper pole moiety, indicating possible obstruction, is most often associated with ureteral ectopia or ureterocele. Dilation of the lower pole moiety is most often associated with high-grade VUR. Rarely, UPJ obstruction of the lower pole may occur.[9]

Radiologic evaluation begins with sonography. A VCUG should be obtained to evaluate the presence of VUR and to evaluate the bladder for any abnormalities. Early bladder filling may reveal a round filling defect in cases of an ectopic ureterocele or VUR during voiding that can indicate an ectopic ureter.[1] In these more complicated duplex disorders, a Tc-99m-MAG3 diuretic renal scan can provide both functional and drainage information for each system. Tc-99m-DMSA is used to assess renal function in duplex systems associated with lower pole VUR.

The ureterocele is a cystic dilation of the distal portion of the ureter (Figure 18-4). Most often, the ureterocele is associated with ureteral duplication (80%) but may also occur with single ureters.[3] When identified on prenatal ultrasound, serial ultrasound studies are obtained to evaluate amniotic fluid volume, bladder volume, hydronephrosis, and echogenicity of the kidney. Ultrasound is the best modality for diagnosing ureteroceles and reveals a round or oval, thin-walled cystic structure that protrudes into the posterolateral side of the bladder[1] (Figure 18-4). Because VUR into the lower pole ureter is not uncommon, a VCUG should also be obtained. On VCUG, ureteroceles appear as smooth, broad-based filling defects positioned near the trigone. The Tc-99m-MAG3 diuretic renal scan is performed to assess the drainage and the degree of dysfunction of the hydronephrotic kidney. Magnetic resonance urography may also be helpful in defining complex anatomical relationships.

Prune-belly syndrome is characterized by deficiency of the abdominal wall musculature, bilateral cryptorchidism, and a dysmorphic urinary tract usually associated with nonobstructive, severe VUR into dilated tortuous ureters. Prenatal ultrasound will reveal severe bilateral hydroureteronephrosis, a dilated posterior urethra, and a large bladder that empties poorly. Increased renal parenchymal echogenicity, cystic changes, and poor corticomedullary differentiation are sonographic signs of renal dysplasia. After birth, a VCUG is performed to evaluate the severity of VUR, the degree of bladder distention, the bladder's ability to empty, and urethral abnormalities. A DMSA scan can be obtained to evaluate renal size and function. Alternatively a Tc-99m-MAG3 diuretic renal scan may provide both functional and drainage information.

Bladder Abnormalities

The exstrophic complex of anomalies of the bladder ranges from epispadias to cloacal exstrophy. The most common anomaly is classic bladder exstrophy. Prenatal ultrasound may suggest bladder exstrophy in a fetus by absence of bladder filling, a low-set umbilicus, and widening of the pubic rami. Although sonography is an excellent imaging modality to evaluate the fetus, factors such as the maternal body habitus and/or oligohydramnios can prevent an adequate assessment of fetal anatomy. Prenatal MRI has become an important imaging study in these and other cases of complex congenital genitourinary anomalies. Children born with any exstrophic complex abnormality will require complex treatment and full evaluation of the skeletal, genitourinary, and reproductive systems.

Anomalies of the urachus, the embryonic remnant of the communication between the bladder and the umbilicus, include urachal sinus, urachal cyst, patent urachus, and urachal diverticulum. Patients most often present with periumbilical discharge, followed by a mass or cyst and abdominal or periumbilical pain. Ultrasonography is the initial diagnostic imaging modality of choice. Routine use of VCUG is not generally warranted. However, in cases of umbilical drainage, some physicians recommend a sonogram or a VCUG to help differentiate a patent urachus that communicates with the bladder from a blind-ending sinus.[46] Computed tomography or MRI may also be used when sonography is nondiagnostic.

Bladder diverticula are found in approximately 1.7% of children.[47] They may or may not be associated with VUR. Bladder ultrasonography may detect bladder diverticula; however, a VCUG with oblique views is the best imaging modality because it provides anatomical detail and can assess emptying of the diverticulum. It is important to evaluate emptying of the diverticulum because stasis may be a risk factor for infection.

The most common cause of neuropathic bladder in children is spina bifida. Neuropathic bladder also may be suspected in children with voiding disorders if plain films reveal significant abnormalities of the spine or sacrum. A renal or bladder ultrasound should be obtained in these children to evaluate the upper tracts for hydroureteronephrosis that can be secondary to a high-pressure bladder. The bladder wall may be thickened or trabeculated, and bladder diverticula may be appreciated. A VCUG will diagnose VUR, if present, and will often reveal trabeculations, sacculations, and diverticula that may not be seen on ultrasound.[9]

Bladder masses in children are rare and may be infectious, benign, or malignant. Bladder lesions can cause irritative voiding symptoms, urinary retention, gross hematuria or, in advanced cases, a palpable mass.[48] The anatomy should be defined with renal and bladder ultrasonography and VCUG. Contrast CT or MRI imaging can help further define a lesion, although these studies are most often used for staging after a diagnosis is obtained. Cystoscopic inspection with biopsy may be indicated.

Fifteen percent to 20% of RMS arise from the genitourinary system, particularly bladder and prostate. The vagina and uterus are relatively unusual sites.[3] On ultrasound, the mass may be heterogenous or homogenous and hypoechoic. If a bladder mass is identified, cystoscopy is warranted because biopsy of the mass will confirm the diagnosis. Proper assessment for determining the extent of disease includes chest radiography and CT scan.[3] Magnetic resonance imaging will provide more detail about tumor extension.

Viral cystitis usually presents with sudden onset of gross hematuria, severe dysuria, and frequency. Sonography often reveals massive bladder wall thickening that may be asymmetrical and simulate a bladder mass. Biopsy results in bleeding and should be avoided.

Bladder stones are more commonly seen in children with significant bladder pathology, such as following bladder augmentation or continent urinary diversions using a segment of bowel to reconstruct the bladder. Bladder stones may be detected by plain film if radiopaque, or by ultrasound or CT. Computed tomography scan is more sensitive in documenting bladder stones in the augmented bladder because small stones may hide in the folds of the bowel and be missed by ultrasound.[9]

Urethral Abnormalities

Posterior urethral valve is a cause of prenatally detected bilateral hydronephrosis in male fetuses. Prenatal ultrasound findings that suggest a PUV include an enlarged bladder with a thickened bladder wall, posterior urethral dilation, unilateral or bilateral hydronephrosis, increased renal echogenicity, and oligohydramnios. Prenatal sonography of the bladder may show the "keyhole" sign, representing the dilated prostatic urethra immediately below the distended bladder. The kidneys may be severely hydronephrotic with increased echogenicity or cystic changes in renal parenchyma suggestive of dysplasia. Postnatal outcomes are worse when these findings are detected before 24 weeks of gestation.

Postnatally, a urethral catheter (or feeding tube) should be placed and urine output monitored closely. Once the infant is stable, a PUV is diagnosed with a VCUG. The posterior urethra is much more dilated than normal, and the anterior urethra is usually only partially filled. The bladder neck is often prominent and may appear as an annular band (Figure 5-14). The bladder can be irregular with trabeculations, diverticula, and bladder wall thickening. Vesicoureteral reflux may be present and is often severe.

The function of each renal unit can vary and may be equal or asymmetrical. In some cases associated with unilateral high-grade reflux, function of one kidney may be sacrificed because that unit acts as a "pop-off" mechanism that allows the contralateral kidney to develop normally. This syndrome of unilateral VUR and renal dysplasia has been well described. Bladder diverticula, a patent urachus, and urinomas may also act as pop-

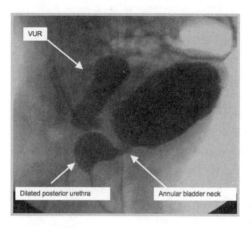

Figure 5-14.
Voiding cystourethrogram in an infant with posterior urethral valve (PUV). Voiding cystourethrogram is used to diagnose PUV. Note the dilated posterior urethra, the narrow annular bladder neck, and the trabeculated bladder wall. In this case, severe vesicoureteral reflux (VUR) is also present.

off mechanisms, preserving renal function by lowering bladder pressures. The presence and number of pop-off mechanisms in the system are directly correlated with favorable renal and bladder outcomes. Renal function may be assessed by nuclear scintigraphy. Tc-99m-MAG3 diuretic renal scintigraphy is used to evaluate function and drainage of the hydronephrotic urinary system. Further evaluation in these children is dictated by renal and bladder function and the presence of other genitourinary abnormalities. A nadir serum creatinine higher than 0.8 mg/dL by 1 year of age indicates a high risk of progressive deterioration in renal function.[49]

Anterior urethral valves are rare causes of obstruction in the male infant. Much like the PUVs, presentation can be antenatally with oligohydramnios, bilateral hydronephrosis, and bladder thickening. Postnatally, patients may present with a weak stream, a midline scrotal bulge with voiding, urinary frequency, or urinary infection. A VCUG will demonstrate an obstructing valve at the penoscrotal, bulbar, or penile urethra.[9] As with all cases of bladder outlet obstruction, VUR is often present. A VCUG or MRI can diagnose other urethral abnormalities, including prostatic utricle, megalourethra, and congenital urethral diverticulum.

Scrotum and Testes

Cryptorchidism
Cryptorchidism, or undescended testis, is the most common disorder of the male endocrine glands in children, occurring in 3.7% of full-term boys. It has been reported to be as high as 30% in premature boys.[50] Currently there is virtually no role for radiologic imaging in children with simple

cryptorchidism. Evaluation by a pediatric urologist has a detection rate of more than 80%.[51] Ultrasound, CT, and MRI can detect testes located in the inguinal region that are easily palpable by an experienced examiner. However, for the intra-abdominal testicle, ultrasound, CT, and MRI are poor imaging studies, with detection rates as low as 0%.[52] Although studies have reported that MRA correctly identifies practically all intra-abdominal testicles, this technique is expensive and requires sedation. Most importantly, imaging does not affect management because surgery is required in any case. Currently, for patients with a nonpalpable testicle, examination under anesthesia followed by scrotal exploration or laparoscopy is the standard of care.[51]

♣ Pearl

Currently, there is virtually no role for radiologic imaging in children with simple cryptorchidism.

Testicular Torsion

The differential diagnosis for the acute scrotum in the absence of trauma includes spermatic cord torsion, torsion of the testicular appendage, epididymitis, hernia and, occasionally, tumor. Accurate diagnosis can often be difficult. Time is of utmost importance. Studies have shown that after 6 hours of spermatic cord torsion, approximately 90% of testicles will be nonviable. This rate approaches 100% after 24 hours.[53]

Acute testicular torsion, which usually occurs in the pubertal boy and less commonly in the younger male, is most often described as a sudden onset of testicular pain. Nausea and vomiting are common and very sensitive symptoms in cases of testicular torsion. Suspicious early physical findings include a high-riding testicle with a horizontal lie, diffuse tenderness, and an absent cremasteric reflex. In boys with this clinical picture, imaging should be avoided and emergent urologic evaluation obtained, particularly if the onset of pain occurred within the previous 6 to 8 hours.

When findings are less equivocal or when the onset of pain was greater than 24 hours, Doppler ultrasound may be used to evaluate testicular blood flow. However, it should never delay surgical exploration in highly suspicious cases of less than 12 hours' duration. The typical grayscale pattern of testicular torsion is nonspecific and can vary from a normal-appearing testicle in early cases to a heterogeneous echo pattern in cases of hemorrhagic infarct. Because grayscale findings are nonspecific, Doppler ultrasound is essential in the examination for testicular torsion. The absence of testicular blood flow on color and power Doppler ultrasound is considered diagnostic for ischemia. The finding of absent testicular blood flow on color Doppler ultrasound is 86% sensitive, 100% specific, and 97% accurate in the diagnosis of torsion.[54]

Testicular scintigraphy is an alternative imaging modality for testis torsion. It is performed with intravenous injection of Tc-99m-pertechnetate and includes a blood flow study and fixed images. The normal examination shows symmetrical blood flow in both testes, whereas unilateral decreased flow is seen with testicular torsion. Intrascrotal hydrocele is a potential pitfall for nuclear scintigraphy. When a central photopenic region is seen, transillumination of the scrotal contents or sonography can help differentiate between hydrocele and testicular torsion.[9]

The absence of testicular enhancement on contrast-enhanced MRI defines testicular torsion. The sensitivity and specificity of MRI in the diagnosis of testicular torsion is 93% and 100%, respectively.[55] Although MRI appears promising, prospective trials are needed. In addition, MRI often requires sedation, is not as readily available as sonography, and continues to be expensive.

Torsion of a testicular appendix can be confused with testicular torsion. Typically the clinical presentation differs. Boys with torsion of the appendix tend to be younger. Pain is often not as severe, and nausea and vomiting are usually absent. The "blue dot" sign seen at the superior pole of the testis represents infarction of the appendix testis and is a pathognomonic physical finding.[53] The cremasteric reflex is usually present with a torsed appendix. On sonography, the ischemic appendix appears as a small, hyperechoic or hypoechoic mass with no evidence of blood flow. However, there may be evidence of an inflammatory response with marked hyperemia around the area of the torsed appendix or diffusely throughout the testis and epididymis.

≈ Pearl

In boys with a 6- to 8-hour clinical picture of testicular torsion, imaging should be avoided and an emergent urologic evaluation should be obtained.

Later the torsed appendage may appear as a small, calcified structure.

Epididymitis is commonly associated with a more gradual onset of pain. Tenderness is usually localized to the superior pole of the testis and is often associated with fever and pyuria. Sonography reveals epididymal enlargement. Color Doppler shows increased blood flow. The cremasteric reflex is usually present in the early stages of infection. Urine culture is mandatory, and bacterial infection should raise suspicion in prepubertal boys for an ectopic ureter into the seminal vesicles.

Testicular Masses

Scrotal masses can be cystic or solid, extratesticular or intratesticular. A common scrotal mass is the hydrocele. Hydroceles are located at the anterolateral aspect of the testicle. They are fluid filled and thus are anechoic on sonography, appearing as a black area around the testicle. Loculations can be seen when an inflammatory process, such as epididymitis or orchitis, is present. In most cases, the diagnosis of a hydrocele can be confirmed in the office using simple and inexpensive transillumination rather than sonography. Varicoceles are an abnormal dilation of the veins in the pampiniform plexus located in the spermatic cord. Almost all cases of varicoceles are left sided due to a longer left testicular vein and its right angle of entry into the left renal vein. Although ultrasound examination with the patient standing and lying will help to identify varicoceles, physical examination that reveals a soft, nontender scrotal mass described as a "bag of worms" is usually all that is needed to establish the diagnosis in adolescents.

Testicular tumors are uncommon, accounting for 1% to 2% of all pediatric solid tumors.[3] Benign lesions represent a greater percentage of cases in children than in adults. However, any solid testicular mass should be considered a neoplasm, and urgent evaluation should be implemented. Testicular ultrasound provides important information in the evaluation of testicular masses in children. Sonography has been shown to reliably differentiate intratesticular from extratesticular masses. Color Doppler ultrasound is even more effective than grayscale ultrasound in detecting intratesticular neoplasms in the pediatric population. Any suspicious solid scrotal mass should be evaluated with sonography and the patient referred to a pediatric urologist for further evaluation.

Masses in the Female

Interlabial masses include Gartner duct cyst, imperforate hymen with hydrocolpos or hydrometrocolpos, prolapsed urethra or ureterocele, and tumors such as sarcoma botryoides. Physical examination may be adequate for diagnosis; however, imaging can often be useful.

Vaginal atresia or imperforate hymen results in hydrocolpos or hydrometrocolpos. This is the most common midline suprapubic cystic mass in girls. In hydrocolpos, ultrasound will reveal echogenic material filling a dilated vaginal vault.[9] The mass can compress the ureters and result in hydronephrosis. Sonography of the kidneys is indicated if the diagnosis is suspected.

Sarcoma botryoides (RMS of the vagina) may present as an interlabial mass, classically described as a "cluster of grapes," extruding from the vaginal introitus. Renal-bladder sonography is appropriate when this diagnosis is considered. Sonography can visualize the botryoid form well and can identify signs suggestive of bladder outlet obstruction. It may demonstrate hydronephrosis secondary to ureteral compression by the tumor. Computed tomography scanning is an important part of the diagnostic workup and can provide useful information regarding the extent of tumor, site of origin, and lymphatic involvement. Magnetic resonance imaging can be helpful also. Histologic evaluation is necessary for definitive diagnosis.

Intersex

Although prenatal ultrasound can raise suspicion for intersex, it does not provide a definite diagnosis. Sonography is the initial imaging modality. Although it is only 50% accurate in detecting intra-abdominal testes, it can detect gonads in the inguinal region and can assess Müllerian anatomy. If a gonad is palpable, ultrasound may distinguish testicle from ovary by its oval shape, larger size, and the presence of an epididymis. An ovary is more echogenic and may have follicular cysts.[9] Pelvic ultrasound may detect a uterus, which can be identified as an oval, midline echogenic structure with a prominent endometrial stripe.

Genitography, a fluoroscopic contrast study, is important in the evaluation of a child whose sexual differentiation is indeterminate. It is used to detail the anatomy of the urethra and vagina. Ultrasound should be the initial screening study to evaluate the pelvis, uterus, ovaries, and testes. Magnetic resonance imaging is reserved for cases with equivocal ultrasound findings.

Summary

Imaging in the pediatric patient is important in diagnosis, management planning, and follow-up of many genitourinary malformations. However, one must be familiar with the differential diagnosis and the various imaging modalities available, including the benefits, risks, and limitations of each. Combined with a good history, a complete physical examination, and appropriate laboratory studies, radiologic imaging is an invaluable resource to physicians in the diagnosis and management of genitourinary abnormalities in the pediatric population.

References

1. Belman AB, King LR, Kramer SA. *Clinical Pediatric Urology.* 4th ed. New York, NY: Taylor and Francis; 2002

2. Morey AF, McAninch JW, Tiller BK, Duckett CP, Carroll PR. Single shot intraoperative excretory urography for the immediate evaluation of renal trauma. *J Urol.* 1999;161:1088–1092

3. Campbell MF, Walsh PC, Retik AB. *Campbell's Urology.* 8th ed. Philadelphia, PA: Saunders; 2002

4. Sty JR, Pan CG. Genitourinary imaging techniques. *Pediatr Clin North Am.* 2006; 53:339–361

5. Singer EA, Golijanin DJ, Davis RS, Dogra V. What's new in urologic ultrasound? *Urol Clin North Am.* 2006;33:279–286

6. Cromie WJ, Lee K, Houde K, Holmes L. Implications of prenatal ultrasound screening in the incidence of major genitourinary malformations. *J Urol.* 2001;165:1677–1680

7. Levi S. Ultrasound in prenatal diagnosis: polemics around routine ultrasound screening for second trimester fetal malformations. *Prenat Diagn.* 2002;22:285–295

8. Gloor JM. Management of prenatally detected fetal hydronephrosis. *Mayo Clin Proc.* 1995;70:145–152

9. Palmer LS. Pediatric urologic imaging. *Urol Clin North Am.* 2006;33:409–423

10. Grignon A, Filion R, Filiatrault D, et al. Urinary tract dilatation in utero: classification and clinical applications. *Radiology.* 1986;160:645–647

11. Fernbach SK, Feinstein KA, Schmidt MB. Pediatric voiding cystourethrography: a pictorial guide. *Radiographics.* 2000;20:155–168; discussion 168–171

12. Goldfarb CR, Srivastava NC, Grotas AB, Ongseng F, Nagler HM. Radionuclide imaging in urology. *Urol Clin North Am.* 2006;33:319–328

13. Moog R, Becmeur F, Dutson E, Chevalier-Kauffmann I, Sauvage P, Brunot B. Functional evaluation by quantitative dimercaptosuccinic acid scintigraphy after kidney trauma in children. *J Urol.* 2003;169:641–644

14. Brant WE, Helms CA. *Fundamentals of Diagnostic Radiology.* 2nd ed. Baltimore, MD: Williams & Wilkins; 1999

15. Kawashima A, Vrtiska TJ, LeRoy AJ, Hartman RP, McCollough CH, King BF Jr. CT urography. *Radiographics.* 2004;24(suppl 1):S35–S54; discussion S55–S38

16. Caire JT, Ramus RM, Magee KP, Fullington BK, Ewalt DH, Twickler DM. MRI of fetal genitourinary anomalies. *AJR Am J Roentgenol.* 2003;181:1381–1385

17. Hoberman A, Charron M, Hickey RW, Baskin M, Kearney DH, Wald ER. Imaging studies after a first febrile urinary tract infection in young children. *N Engl J Med.* 2003;348:195–202

18. American Academy of Pediatrics Committee on Quality Improvement, Subcommittee on Urinary Tract Infection. Practice parameter: the diagnosis, treatment, and evaluation of the initial urinary tract infection in febrile infants and young children. *Pediatrics.* 1999;103:843–852

19. Rushton HG. Urinary tract infections in children. Epidemiology, evaluation, and management. *Pediatr Clin North Am.* 1997;44:1133–1169

20. Rushton HG, Majd M. Dimercaptosuccinic acid renal scintigraphy for the evaluation of pyelonephritis and scarring: a review of experimental and clinical studies. *J Urol.* 1992;148:1726–1732

21. Hansson S, Dhamey M, Sigstrom O, et al. Dimercapto-succinic acid scintigraphy instead of voiding cystourethrography for infants with urinary tract infection. *J Urol.* 2004;172:1071–1073; discussion 1073–1074

22. Rodriguez LV, Spielman D, Herfkens RJ, Shortliffe LD. Magnetic resonance imaging for the evaluation of hydronephrosis, reflux and renal scarring in children. *J Urol.* 2001;166:1023–1027

23. Farhat W, McLorie G, Geary D, et al. The natural history of neonatal vesicoureteral reflux associated with antenatal hydronephrosis. *J Urol.* 2000;164:1057–1060

24. Jaswon MS, Dibble L, Puri S, et al. Prospective study of outcome in antenatally diagnosed renal pelvis dilatation. *Arch Dis Child Fetal Neonatal Ed.* 1999;80:F135–F138

25. Skoog SJ, Belman AB, Majd M. A nonsurgical approach to the management of primary vesicoureteral reflux. *J Urol.* 1987;138:941–946

26. Smellie JM, Normand ICS. Reflux nephropathy in childhood. In: Hodson J, Kincaid-Smith P, eds. *Reflux Nephropathy.* New York, NY: Masson Publishing USA; 1979:14–20

27. Bajpai M, Chandrasekharam VV. Nonoperative management of neonatal moderate to severe bilateral hydronephrosis. *J Urol.* 2002;167:662–665

28. Dhillon HK. Prenatally diagnosed hydronephrosis: the Great Ormond Street experience. *Br J Urol.* 1998;81(suppl 2):39–44

29. Merrot T, Lumenta DB, Tercier S, Morisson-Lacombes G, Guys JM, Alessandrini P. Multicystic dysplastic kidney with ipsilateral abnormalities of genitourinary tract: experience in children. *Urology.* 2006;67:603–607

30. Hildebrandt F. Genetic renal diseases in children. *Curr Opin Pediatr.* 1995;7:182–191

31. Avner ED, Sweeney WE Jr. Renal cystic disease: new insights for the clinician. *Pediatr Clin North Am.* 2006;53:889–909

32. Weber TM. Sonography of benign renal cystic disease. *Radiol Clin North Am.* 2006;44:777–786

33. Bleyer A. Older adolescents with cancer in North America deficits in outcome and research. *Pediatr Clin North Am.* 2002;49:1027–1042

34. SEER. Cancer Incidence and Survival among Children and Adolescents: United States SEER Program 1975–1995. http://seer.cancer.gov/publications/childhood/adolescents/pdf. Accessed April 3, 2007

35. Leslie JA, Cain MP. Pediatric urologic emergencies and urgencies. *Pediatr Clin North Am.* 2006;53:513–527

36. Uchiyama M, Iwafuchi M, Yagi M, et al. Treatment of childhood renal cell carcinoma with lymph node metastasis: two cases and a review of literature. *J Surg Oncol.* 2000;75:266–269

37. Jalil ND, Pattou FN, Combemale F, et al. Effectiveness and limits of preoperative imaging studies for the localisation of pheochromocytomas and paragangliomas: a review of 282 cases. French Association of Surgery (AFC) and The French Association of Endocrine Surgeons (AFCE). *Eur J Surg.* 1998;164:23–28

38. Chandler JC, Gauderer MW. The neonate with an abdominal mass. *Pediatr Clin North Am.* 2004;51:979–997

39. Elder JS. *Management of Antenatally Detected Hydronephrosis.* Oxford, UK: Butterworth-Heinemann; 1996

40. Grotewold Chelimsky G, Gonzalez R. *Abnormalities of the Kidney.* Oxford, UK: Butterworth-Heinemann; 1997

41. Srivastava T, Alon US. Urolithiasis in adolescent children. *Adolesc Med Clin.* 2005; 16:87–109

42. Fielding JR, Steele G, Fox LA, Heller H, Loughlin KR. Spiral computerized tomography in the evaluation of acute flank pain: a replacement for excretory urography. *J Urol.* 1997;157:2071–2073

43. McLellan DL, Retik AB, Bauer SB, et al. Rate and predictors of spontaneous resolution of prenatally diagnosed primary nonrefluxing megaureter. *J Urol.* 2002;168:2177–2180; discussion 2180

44. Shukla AR, Cooper J, Patel RP, et al. Prenatally detected primary megaureter: a role for extended followup. *J Urol.* 2005;173:1353–1356

45. Ismaili K, Hall M, Donner C, Thomas D, Vermeylen D, Avni FE. Results of systematic screening for minor degrees of fetal renal pelvis dilatation in an unselected population. *Am J Obstet Gynecol.* 2003;188:242–246

46. Little DC, Shah SR, St. Peter SD, et al. Urachal anomalies in children: the vanishing relevance of the preoperative VCUG. *J Pediatr Surg.* 2005;40:1874–1876

47. Blane CE, Zerin JM, Bloom DA. Bladder diverticula in children. *Radiology.* 1994; 190:695–697

48. Defoor W, Minevich E, Sheldon C. Unusual bladder masses in children. *Urology.* 2002;60:911

49. Denes ED, Barthold JS, Gonzalez R. Early prognostic value of serum creatinine levels in children with posterior urethral valves. *J Urol.* 1997;157:1441–1443

50. Berkowitz GS, Lapinski RH, Dolgin SE, Gazella JG, Bodian CA, Holzman IR. Prevalence and natural history of cryptorchidism. *Pediatrics.* 1993;92:44–49

51. Kolon TF, Patel RP, Huff DS. Cryptorchidism: diagnosis, treatment, and long-term prognosis. *Urol Clin North Am.* 2004;31:469–480

52. Hrebinko RL, Bellinger MF. The limited role of imaging techniques in managing children with undescended testes. *J Urol.* 1993;150:458–460

53. Jayanthi VR. Adolescent urology. *Adolesc Med Clin.* 2004;15:521–534

54. Burks DD, Markey BJ, Burkhard TK, Balsara ZN, Haluszka MM, Canning DA. Suspected testicular torsion and ischemia: evaluation with color Doppler sonography. *Radiology.* 1990;175:815–821

55. Terai A, Yoshimura K, Ichioka K, et al. Dynamic contrast-enhanced subtraction magnetic resonance imaging in diagnostics of testicular torsion. *Urology.* 2006;67:1278–1282

■ *Urinary Tract Infection*

Billy S. Arant, Jr

Abbreviations

DMSA	Dimercaptosuccinic acid
IVP	Intravenous pyelography
UTI	Urinary tract infection
VCUG	Voiding cystourethrogram
VUR	Vesicoureteral reflux

Introduction

Urinary tract infection in children may cause more long-term morbidity than any other bacterial infection. Yet the management of UTI may also be the most argued topic in pediatrics. The only treatment guideline or practice parameter for managing UTI in children was published by the American Academy of Pediatrics in 1999,[1] but it applies only to febrile infants and young children—there is no such guideline for older children who suffer similar consequences with UTI. It is generally agreed that it is appropriate to treat a child with symptoms of a UTI with an antimicrobial agent. Usually, but not always, decisions are based on culture results of a properly obtained urine specimen. Once the infection is controlled, however, the controversy begins with what, if anything, should be done next. How and for how long should the patient be followed? Did this episode of UTI represent cystitis or pyelonephritis? Is diagnostic imaging really necessary and, if so, which test is best? Is there a different plan for boys and girls? What about younger versus older children, and if there is a difference, at what age does the recommendation change? Is this something a general pediatrician can manage, or is referral to a nephrologist or urologist indicated?

When looking for answers to these questions, one must consider the source of information—not only the expert opinion of an experienced investigator, but also the existence of evidence from clinical trials designed to answer a specific question. The clinical bias of the advisor should also be considered. A general pediatrician, even one who participated in clinical studies, may be very knowledgeable about the first UTI in a child but not have the long-term perspective of a physician who deals with complications that may have been anticipated. An infectious disease expert, for instance, may be interested only in the "bug" or the drug for each episode but have no long-range perspective for a disease that will most likely recur. A radiologist may have proprietary interests and recommend multiple tests that provide very similar information, whereas another may dislike the inconvenience of doing some procedures, such as a VCUG, in uncooperative children with anxious parents. A surgeon or urologist may

❧ Pearl

Urinary tract infection is a potentially serious disease that can cause severe morbidity if not recognized and treated appropriately.

be focused on performing some corrective procedure rather than adopting a "watch and wait" approach. A nephrologist may overreact because of the consequences of hypertension or chronic renal insufficiency often seen in children whose UTIs were poorly managed. Perhaps the greatest error a young physician can make in this regard is seeking the opinion of anyone, expert or not, without asking for the source of evidence used in support of the advice. After all, the question asked during malpractice litigation associated with a poor outcome is, "Doctor, what was the basis for your decision, and where can I read about it?" The casual recommendation of a colleague or teacher will not satisfy a deposing attorney or a jury. The advising colleague or teacher will not be available to share the responsibility of the situation, whereas evidence used to make the decision will always be there.

Epidemiology

Urinary tract infection will occur in up to 2% of boys[2] and 8% of girls prior to sexual activity,[3] and 20% to 50% of these will have VUR if examined.[4] Seven percent of febrile infants will have UTI, making the urinary tract second only to the respiratory tract in areas affected by bacterial infection at this age.[5] During the first 3 months of life, uncircumcised boys have the highest incidence of UTI at any age, which has been estimated as 20 to 30 times higher than in circumcised boys and higher than in female infants.[6] The female/male ratio of UTI in children of all ages is 5:1 in populations in which most boys are circumcised at birth but only 3:1 in populations in which boys are usually not circumcised. There is no plausible explanation for why UTI is observed less commonly in black children (both boys and girls) in Africa or North America, but all other races are affected similarly. The risk of UTI is higher when siblings have already experienced a UTI, which may be related more to the genetics of VUR than to UTI.[7]

Most UTIs are caused by Gram-negative bacteria representing the usual colorectal flora: *Escherichia coli* predominates, followed by *Klebsiella, Enterobacter, Pseudomonas,* and *Proteus; Enterococcus* is the only Gram-positive organism considered a urinary pathogen in a normal urinary tract. Bacteria gain access to the urinary tract either by blood (rarely) or the bladder (usually). Bacteria gain entry into the bladder through the urethral meatus, which accounts for the higher rate of UTI in the girl whose bladder is relatively less well protected due to a short urethra. Fortunately, most girls do not develop UTI unless they empty their bladders infrequently or incompletely. Obstruction to urine flow anywhere in the urinary tract, but especially in the bladder outflow tract, results in residual urine, which provides a medium conducive to bacterial growth. Relative obstruction occurs with VUR when the bladder urine refluxes into the ureter during micturition and subsequently returns to the empty bladder. When the infected urine reaches the papilla, pyelitis, and the papillary collecting duct, pyelonephritis may develop. P-fimbriated *E coli* attach to uroepithelial cells in the urethra and bladder and have been reported to cross the UVJ, even in the absence of VUR, to cause pyelonephritis. In the urinary tract, bacteria double in number every 20 minutes but must reach about 100,000 organisms/mL of urine before the inflammatory response produces symptoms. A single organism remaining undisturbed in bladder urine would exceed 100,000 organisms in less than 6 hours or even more overnight in a person who fails to empty the bladder completely before going to sleep. This is primarily the case in girls.

Although much has been made over the causality of cystitis due to bubble bath, there is no direct evidence for this. There are 2 more likely explanations. First, the chemical in bubble bath remains on the vaginal or urethral mucosa when a girl gets out of a bath and dries off without rinsing her skin and genitalia with clean water. Later, dysuria is experienced as urine flows over the irritated mucosa, but in this case, the urine remains sterile. Unless dysuria leads to micturition avoidance or partial urinary retention, UTI more likely results from the prolonged time that girls spend in dirty bath water enjoying the bubbles and allowing dirty bath water to enter the urethra and bladder. If a girl does not empty her bladder soon after a bubble bath, bacterial growth may occur.

> ### ᕲ Pearl
>
> Urinary tract infection is the most common bacterial disease responsible for long-term morbidity in children.

Presenting Symptoms

There is no one complaint specific for UTI (Table 6-1). When most physicians or parents think of UTI, the complaints of dysuria, frequency, urgency, and urinary incontinence in a child who was previously toilet trained come to mind. This usually is true for children when the lower urinary tract is inflamed but not necessarily infected. In children who can cooperate, a careful history may determine the timing of the dysuria—before, during, or after micturition is initiated. Cystitis hurts before micturition, whereas pain from urethritis begins with initiation of urine flow; and when only the external genitalia or perineum are irritated, dysuria begins after the stream is initiated when acid or saline urine wets the irritated mucosa or skin and may continue even after micturition ceases.

Fever is either not present or very low grade in cystitis, but either fever or an abnormal imaging study is required to affirm the diagnosis of pyelonephritis. However, up to 26% of children with VUR may have remained afebrile.[8] Unless a child has or had lower tract symptoms, pyelonephritis has to be suspected in any febrile child unless there is another clear explanation for the fever. The second complaint elicited most often with pyelonephritis is vomiting or diarrhea, which may be associated with abdominal discom-

Table 6-1. Differential Findings in Urinary Tract Infection		
	Cystitis	Pyelonephritis
History of present illness		
Fever	±	+
Dysuria	+	–
Frequency	+	–
Urgency	+	–
Incontinence	+	–
Dysfunctional voiding	+	+
Abdominal pain	±	+
Vomiting	–	+
Physical examination		
Fever	±	+
Suprapubic tenderness	+	–
CVA tenderness	–	+
Laboratory findings		
Hematuria	+	+
Pyuria	+	+
Proteinuria	–	+
Leukocyte esterase	+	+
Nitrite	+	+
Gram stain	+	+
Leukocytosis	–	+
Neutrophilia	–	+
Elevated ESR/CRP	–	+
Urine culture >10^5 colonies/mL	–	+

Abbreviations: ±, inconsistently found; +, usually present; -, ususally absent; CVA, costovetebral angle; ESR, erythrocyte sedimentation rate; CRP, C-reactive protein.

fort. So the febrile child is often suspected of having something other than UTI—gastroenteritis or the perennial favorite "red ears"—an excuse for initiating treatment and obviating the need to wait for a urine specimen. Fortunately, antibiotics prescribed for otitis media are usually effective against urinary pathogens. However, the real diagnosis is overlooked. When a child subsequently presents with similar symptoms and UTI is discovered, the physician may have the impression that this represents the first UTI. The opportunity to prevent a subsequent UTI and reduce the risk of further renal injury can be missed in this case.

It is important to know the voiding pattern in each child in whom UTI is suspected. In a continuity setting, this should be part of the well-child information recorded at least by the time toilet training is achieved. This includes the number of voidings per 24 hours and whether the child is continent of urine between voidings, regardless of toilet training. An infant who is still in diapers, even from birth, should have a dry diaper between voidings and bowel movements. If urine leaks constantly, abnormal insertion of a ureter into the urethra or vesico-vaginal fistula must be considered. If a child is toilet trained but has only enuresis, especially if there is a family history of enuresis, there should be no increased concern for UTI. However, if before acute illness a child exhibits an aversion to micturition, complains of suprapubic or perineal pain during micturition, interrupts the urinary stream several times while voiding, has difficulty initiating a stream, voids small volumes of urine more frequently than expected, or has daytime urinary incontinence, dysfunctional micturition should be suspected. This rather common condition, which often presents with cloudy urine and alkaline pH with the noxious odor of ammonia when urine remains in the bladder longer than normal, may be mistaken for UTI when symptoms are long standing rather than acute. However, incomplete bladder emptying or residual urine in this condition may predispose developing the first or recurrent UTI, especially in girls. Constipation is often a comorbid problem with these children. Constipation can obstruct the bladder outlet, and contracting the anal sphincter to inhibit defecation causes the bladder to contract against a closed bladder sphincter or sphincter dyssynergia, referred to also as *dysfunctional elimination syndrome.*

> ### ᴥ *Pearl*
> Abnormal voiding patterns identified by clinical history are associated with UTI.

Physical Examination

A child presenting with UTI may appear nearly well, moribund with Gram-negative sepsis or renal abscess, and anything in between. The only physical findings that support the suspicion of UTI are tenderness to suprapubic palpation in cystitis, bladder distention in an atonic or obstructed bladder, and discomfort or pain to percussion at the costovertebral angle with pyelonephritis. These more specific findings are not uniformly found in UTI even after careful examination. The perineum and genitalia must be inspected for signs of irritation, inflammation, and discharge. In boys, the foreskin (if present) should be retracted gently when possible and the urethral meatus and glans inspected. Phimosis, foreign body, trauma, and drainage should be noted. In girls, vaginal discharge or odor should be pursued. A foreign body (eg, toilet paper or feces) may be found, or perhaps vaginosis is the cause. The anus should be inspected, and sphincter tone or anal wink noted. Findings of constipation—encopresis, fecal soiling, or abdominal mass consistent with feces in the colon—should be recorded and the neurologic enervation of the perineum tested for the possibility of a neurogenic bladder owing to spina bifida occulta.

Diagnosis

The diagnosis of UTI can be suspected on clinical findings alone or an abnormal screening urinalysis of a routinely voided or bagged urine specimen (see Table 6-1). Abnormal semiquantitative findings in the urinary sediment done routinely in clinical laboratories correlate poorly with culture results.[1] Isolated microscopic hematuria is rarely associated with UTI (B. S. Arant, unpublished observations, 2007), but gross hematuria, suprapubic tenderness, and high fever are consistent with viral hemorrhagic cystitis in which the urine culture is negative for bacteria. However, infected urine may contain one or more abnormal dipstick findings—blood, pus, protein, leukocyte esterase, or nitrite—which are more reliable in predicting UTI.[1,9] Because the culture result is not known before the decision to treat a febrile child, the single best indicator that the culture will be positive is the finding on Gram stain of uncentrifuged urine one or more organisms per oil immersion field. This examination can be done even on a voided specimen in several minutes in an office or hospital laboratory. Although the organism cannot be identified other than Gram-positive or -negative in this way, this simple test allows limitation or redirection of the search for another focus of infection.

Diagnosis of UTI depends entirely on the results of a culture limited usually to a single urine specimen owing to the urgency to treat. Moreover, there must be significant bacteriuria, defined as at least 100,000 ($\geq 10^5$) bacteria of a single strain in 1 mL of urine. More recently, 50,000 or more colonies were accepted for certain prospective studies using carefully collected or catheterized specimens in a research setting when the cells in the urine were quantitated rather than estimated—a technique with no practical use.[10] As a rule, there are actually more than 10^6 organisms per milliliter of infected urine, but the standard reporting is only 10^5 or more when, on inspection—

not by actual count—the technician observes "significant" bacterial growth. Please note that significant colony counts, not microorganism identification or antibiotic sensitivities, can be estimated after only 12 to 18 hours following inoculation. So there is no need to wait for the laboratory to report the results at 24 or 48 hours to plan for further evaluation or treatment.

When done appropriately, a urine culture will identify the organism, provide a list of effective antimicrobials, and determine whether further evaluation is required. If the tested urine is sterile, there was no UTI, and antibiotic treatment, if started, can be stopped. Imaging study and follow-up for UTI are not necessary. Once treatment has been initiated, however, one may learn that the original urine specimen was mishandled or allowed to remain at or about room temperature while inoculation was delayed. Warm urine is nearly an ideal medium for bacterial growth. What would have been insignificant bacteriuria originally may now be reported as significant. The number of colonies reported will be the number of organisms in 1 mL of urine at the time of inoculating the culture medium. In this situation the diagnosis of UTI has been made, treatment initiated, and the patient committed to further evaluation and follow-up, which may have been unnecessary. Remember, it is the result of the urine culture that confirms the diagnosis of UTI, and it is the relatively high risk of sepsis or renal injury with UTI that mandates further consideration.

When more than one organism grows from the urine, which may occur in any specimen collected by a method other than the suprapubic technique, the result must be interpreted in light of clinical findings. This is easier when one organism has significant growth ($>10^5$/mL), whereas others have less than 10^4/mL—one may be the pathogen and the others contaminants. It also helps to remember that most organisms causing UTI are Gram-negative—*Enterococcus* is the exception. *Staphylococcus* of any species is not considered a pathogen unless urinary tract obstruction or renal abscess is suspected.

Although there are a few situations other than a suprapubic aspirate that artificially lower the colony count, such as a very dilute urine in a person with a renal concentrating defect or high-volume fluid intake with frequent bladder emptying—these conditions are unusual. Newborns have been falsely represented as unable to concentrate their urine, and thus have low colony counts when UTI is present. However, even preterm neonates concentrate their urine appropriately and nearly always exhibit significant bacteriuria with UTI. So the urine volume and specific gravity should be considered when deciding to accept a colony count of less than 10^5/mL. The only other condition in which a compromised colony count would be valid is when a patient is taking an antibiotic at the time the culture specimen is obtained. Urine is usually rendered sterile within hours of administration of the first dose of an effective antibiotic. Prior or concurrent therapy with an antibiotic to which the organism in the urine is resistant may suppress but not inhibit bacterial growth, and thus the colony count would be less than 10^5/mL.

To minimize clinical angst, collecting a nearly ideal urine specimen for evaluation is important. A voided specimen is always a good choice for screening and, when collected correctly in cooperating children, may be used for culture as well. It is easy to request that a clean-catch midstream urine sample be obtained, but too few concerned individuals know exactly what that means. Collection of urine usually falls to persons with no understanding of the consequences of an improperly collected urine specimen. When a child is able to cooperate, a urine sample can be collected after the urinary stream is initiated and before it ends (ie, midstream). This requires the assistance of an informed second person for most children—a parent instructed in the technique is often better than a stranger. There is no need for cleansing first—the initial urine clears the urethra and meatus better than sponges if collected in a container whose interior and cap are not contaminated with fingers or clothing (ie, clean catch). This is possible in circumcised boys and in those who are uncircumcised when the foreskin can be retracted. Girls can do this easily if they sit backwards on the toilet seat facing the wall or tank. The awkwardness of this position forces the thighs apart and the labia to spread, allowing placement of the sterile container in a dependent position between the thighs for collecting the specimen midstream. Cleansing the urethral meatus is advantageous when the initial urinary stream is collected, which is likely when instructions for midstream clean-catch urine are not communicated effectively or supervised correctly. Infants and uncooperative children present another dilemma. If there is only one chance to make a correct diagnosis before treatment is started, a voided specimen is the least desirable option.

More often than not, transurethral catheterization is performed to expedite a diagnosis or patient flow. The expense associated with bladder catheterization is overlooked and will not be recouped in its entirety. This includes the cost of the sterile catheter, the catheter tray or prep kit, the sterile gloves, and the time of 2 employees. Although it is assumed that a catheter placed under sterile conditions has minimal morbidity, contamination of urine with organisms introduced by the catheter occurs in 12% to 15% of patients. This problem is not apparent because most patients will be placed on antibiotic therapy immediately afterward. To place a catheter safely, the urethral meatus must be cleansed and the sterile catheter tip should only touch the meatus before or during the insertion. If the catheter tip touches any structure other than the urethral meatus, sterile technique requires that the catheter be discarded. Moreover, if any part of the catheter expected to penetrate the urethra is contaminated during the procedure, the catheter must not be used. To avoid contamination, the meatus must be adequately exposed with good lighting and a second person assisting—preferably not a parent. If the ordering physician is required to observe the technique used by the person placing the catheter or, better still, to perform the catheterization, fewer catheterizations might be done in outpatient settings. Inserting a catheter in an uncircumcised boy without contamination when the foreskin cannot be retracted or the meatus exposed is also difficult, even in experienced hands. Those who advocate casual catheterization of the bladder usually are unaware of the rates of bladder contamination and consequent urosepsis experienced before the antibiotic era—the availability of antibiotics is no excuse for poor technique.

The best option for obtaining uncontaminated urine in difficult patients, regardless of age, is suprapubic aspiration. Although first used in adults, some have assumed that this technique is reserved only for infants and that it is painful or more stressful than transurethral catheterization. Older girls with prior experience of catheterization and suprapubic aspiration usually choose the suprapubic approach. The only contraindications are bleeding disorders, skin lesions in the suprapubic area, and an empty bladder. If the bladder cannot be identified by palpation or percussion and it has been less than 1 hour since micturition last occurred, ultrasonography can be used to identify the bladder. The procedure is quick and cheap, requiring only an antiseptic sponge, sterile 3-mL syringe, 22-gauge/1½-inch hypodermic needle, a physician, an assistant, and a few minutes. Most important, the urine will not be contaminated and no colony count criterion is needed—any bacterial growth is diagnostic of UTI.

The diagnosis of pyelonephritis, in fact, requires significant bacteriuria plus the finding of fever or an imaging study consistent with renal parenchymal inflammation. There is usually only one chance to make the diagnosis of UTI correctly owing to the fact that there is a desire to alleviate discomfort and reduce fever, as well as eliminate further bacterial growth. Urgency in considering a diagnosis of UTI in a febrile child is best explained by the presence of purulence in the highly vascular renal parenchyma, which has the potential for entering the blood and causing urosepsis, usually with a Gram-negative organism, which may prove fatal.

Pearl

The diagnosis of UTI requires a urine culture on an appropriately collected specimen. There is no absolute rule for when to order a catheterized urine specimen.

Diagnostic Imaging

Diagnostic imaging of the infected urinary tract has always been and remains controversial. By 1975 there was a strong recommendation for studying all children following the first UTI to detect urinary tract abnormalities, including VUR, and to provide adequate treatment and follow-up. Recently, performing imaging studies has become more accepted.[11] There is no single controversy but rather different opinions among physicians that are not necessarily based on evidence but on personal experience, absence of convincing evidence, ignorance of existing evidence and, in many cases, myth emerging from long-standing traditions of clinical practice. For instance, it has long been held that a VCUG should be delayed 4 to 6 weeks after an acute UTI to avoid detecting VUR in patients who only had VUR as a result of the inflammatory changes in the bladder mucosa near the UVJ. The only evidence in support of this concept was the initial animal studies in the late 1930s, in which the contrast material was caustic to the bladder mucosa and VUR was observed in animals not prone to VUR. Another influence was what some considered an overaggressive approach prior to 1980 to open surgical repair of VUR of any grade based on the assumption that all VUR was harmful and could easily be eliminated. By waiting for inflammation to subside, it was thought that VUR would be identified less frequently and, therefore, many children spared an operation. This myth was so firmly entrenched in the nephrology and urology communities that it persisted even when a widely respected pediatric radiologist reported no difference in the incidence of VUR when the urine was sterile or infected.[12] Recently, several studies have compared the prevalence of VUR in children studied in the first week after diagnosis with those studies performed 4 to 6 weeks after diagnosis, and no difference was found.[13,14] Although the evidence clearly shows no advantage to waiting, rather a disadvantage because many patients do not show up for their VCUG when it is postponed, the recommendation to delay the study still prevails. The latest challenge to the value of any imaging study following UTI is based on a single study peculiar in the literature[11] and unfounded speculations by those who have reported no reasonable evidence for such an opinion.

The morbidity of pyelonephritis is strongly related to the number of acute episodes experienced by a child.[15] Eliminating a structural abnormality may reduce or eliminate the risk of recurrent pyelonephritis. Identifying a relative obstruction, such as VUR, which is associated with UTI and renal parenchymal injury in the absence of infection when voiding pressures are high,[16] should be followed with a careful plan of management to minimize and aggressively treat recurrent UTI, which has been shown to prevent further renal injury.[17]

The recommendations for imaging studies in this chapter are based mainly on the observation that careful evaluation of infants and children after a first UTI and urinary surveillance to ensure a sterile urine and normal intravesical pressure for those in whom abnormalities were detected have been associated with a reduction in the prevalence of end-stage renal disease in children from 19% in 1987[18] to less than 8% in 2006.[19] Those who recommend contrarily should be asked to support their suggestions with confirmed data. Imaging of the kidney and urinary tract is discussed in Chapter 5.

❧ Pearl

Between 30% and 50% of infants and young children with a first UTI will have an abnormality identified when imaging studies are performed.

Renal Ultrasonography

Renal ultrasonography can be performed at any time once the diagnosis of UTI is confirmed by culture. It is recommended for any child with a first or subsequent UTI, regardless of age, if not previously evaluated by imaging studies (see also Chapter 5 for additional information). Justification for this examination is mainly to rule out an anatomical problem that would confound treatment of the UTI, such as anatomical obstruction, urolithiasis, or abscess. The size and appearance of the kidneys are important, especially if there is a discrepancy in size to suggest prior renal insult or deformity or absence of a kidney. A ureteral duplication may be identified, which can be a normal variant in the absence of obstruction, VUR, or abnormal bladder insertion. Depending on the sophistication of the equipment and the examiner, it is possible, on occasion, to identify debris in the collecting system or bladder typical in pyelonephritis, note renal parenchymal inflammation and, when the bladder is full, real-time evidence of intermittent distention of the ureter or renal pelvis suggesting VUR. Bladder capacity, trabeculation of the bladder, and ureteral jets may be noted.

≥● Pearl

A normal renal ultrasound examination does not necessarily mean that no abnormality exists, and it should be considered a screening tool rather than a definite examination of the urinary tract.

Voiding Cystourethrogram

Voiding cystourethrogram is recommended following a first episode of UTI to detect VUR, bladder obstruction, bladder structure, and capacity, as well as congenital abnormalities (see also Chapter 5 for additional information). The yield of this study is probably greater than any other diagnostic test ordered in children. A VCUG is recommended in every child to at least 7 years of age and even older if voiding patterns or renal ultrasound is abnormal. Failing to identify VUR with a single VCUG does not mean VUR is not present—it is just not identified during that examination. A second VCUG may be warranted in a child who did not have VUR in the past but who now has recurrent UTI despite appropriate precautions to prevent it. A radionuclide VCUG has been demonstrated up to 25% more sensitive in picking up VUR than a contrast study. The only disadvantage to radionuclide VCUG is the limited potential for identifying a structural abnormality of the bladder. Therefore, a radionuclide VCUG (where available) should be considered a better choice than a second VCUG performed in a child with recurrent UTI but for whom VUR was not detected on a contrast study.

Depending on the sophistication of the facility, VCUG is performed after placement of a transurethral catheter through which a volume of radiopaque contrast material, or radionuclide, is instilled up to a pressure of 70 cm water. Radionuclide VCUG has been shown more sensitive in identifying VUR than contrast studies. The volume of material used is noted as an assessment of bladder capacity. Vesicoureteral reflux is detected in fewer than 0.5% of people at any age in the absence of prior UTI.[16] On the other hand, 50% of infants, 20% of 12-year-olds, and 4% of adults with a history of UTI will exhibit VUR. Moreover, 30% to 50% of siblings of patients with VUR will have VUR as well.[7] When detected, VUR is usually graded according to the 5 grades established by the International Reflux Study in Children.[20] In general, the collecting system is not dilated in grades I and II, but progressive dilation of the ureter, calyces, or renal pelvis is exhibited between grades III to V. The degree of dilation depends on 2 things. First, the intravesical pressure generated during bladder contraction, which can transform a normal caliber ureter on ultrasound (grade I) to a much dilated ureter (grade IV or V); and second, any prior injury to the collecting system in which the elastic fibers in the ureter have been replaced by fibrous tissue. The latter has a static appearance on ultrasound when the bladder is empty and the ureter remains dilated regardless of intravesical pressure.

There is a fair amount of hesitation in doing a VCUG in a child, and this is based mainly on the parental perception of a child's reaction to having a catheter placed. In the hands of an experienced pediatric radiologist, the procedure is minimally frightening. Some parents and pediatricians have expressed interest in sedating children prior to VCUG, even though this is rarely considered when a urine specimen is obtained by transurethral catheterization in the office or emergency department. Any child will resist being held down by strangers—VCUG may be stressful but should not be painful. Sedation alters the bladder forces that maintain competence of the UVJ

❧ Pearl

The abnormal yield of a VCUG in a child after the first UTI is probably greater than any other diagnostic test ordered in children.

and control micturition (bladder contraction and sphincter relaxation are functions of the autonomic nervous system) and renders a patient unable to cooperate. Cooperation by the patient is important to grading VUR, which should be done at peak voiding pressure, usually 30 seconds after micturition is initiated.

Renal Cortical Scintigraphy

This test may be performed by the intravenous injection of a radiolabeled isotope, which attaches to the proximal tubular epithelium located in the renal cortex. The most widely used material is Tc-99m-DMSA. A reduction in uptake of the isotope in one area of the cortex can be interpreted either as acute inflammation with altered parenchymal function, as a nonfunctioning segment of renal parenchyma resulting from prior injury now scarred and nonfunctioning, or as an area of failed embryologic development. When performed acutely with UTI, the cortical defect may be labeled *pyelonephritis*. Importantly, only 50% of patients with pyelonephritis will have any other abnormality—including VUR—detected during their evaluation.[21] If repeated 3 to 6 months later in the absence of a subsequent UTI and the defect is no longer present, one can conclude that the pyelonephritis resolved without scarring. If the cortical defect remains, the conclusion is a scar from a previous episode of pyelonephritis—not necessarily the most recent one. The reason for ordering renal cortical scintigraphy is an effort to identify potential or existing renal injury, which raises the risk of subsequent morbidity. An argument against performing the scintigraphy routinely, especially after a recent febrile UTI, is that if positive, a second study will be needed. In addition to the expense of the study, there is no additional recommendation for management. Finally, radiation exposure must be considered because the isotope remains in the kidney for hours, which may pose significant radiation exposure to the ovaries because they lie in close proximity to the kidneys. This kind of study can be done at any age because renal scarring may occur as frequently in adolescents as it does in young children.[22]

⸭ Pearl

Renal scarring caused by pyelonephritis can occur in a child or adolescent of any age, not just young children.

Intravenous Contrast Urography

This test, performed as IVP or computed tomography scan, may be useful in detecting anatomical abnormalities or even pyelonephritis on occasion. If one of these studies has been done already to rule out urolithiasis or identify the cause of abdominal pain, there may be no need for the ultrasound examination or scintigraphy.

Treatment Options

The goal of UTI treatment is to render the urine sterile with an appropriate antibiotic, identify anatomical or functional factors that predispose to UTI, and prevent another UTI. A management algorithm for UTI in children is presented in Figures 6-1 and 5-11.

Managing Acute Urinary Tract Infection

Once the diagnosis is established by culture, UTI requires antibiotic therapy. If an appropriate antimicrobial agent is selected by chance and confirmed by sensitivity testing on the organism cultured, it is usually continued for 10 to 14 days. The duration of treatment is entirely arbitrary. With the correct drug, the urine is rendered sterile within hours. Single oral dose therapy with amoxicillin (1.0 g) has been studied and found successful in more than 80% of children with uncomplicated UTI, but this was done when most uropathogens were predictably sensitive to that drug. A single intramuscular injection of gentamicin (80 mg) cured pyelonephritis in women. The main reason for continuing treatment for 10 days has been the traditional recommendation for antibiotic therapy ever since it was determined that a 10-day course of penicillin (600,000 U intramuscularly daily for 10 days) was needed to prevent rheumatic fever in patients infected with a rheumatogenic strain of group A β-hemolytic streptococcus. The main advantage of 10 days of antibiotic treatment in UTI is that it allows sufficient time to do a VCUG and still have 2 or 3 days of treatment to prevent any infection introduced by the transurethral catheterization.

The initial choice of the antimicrobial agent should be based on drug resistance generated in each community for common urinary pathogens. The resistance of *E coli* to amoxicillin may vary from one region to another. By comparison, *Enterococcus* responds only to ampicillin (±gentamicin) and not to the usual oral or parenteral drugs chosen to treat acute UTI. For

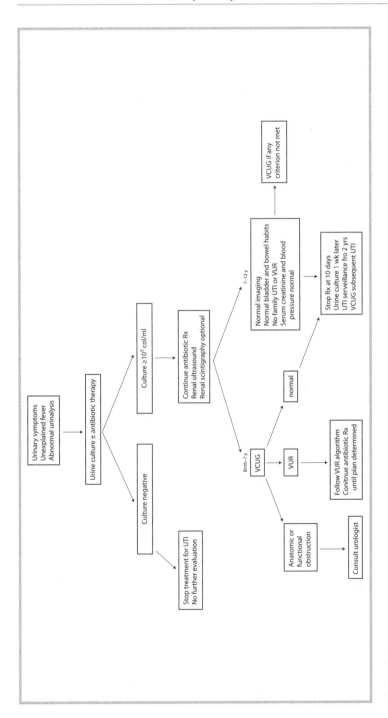

Figure 6-1.

Management algorithm for UTI in a child. UTI indicates urinary tract infection; Rx, treatment; VCUG, voiding cystourethrogram; VUR, vesicoureteral reflux.

all other organisms, a third-generation cephalosporin is the best antibiotic choice prior to obtaining results of the antibiogram. When a patient does not respond promptly to initial treatment, a second drug should be added; or if sensitivities are available, a single new drug should be adequate. Do not be misled by what appears to be a clinical response to initial treatment. The natural history of UTI reported in the preantibiotic era is that within 7 days of the onset of clinical symptoms, the untreated patient will either improve or die—continued treatment with an inappropriate antibiotic may follow the same course. When a patient appears too ill or if emesis is a presenting complaint, parenteral antibiotic treatment is always warranted. This is important for any child with pyelonephritis because an oral agent may not be retained long enough to be absorbed. A single daily dose of ceftriaxone (75 mg/kg) may be given intramuscularly or intravenously. An aminoglycoside can be given instead, but only if overall renal function is normal, the patient is adequately hydrated, and nonsteroidal anti-inflammatory drug therapy has not been given recently—alone or together these factors contribute to aminoglycoside nephrotoxicity. Although it has been traditional to admit a child with pyelonephritis to the hospital for observation, particularly infants and young children, one study found that these patients could be managed as outpatients when follow-up was ensured. This is inadvisable for physicians treating unfamiliar patients.

If no urinary tract abnormality is identified during the evaluation for the first UTI, effective treatment may be discontinued after 10 days. It is suggested that a follow-up urine culture be done 7 to 10 days later to ensure the urine has remained sterile. Continued surveillance for bacteriuria should be continued for at least 6 months and up to 2 years, which is the time recurrences will most likely occur.[3]

> ### ஐ Pearl
>
> Aggressive management of UTI reduces renal injury.

Preventing Recurrent Urinary Tract Infection

Prevention must be planned thoughtfully once the anatomy of the urinary tract has been assessed by imaging studies and acute UTI cured. The recurrence rate of UTI is high—up to 80% in school-aged girls—and recurrence is usually seen within 6 months.[3] Even with diligent urinary surveillance or antibiotic prophylaxis, 20% of children with VUR will have breakthrough

UTI[8]—recurrence is higher without close follow-up. With each recurrence, the risk of renal scarring increases exponentially—5% with the first episode and 60% with the fourth.[15]

The follow-up management of the first UTI is to prevent any subsequent infection of the urinary tract (Box 6-1). The approach is to establish good hygiene of the perineum, especially in girls, and the foreskin and glans in uncircumcised boys. These areas harbor the organism that will start the next UTI. Teaching parents good hygienic practice should be included in newborn discharge instructions and should be reviewed at each well-child visit until a boy knows (when lysis of adhesions permit) to retract his foreskin during micturition and for daily bathing. In a male infant with an abnormal urinary tract prone to infection, such as posterior urethral valves or neurogenic bladder, circumcision may be seriously considered because urinary pathogens, especially P-fimbriated *E coli,* can attach to the underside of the foreskin and uroepithelium of the urethra and bladder.

Normal bladder and bowel habits must be established. The bladder should be emptied at least every 2 to 3 hours while awake, immediately before bedtime, and at awakening. The consequences of bladder dysfunction have been addressed previously. Stool holding or constipation can partially obstruct the bladder outlet causing incomplete emptying. Perineal soiling provides a continuous supply of urinary pathogens to perimeatal skin and mucosa. It is desirable that the rectum be emptied daily in children with UTI by means of regular lubricants or laxatives.

Daily antibiotic prophylaxis in an attempt to maintain sterile urine has been the standard recommendation for many years. Daily administra-

---

Box 6-1. Preventing the Next Urinary Tract Infection— Goal: Maintaining a Sterile Urine

- Voiding schedule: complete bladder emptying >6 times/24 hours
- Bladder pressure remains normally low at all times
- No urinary incontinence while awake once toilet trained
- Bowel habits: prevent constipation and its consequences
- Daily antibiotic prophylaxis with recommended drugs or urinary surveillance with home dipstick weekly and with symptoms
- Urine culture with unexplained fever, urinary symptoms, positive dipstick
- When UTI suspected, initiate antibiotic therapy pending culture result

tion of trimethoprim alone (1–2 mg/kg), trimethoprim-sulfasoxazole (1–2 mg/kg or 5–10 mg/kg), or nitrofurantoin (1–2 mg/kg) is recommended for children with persistent VUR and may be considered for those with recurrent UTI in the absence of VUR. These drugs have a low rate of side effects, are concentrated mainly in the urine, and have been given safely for up to 20 years to patients with VUR. No other antibiotic is recommended for prophylaxis unless there is an allergy or intolerance to 1 of these 3 drugs. In a child continent of urine during sleep, a single dose of the antibiotic is given at bedtime after the bladder is emptied. These drugs are effective because they are excreted promptly into the urine in concentrations sufficient to inhibit bacterial growth of usual urinary pathogens without altering bowel flora. During the day, regular micturition provides a natural reduction in bacterial growth. For all infants and children not yet continent overnight, the antibiotic dose is halved and given twice daily. Otherwise, the drug would remain in the bladder less than 2 hours. Breakthrough infections when this regimen is followed are usually associated with resistant or unusual organisms. This practice is questioned as well. A recent review of a large patient database concluded antibiotic prophylaxis was not effective.[23] There were many flaws in the study design, and assumptions made by the investigators rendered the data unreliable in making any such conclusion. Because the database was large does not guarantee a reliable population sample. From the outset, only 0.8% of young children had at least one UTI identified—the literature is consistent in reporting a much higher incidence in this age group. Failure to administer an antibiotic appropriately in a compliant fashion without attention to other problems associated with recurrence may be the reason for failing to prevent recurrent UTI altogether—not antibiotic prophylaxis alone. Intermittent antibiotic treatment for each recurrent UTI was associated with new renal scarring in 21% of children with VUR[24]; whereas new scars were seen in fewer than 2% of patients on continuous prophylaxis.[17] Only a prospective study, such as the one funded by the National Institutes of Health and currently underway in which a strict protocol is followed for every patient, will answer this question. Until this study is completed, antibiotic prophylaxis is still recommended in patients with VUR and may be considered in patients with recurrent pyelonephritis but in whom VUR was never demonstrated. Management of VUR is presented in Figure 18-5.

For cases in which patients or parents refuse prophylaxis and physicians reject the benefit and embrace unproven strategies, every effort must still be made to prevent another UTI. An alternative to antibiotic prophylaxis is routine surveillance of the urine once or twice weekly by dipstick in the asymptomatic child. However, all recommendations to prevent UTI, except for the antibiotic

❧ Pearl

Continuous antibiotic prophylaxis to prevent recurrent UTI has been associated with important reductions in the risk of renal scarring compared with other studies in which antibiotic therapy was only given for symptomatic UTI.

therapy, must be in place. A positive finding of leukocyte esterase or nitrite, urinary symptoms, or unexplained fever should prompt a urine culture and immediate antibiotic treatment pending the culture result. Prompt treatment of pyelonephritis in animal models has been shown to reduce the risk of renal injury.

Natural History and Prognosis

Prior to the introduction of antibiotics, the most frequent abnormal finding at autopsy was pyelonephritic scarring.[25] Pyelonephritis has been the traditional cause of more than 20% of cases of chronic renal failure in Europe and Australia–New Zealand.[16] In the United States during the 1980s, primary VUR and obstructive uropathy, both associated with UTI, with tissue or radiologic confirmation of renal scarring accounted for 33% of children and adolescents needing dialysis or renal transplantation at a single center.[18] Renal scarring associated with one or more UTI also accounted for 23% of patients 18 years of age or younger with sustained hypertension.[26] In fact, renal scarring is identified in up to 30% of young women with hypertension, and these individuals have significant risk of developing worsening hypertension and deterioration of renal function during pregnancy, from which many do not recover renal function postpartum.[27]

Since 1970 there has been an effort, mainly in the industrialized world, to reduce the number of patients with consequential pyelonephritis. At first there was an aggressive approach to early identification and accurate diagnosis of UTI in children, followed with initial and serial radiologic imaging. Those identified with VUR or obstructive uropathy frequently had the abnormality treated surgically on the notion—not evidence—that elimination of the lesion would avoid further problems. Some attempted compulsive medical management to prevent recurrent UTI and renal scarring and did so with good results, but few physicians or patients achieved the degree of compliance needed to match such good outcomes.[17] The argument over which treatment was superior, surgical or medical, was answered finally with prospective, random allocation of patients with VUR to one treatment or the other. At the end of the 5-year follow-up period, neither treatment showed an advantage for preventing renal scarring.[28] Therefore, either treatment was found acceptable.

Parents and physicians alike have voiced objections to serial radiologic studies, frequent urine cultures, and antibiotic prophylaxis. The subsequent argument evolved that VUR can be eliminated successfully by surgery, although this treatment is more expensive, does not benefit those with dysfunctional micturition, and does nothing to help the 50% of children with pyelonephritis who are at risk of renal scarring and have no VUR to correct.[21] Nor does the recently introduced, already popular technique of endoscopic injection of a biocompatible material beneath the UVJ—referred to as the *sting*—offer a proven alternative treatment. This procedure is very attractive to parents, more comfortable than surgery to patients, and does not require an overnight hospital stay. On the other hand, the procedure offers no guarantee that VUR will be eliminated on the first or subsequent attempts, the charge is repeated for each separate procedure, reimbursement is not uniform and, like the dilemma of surgical versus medical treatment, the procedure has not yet been shown to reduce the risk of subsequent UTI or renal injury compared with surgery or conservative management.

Aggressive oversight and management of UTI in children during the past 30 years has reduced the prevalence of end-stage renal disease by more than half according to the latest data. Departure from this approach for unproven methods based on convenience, comfort, and choice seems to risk a reversal of realized success, but it will take another 20 years to know if all was for naught. As George Santayana (*Life of Reason*, 1906) warned, "Those who cannot remember the past are condemned to repeat it."

ह Pearl

Up to 80% of girls will have another UTI within 6 months of the most recent one.

References

1. American Academy of Pediatrics Committee on Quality Improvement and Subcommittee on Urinary Tract Infection. Practice parameter: the diagnosis, treatment, and evaluation of the initial urinary tract infection in febrile infants and young children. *Pediatrics.* 1999;103:843–852

2. Marild S, Jodal U. Incidence rate of first-time symptomatic urinary tract infection in children under 6 years of age. *Acta Paediatr.* 1998;87:549–552

3. Kunin CM. A ten-year study of bacteriuria in schoolgirls: final report of bacteriologic, urologic, and epidemiologic findings. *J Infect Dis.* 1970;122:382–393

4. Baker R, Maxted W, Maylath J, Shuman I. Relation of age, sex and infection to reflux: data indication high spontaneous cure rate in pediatric patients. *J Urol.* 1966;95:27–32

5. Hoberman A, Chao HP, Keller DM, Hickey R, Davis HW, Ellis D. Prevalence of urinary tract infection in febrile infants. *J Pediatr.* 1993;123:17–23

6. Wiswell TE, Hachey WE. Urinary tract infections and the uncircumcised state: an update. *Clin Pediatr.* 1993;32:130–134

7. Noe HN. The long-term results of prospective sibling reflux screening. *J Urol.* 1992; 148:1739–1742

8. Arant BS Jr. Medical management of mild and moderate vesicoureteral reflux: follow-up studies of infants and young children. A preliminary report of the Southwest Pediatric Nephrology Study Group. *J Urol.* 1992;148:1683–1687

9. Gorelick MH, Shaw KN. Screening tests for urinary tract infection in children: a meta-analysis. *Pediatrics.* 1999;104:e54

10. Hoberman A, Wald ER, Reynolds EA, Penchansky L, Charron M. Is urine culture necessary to rule out urinary tract infection in young febrile children? *Pediatr Infect Dis J.* 1996;15:304–309

11. Hoberman A, Charron M, Hickey RW, Baskin M, Kearney DH, Wald ER. Imaging studies after a first febrile urinary tract infection in young children. *N Engl J Med.* 2003;348:195–202

12. Gross GW, Lebowitz RL. Infection does not cause reflux. *Am J Roentgenol.* 1981; 137:929–932

13. McDonald A, Scranton M, Gillespie R, Mahajan V, Edwards GA. Voiding cystourethrograms and urinary tract infections: how long to wait? *Pediatrics.* 2000;105:e50

14. Mahant S, To T, Friedman J. Timing of voiding cystourethrogram in the investigation of urinary tract infections in children. *J Pediatr.* 2001;139:568–571

15. Jodal U. The natural history of bacteriuria in childhood. *Infect Dis Clin North Am.* 1987;1:713–729

16. Arant BS Jr. Vesicoureteric reflux and renal injury. *Am J Kidney Dis.* 1991;17:491–511

17. Smellie JM, Prescod NP, Shaw PJ,Risdon RA, Bryant TN. Childhood reflux and urinary infection: a follow-up of 10–41 years in 226 adults. *Pediatr Nephrol.* 1998;12:727–736

18. Arant BS Jr. Reflux nephropathy. In: Malluche HH, Sawaya BP, Hakim RM, Sayegh MH, eds. *Clinical Nephrology, Dialysis and Transplantation,* Munich, Germany: Dustri-Verlag; 1999;I-13:1–29

19. Smith JM, Stablein DM, Munoz R, Hebert D, McDonald RA. Contributions of the Transplant Registry: the 2006 Annual Report of the North American Pediatric Renal Trials and Collaborative Studies (NAPRTCS). *Pediatr Transplant.* 2007;11:366–373

20. Lebowitz RL, Olbing H, Parkkulainen KV, Smellie JM, Tamminen-Mobius T. International Reflux Study in Children Writing Committee. International system of radiographic grading of vesicoureteric reflux. *Pediatr Radiol.* 1985;15:105–109

21. Rushton HG, Majd M, Jantausch B, Wiedermann BI, Belman AB. Renal scarring following reflux and nonreflux pyelonephritis in children. Evaluation with 99m-technetium dimercaptosuccinic acid scintigraphy. *J Urol.* 1992;147:1327–1332

22. Benador D, Benador N, Slosman D, Mermillod B, Girardin E. Are younger children at highest risk of renal sequelae after pyelonephritis? *Lancet.* 1997;149:17–19

23. Conway PH, Cnaan A, Zaoutis T, Henry BV, Grundmeier RW, Keren R. Recurrent urinary tract infections in children. *JAMA.* 2007;298:179–186

24. Lenaghan D, Whitaker JG, Jensen F, Stephens FD. The natural history of reflux and longterm effects of reflux on the kidney. *J Urol.* 1976;115:728–730

25. Shure NM. Pyelonephritis and hypertension. A study of their relation in 11,898 necropsies. *Arch Int Med.* 1942;70:284–292

26. Arar MY, Arant BS Jr, Hogg RJ, Seikaly MG. Etiology of sustained hypertension in children in the Southwestern United States. *Pediatr Nephrol.* 1994;8:186–189

27. Jacobson SH, Eklof O, Eriksson CG, Lins LE, Tidgren B, Winberg J. Development of hypertension and uraemia after pyelonephritis in childhood—27 year follow-up. *Br Med J.* 1989;299:703–706

28. Olbing H, Claesson I, Ebel DK, et al. Renal scars and parenchymal thinning in children with vesicoureteral reflux: a 5-year report of the International Reflux Study in Children (European Branch). *J Urol.* 1992;148:1653–1656

Chapter 7

Hematuria

Noel M. Delos Santos and Bettina H. Ault

Abbreviations

ANCA	Antineutrophil cytoplasmic antibody
Anti-DNase B	Antideoxyribonuclease B titers
APSGN	Acute poststreptococcal glomerulonephritis
C-ANCA	Cytoplasmic staining of antineutrophil cytoplasmic antibody
CKD	Chronic kidney disease
CT	Computed tomography
GBM	Glomerular basement membrane
GN	Glomerulonephritis
hpf	High-power field
HSP	Henoch-Schönlein purpura
HUS	Hemolytic uremic syndrome
IgA	Immunoglobulin A
IgAN	Immunoglobulin A nephropathy
NS	Nephrotic syndrome
P-ANCA	Perinuclear antineutrophil cytoplasmic antibody
PR3-ANCA	Proteinase 3 antineutrophil cytoplasmic antibody
RBC	Red blood cell
RPGN	Rapidly progressive glomerulonephritis
SLE	Systemic lupus erythematosus
UPJ	Ureteropelvic junction
UTI	Urinary tract infection

Introduction

Hematuria is the presence of blood in urine. Gross or macroscopic hematuria is blood that is evident to the naked eye, whereas microscopic hematuria requires a urine reagent or dipstick screening and visualization of 5 RBCs/hpf or more on microscopy. Persistent hematuria occurs in about 2% of children and adults in the community. Often, hematuria in children is benign, with unknown etiology and good prognosis; nonetheless, it can be a distressing problem for patients, parents, and physicians alike. Therefore, an approach to hematuria should provide a means of detecting kidney or urinary disease while providing reassurance for less serious conditions.

Detecting Hematuria

Macroscopic hematuria ranges in color from bright red to dark brown. Microscopic hematuria can be detected by urine reagent dipsticks, which are capable of detecting as little as 3 to 5 RBCs/hpf (Chapter 3). Not all red urine is hematuria. Urine substances other than RBCs can discolor urine or cause a positive reaction with reagent dipsticks for blood, such as free hemoglobin or myoglobin, food pigments (such as vitamin C, beets, dyes), or medicines (such as Pyridium) (Boxes 7-1 and 7-2). Both macroscopic and microscopic hematuria, therefore, require confirmation with a microscopic examination of the urine. Ten milliliters of urine is placed in a centrifuge tube and centrifuged for 5 minutes at 2,000 revolutions per minute, urine supernatant is decanted, and the urine sediment is resuspended in the 0.5 mL of urine that remains within the tube. The sediment is visualized using a slide and cover slip with a light microscope 40× objective lens. The

---

Box 7-1. Some Causes of Red or Dark Urine

Antipyrine	Lead
Beets (beeturia)	Myoglobin
Benzene	Phenolphthalein
Bile pigments	Phenothiazines
Blackberries	Rifampicin
Diphenylhydantoin	*Serratia marcescens*
Hemoglobin	Uric acid

Box 7-2. Some Agents That Cause Hemoglobinuria

Aniline dyes	Oxalic acid
Carbon monoxide	Phenacetin
Chloroform	Phenol
Fava beans	Phosphorus
Mushrooms	Quinine
Naphthalene	Sulfonamides

RBCs counted are averaged among 10 fields. A count of 5 RBCs/hpf or more is significant for hematuria.

The morphology or shape of RBCs can be an important clue to the source of bleeding.[1] Dysmorphic RBCs exhibit plasma membrane blebs and may be accompanied by RBC casts. This is a herald sign for GN. The sensitivity and specificity of using dysmorphic RBCs to detect GN increases as greater percentages of the RBCs are involved. Dysmorphic RBCs, therefore, should direct the differential diagnosis to include the upper urinary tract (ie, renal parenchyma) (Figure 7-1B).

ஃ *Pearl*

Hematuria detected by dipstick should be confirmed by urine microscopy. Dysmorphic RBCs point to glomerular disease.

Eumorphic RBCs in urine are round with central concavity and resemble RBCs seen in peripheral blood smears (Figure 7-1A). A eumorphic RBC morphology should direct the differential diagnosis to the lower urinary tract (ie, renal tubules, renal pelvis, ureter, bladder, and urethra).

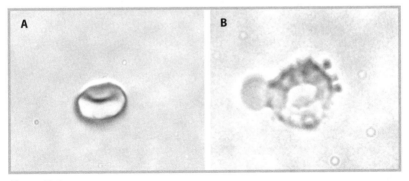

Figure 7-1.
A. Eumorphic red blood cell (RBC). **B.** Dysmorphic RBC showing blebs. (Courtesy of Dr Patrick Walker.)

Causes of Hematuria

A differential diagnosis that encompasses glomerular disease, infections, strenuous exercise, urolithiasis, hypercalciuria, hematologic disorders, anatomical abnormalities, and drugs should be kept in mind when obtaining patient history, performing a physical examination, and considering ancillary tests. Common causes of hematuria are presented in Boxes 7-3 and 7-4.

Infections of the urinary tract may cause hematuria. Bacterial cystitis can present with frequency, urgency, dysuria, enuresis, and microscopic or macroscopic hematuria with pyuria. Adenovirus may cause hemorrhagic cystitis in children. Pyelonephritis can present with high fever, flank pain, microscopic or macroscopic hematuria with pyuria, leukocytosis, and C-reactive protein (Chapter 6). Urine reagent strips undergo a color reaction by leukocyte esterase. Some bacteria are capable of converting urine nitrate to nitrite, which is also detectable by reagent strip. This is generally quite specific for UTI (however, in cases of gross hematuria, the heme pigment may stain the reagent strip and cause a false-positive for nitrite). Moderate to heavy exercise may cause transient hematuria, which should resolve after refraining from exercise for 2 days.

Box 7-3. Causes of Macroscopic and Microscopic Hematuria

Macroscopic Hematuria

More common
- Cystitis
- Hypercalciuria
- IgA nephropathy
- Poststreptococcal GN

Less common
- Urinary tract malformation
- Wilms tumor
- Polycystic kidney disease
- SLE
- Exercise
- Coagulopathy

Rare
- Bladder parasite
- Tuberculosis

Microscopic Hematuria

More common
- Hypercalciuria
- Glomerulopathy
- Unknown etiology

Less common
- Vasculitis
- Exercise
- Hematologic disorder
- Drugs
- Tubulointerstitial nephritis

Rare
- Bladder parasite
- Tuberculosis
- Loin-pain syndrome

Abbreviations: GN, glomerulonephritis; SLE, systemic lupus erythematosus.

Box 7-4. Common Causes of Hematuria at Different Ages^a

Newborn
- Congenital abnormalities of the kidney and urinary tract
- Renal vascular disorders
- Renal cortical necrosis

Infancy
- Renal vein thrombosis
- Hemolytic uremic syndrome
- Acute infections
- Wilms tumor

Early childhood
- Acute glomerulonephritis
- Hemorrhagic cystitis
- Trauma
- Henoch-Schönlein purpura

Late childhood
- Menstruation
- Trauma
- Glomerulonephritis
  — Acute glomerulonephritis
  — Henoch-Schönlein purpura
  — Systemic lupus erythematosus
- Recurrent benign hematuria
- IgA nephropathy
- Hypercalciuria

^aFrom Tina LU, Fildes RD. Hematuria and proteinuria. In: Barakat AY, ed. *Renal Disease in Children: Clinical Evaluation and Diagnosis*. New York, NY: Springer-Verlag; 1990.

Urolithiasis may present with abdominal or flank pain (renal colic) with microscopic or macroscopic hematuria. Urine microscopy may show crystals. Macroscopic hematuria with severe flank or abdominal pain should be evaluated urgently to control pain and ensure that there is no urine outflow obstruction. Urolithiasis may be due to anatomical abnormalities, infection, or metabolic abnormalities (Chapter 19), but the most common etiology in children is hypercalciuria. Hypercalciuria is a common cause of gross and microscopic hematuria in children as well. In the so-called stone belt (the Southern states), approximately 10% of white children are affected, whereas it is a rare finding in black children. Hypercalciuria, which is defined as random urine calcium/creatinine ratio greater than 0.2, or 24-hour urine calcium of greater than 4 mg/kg body weight/24 hours, may be associated with hematuria. This may be exacerbated by a high sodium intake (>1,500–2,000 mg/d). Patients may give a history of dysuria and/or frequency. Calcium oxalate crystals may be detected on microscopic examination of the urine. A family history of urolithiasis is variable. Ten percent to 15% of children with hypercalciuria are at risk for developing kidney stones or renal colic.[2]

Anatomical abnormalities also can cause hematuria. A history of abdominal trauma with hematuria or blood at the urethral meatus should be evaluated with a CT scan of the abdomen and pelvis in consultation with a urologist. Urinary tract trauma can also result from catheterization of the urinary bladder. Wilms tumor and UPJ are 2 uncommon but important causes of macroscopic hematuria.[3] Autosomal dominant or autosomal recessive polycystic kidney disease may present with hematuria and a familial inheritance pattern.[4] Autosomal dominant polycystic kidney disease is the most common form of polycystic kidney disease, occurring in 1 in 800 live births. Autosomal recessive polycystic kidney disease, which is much rarer (1 in 20,000 live births), may also present with hematuria. Tuberous sclerosis is characterized by a cystic kidney disease similar to autosomal dominant polycystic kidney disease and may have severe and even life-threatening hematuria because of the characteristic angiomyolipomata found in this disorder.[5] In cases of cystic kidney disease with hematuria, infection and nephrolithiasis should be ruled out. Renal artery or vein thrombosis, which occurs mainly in the neonatal period in association with umbilical catheters and patent ductus arteriosus, may present with microscopic or macroscopic hematuria, oliguria, thrombocytopenia, and hypertension. An enlarged affected kidney may be seen on ultrasound. Neonatal renal vein thrombosis is often associated with polycythemia and dehydration and is more common in infants of diabetic mothers. Alternatively, microscopic or macroscopic hematuria and hypertension in a newborn with perinatal anoxia may be a manifestation of renal cortical necrosis. Renal vein thrombosis can be seen in older children and teenagers with NS, usually as a result of membranous nephropathy. This is often associated with SLE. Antiphospholipid antibodies may be present. Affected children typically have hematuria and flank pain.

Hematologic diseases should be kept in mind in a child with hematuria. Children with sickle cell anemia or trait may have macroscopic or microscopic hematuria. Bleeding usually originates from the left kidney. Red blood cell sickling is thought to result in vascular obstruction and focal infarcts. Renal papillary necrosis may be seen as calyceal clubbing on imaging. Renal medullary carcinoma is an aggressive tumor that may occur in children with a sickle cell hemoglobinopathy and should be excluded in those children who develop hematuria with flank or abdominal pain.[6] Coagulopathy and thrombocytopenia are uncommon causes of gross hematuria.

Cyclophosphamide is one of the best-known drugs causing hematuria. Hemorrhagic cystitis is a painful disorder in patients receiving cyclophosphamide for treatment of malignancy or glomerular disease. Nonsteroidal anti-inflammatory drugs inhibit prostaglandin synthesis in the kidneys, which affects blood flow. Nonsteroidal anti-inflammatory drugs may cause hematuria, either because of papillary necrosis or as a result of tubulo-interstitial nephritis.[7]

Acute poststreptococcal glomerulonephritis peaks in occurrence at 4 to 5 years of age.[8] Typically, there is a history of preceding pharyngitis or impetigo infection, macroscopic hematuria, volume overload, hypertension, and edema (Chapter 9). Microscopic hematuria persists for months; therefore, prolonged follow-up is necessary to ensure a normal urinalysis and blood pressure. Acute renal failure may be present with increased serum creatinine and hyperkalemia. Proteinuria and pyuria may be present. Antistreptolysin-O titer is elevated in most cases of pharyngitis-associated APSGN, whereas elevated anti-DNAse B titers occur with most impetigo-associated cases. The serum C3 complement is depressed during the acute illness and normalizes by 8 weeks. If a patient with APSGN continues to exhibit depressed C3 levels longer than 8 weeks, other kidney diseases must be considered (SLE, nephritis, membranoproliferative GN, hepatitis B GN, and nephritis of chronic bacteremia (shunt or endocarditis). Treatment is usually supportive. A primary care physician can treat most cases of APSGN. A nephrology consultation should be obtained for patients with oliguria, hyperkalemia, NS, cardiac overload, and renal insufficiency.

Immunoglobulin A nephropathy is the most common GN worldwide (Chapter 9). Macroscopic hematuria is a common presenting feature in these patients during an upper respiratory illness (so-called synpharyngitic hematuria). The timing of the macroscopic hematuria and normocomplementemia in IgAN helps to distinguish it from APSGN. There is no routine diagnostic laboratory test for IgAN. A renal biopsy is required for a definitive diagnosis (mesangial IgA deposits on biopsy). These children may also have microscopic hematuria and/or proteinuria, hypertension, and chronic renal insufficiency.

Another group of illnesses producing hematuria are small blood vessel vasculitides with renal involvement.[9] This includes HSP, SLE, Wegener granulomatosis, microscopic polyangiitis, Churg-Strauss disease, and anti-GBM disease in which the glomerular capillaries are affected and clinically exhibit GN. Renal biopsy findings are identical in HSP nephritis and IgA nephritis (mesangial IgA deposits). But unlike IgA nephritis, HSP is a systemic vasculitis with skin (purpuric rash), gastrointestinal (abdominal colic, hematochezia), joint (arthralgia or arthritis), and kidney involvement (macroscopic or microscopic hematuria with or without proteinuria). Not all children with HSP will have renal involvement, but any child with HSP should have a urinalysis on a daily basis for at least the first week of the initial symptoms and periodically thereafter for the following 3 months to detect nephritis.[10]

Systemic lupus erythematosus is an autoimmune disorder with systemic consequences of autoantibody production and immune complex deposition. Kidney involvement ranges from normal to CKD (Chapter 20). Patients may have nephrosis (proteinuria), nephritis (hematuria and proteinuria), or RPGN. Diagnosis of SLE requires 4 or more of the 11 diagnostic criteria established by the American College of Rheumatology: malar rash, discoid rash, photosensitivity, oral ulcers, arthritis, serositis, renal disorder, neurologic disorder, hematologic disorder, immunologic disorder, and antinuclear antibody.[11]

Wegener granulomatosis is a small-vessel vasculitis that should be considered when respiratory tract symptoms do not resolve spontaneously or with antibiotic therapy. In this condition, there is granulomatous inflammation of the respiratory tract. C-ANCA or PR3-ANCA (cytoplasmic-pattern antineutrophil cytoplasmic autoantibodies) are antibodies specific for proteinase 3 and are a very sensitive serologic marker for Wegener granulomatosis. Necrotizing vasculitis affects the small- to medium-sized vessels.

Microscopic polyangiitis is a small-vessel necrotizing vasculitis with myriad features including pulmonary (hemoptysis, pulmonary hemorrhage, respiratory failure), upper respiratory (chronic sinusitis, otitis media, nasal passage ulcers), musculoskeletal (arthralgia, arthritis, myalgia, muscle weakness), and dermatologic (purpuric rash, leukocytoclastic angiitis) symptoms. Patients with microscopic polyangiitis involving the lungs may be positive for C-ANCA (PR3-ANCA). Microscopic polyangiitis patients may also be positive for P-ANCA or MPO-ANCA (perinuclear pattern ANCA antibody specific for myeloperoxidase).

Churg-Strauss disease is characterized by eosinophil-rich and granulomatous inflammation involving the respiratory tract. It is associated with asthma and eosinophilia.

Antiglomerular basement membrane disease is one of many causes of Goodpasture syndrome (RPGN and lung hemorrhage). In this condition autoantibodies are directed at specific antigenic targets within the glomerular and/or pulmonary basement membrane. These antibodies are specific for the α-3 chain of type IV collagen found in certain basement membranes.[12]

Nephrotic syndrome is characterized by edema, proteinuria, hypoalbuminemia, and hypercholesterolemia. Approximately one-third of patients with NS will have microscopic hematuria. Alport syndrome and familial benign hematuria (thin basement membrane disease) are discussed in detail in Chapter 16.

Shiga-toxin associated HUS should be considered in those patients who develop thrombocytopenia, anemia with evidence of hemolysis (schistocytes), and acute kidney injury after a prodrome of infectious colitis[13] (Chapter 20). Shiga-toxin–producing *Escherichia coli* (typically of the O157:H7 strain) is a common agent in hemorrhagic colitis and is responsible for most cases of HUS. Other infectious agents associated with HUS include other serotypes of *E coli*, *Shigella dysenteriae* type 1, *Streptococcus pneumoniae*, and human immunodeficiency virus.

Evaluation of Patients With Hematuria

A physician is typically prompted to evaluate hematuria in 3 clinical settings: (1) asymptomatic hematuria, (2) macroscopic hematuria, and (3) symptomatic microscopic hematuria. Investigations can be directed along these 3 basic categories. The initial history should characterize the hematuria: frequency, severity, and clots. Concurrent and preceding symptoms should be elicited in consideration of the preceding differential diagnosis. Questions in the family history should include renal failure, hearing loss, sickle cell anemia, nephrolithiasis, or hematuria. Important physical examination findings include hypertension, respiratory findings of volume overload, abdominal mass, edema, arthritis, and rashes.

₴ Pearl

Physicians are confronted with 3 clinical settings in hematuria: asymptomatic, macroscopic, and symptomatic microscopic hematuria.

Asymptomatic Hematuria

The American Academy of Pediatrics recommends a routine health maintenance urine analysis screen at 2 different periods: school age and adolescence.[14] It is during these well-child visits or during sports participation evaluations that incidental microscopic hematuria is discovered. Asymptomatic microscopic hematuria occurs in 0.5% to 2.0% of school-aged children.[15,16] A thorough history of patient and family, as well as an accurate physical examination, should be performed. A urinalysis should be repeated 3 times every 1 to 2 weeks. Because isolated hematuria can occur with strenuous exercise, patients should refrain from exercising for 48 hours before the test. The urinalysis should evaluate for the presence of hematuria, proteinuria, leukocyte esterase, and nitrites. A microscopic examination of the urine should evaluate RBC count and morphology, casts, crystals, bacteria, and parasites. The presence of leukocytes, nitrites, bacteria, or proteinuria should prompt a urine culture. Significant proteinuria detected by reagent dipstick (>2+) should be further quantified by random urine protein and creatinine. A random urine calcium and creatinine should be performed on all children with asymptomatic microscopic hematuria to evaluate for hypercalciuria. Urinalysis should also be performed on parents and siblings to evaluate for a hereditary pattern of microscopic hematuria. An evaluation plan for asymptomatic microscopic hematuria is presented in Figure 7-2.

Macroscopic Hematuria

Macroscopic hematuria occurs in 1.3 per 1,000 visits to a pediatric emergency walk-in clinic.[17] Hypercalciuria and UTI are 2 common causes of gross hematuria. Glomerulonephritis is less common, and anatomical abnormalities including Wilms tumor and UPJ obstruction are even less so. Quantification of calcium excretion (random urine calcium/creatinine) and urine culture should be obtained. All patients with gross hematuria should undergo ultrasound imaging of the kidneys and bladder to evaluate for tumors, cysts, hydronephrosis, or renal vessel thrombosis. Proteinuria should be quantified also (random urine protein or creatinine). Patients with hypertension, significant proteinuria, or urine microscopic examinations

₴ Pearl

Renal and bladder ultrasound should be performed on every child with macroscopic hematuria.

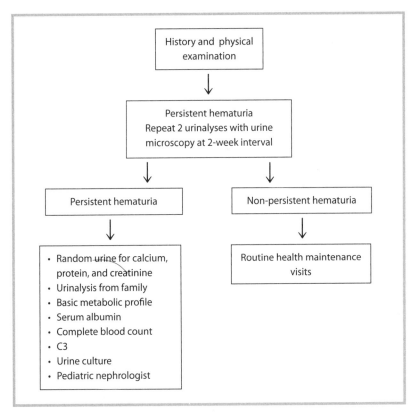

Figure 7-2.
Evaluation of asymptomatic hematuria.

suggestive of GN (dysmorphic RBCs with or without RBC casts) should be evaluated with a basic metabolic profile, serum albumin, cholesterol, antistreptolysin-O titer, anti-DNAse B titer, complement C3, and complete blood count. If the history is suggestive of SLE, an antinuclear antibody titer, complement C4, erythrocyte sedimentation rate, and anti–double-stranded DNA antibody titer should be ordered as well. A family history of sickle cell anemia should prompt a hemoglobin electrophoresis. A history of hemoptysis, rapidly declining renal function (oliguria or a rising daily serum creatinine), or persistent pulmonary symptoms should prompt an anti-GBM antibody titer, C-ANCA, and P-ANCA. Evaluation of patients with macroscopic hematuria is presented in Figure 7-3.

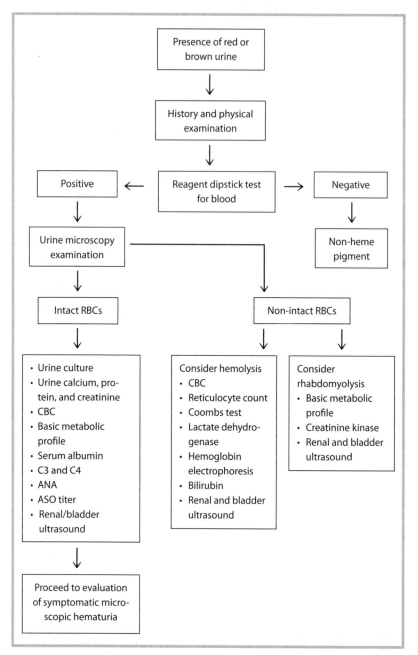

Figure 7-3.

Evaluation of macroscopic hematuria. RBCs indicates red blood cells; CBC, complete blood count; ANA, antinuclear antibodies; ASO, antistreptolysin-O.

Symptomatic Microscopic Hematuria

Features of distinct clinical entities, such as HSP or APSGN, should be considered when evaluating a patient with hematuria. However, many patients will present with nonspecific symptoms and/or abnormal findings on the physical examination that do not easily fit a diagnosis. These patients should undergo a laboratory evaluation that includes a basic metabolic profile, serum albumin, cholesterol, complements C3, and C4. Antistreptolysin-O titer, anti-double-stranded DNA antibody titer, hepatitis serologies, hemoglobin electrophoresis, C-ANCA, P-ANCA, anti-GBM antibody titer, and renal ultrasound or CT scan may be considered. Kidney biopsy is indicated with persistent heavy proteinuria, CKD, recurrent macroscopic hematuria, and suspected SLE. Evaluation of symptomatic microscopic hematuria is presented in Figure 7-4.

ᕉ *Pearl*

Patients with symptomatic hematuria who do not clearly fit a recognizable diagnosis should be referred to a pediatric nephrologist.

When Should a Patient Be Referred?

Patients with persistent hematuria, significant persistent proteinuria, persistent depression of serum complement, oliguria, hypertension, pulmonary symptoms, RPGN, CKD, or who do not easily fit into a diagnosis should be referred to a pediatric nephrologist.[18] Parental anxiety and the need for a nephrology team are also indications for referral. A pediatric urology consultation should be obtained when trauma, obstructing urolithiasis, or urinary tract abnormality are suspected.

Abnormal Findings: History and Physical Examination

↓

Urinalysis/microscopy
Urine protein/Cr
Basic metabolic profile
Serum albumin
CBC
C3

↓

Are features consistent with a familiar clinical entity?

↓

Consider Diagnosis	Suggestive Features	Ancillary Evaluation
Hypercalciuria	Lower UT symptoms; family history of stones; Ca crystals	Urine Ca^{+2}/Cr
Urolithiasis	Abdominal pain, family history of stones	BMP, urine Ca^{+2}/Cr
Urinary tract infection	Lower UT symptoms (cystitis), fever (pyelonephritis)	Urine culture
Glomerulonephritis	Pharyngitis, HT, volume overload, dysmorphic RBCs, RBC casts, proteinuria	ASO titer, streptozyme, C3, urine protein/Cr, CBC
Idiopathic nephrotic syndrome	Pitting edema, proteinuria, oval fat bodies on urine microscopy	BMP, serum albumin, CBC, cholesterol, urine protein/Cr
Systemic lupus erythematosus	Rash, oral ulcers, arthritis, serositis, hematuria, proteinuria	Urine protein/Cr, ANA, ESR, C3, C4, anti-double-stranded DNA antibody
Sickle cell hemoglobinopathy	Enuresis, isosthenuria, family history of sickle cell disease	Urine protein/Cr, CBC, hemoglobin electrophoresis, reticulocyte count, renal ultrasound
Hemolytic uremic syndrome	Prodrome of colitis, pallor and fatigue, oliguria, petechiae	CBC, blood smear for schistocytes, reticulocyte count, lactate dehydrogenase, stool culture

↓

Figure 7-4.

Evaluation of symptomatic microscopic hematuria. Cr indicates creatinine; CBC, complete blood count; UT, urinary tract; Ca, calcium; BMP, basic metabolic profile; HT, hypertension; RBC, red blood cell; ASO, antistreptolysin-O; ANA, antinuclear antibody; ESR, erythrocyte sedimentation rate; IgA, immunoglobulin A.

	Abnormal Findings: History and Physical Examination, continued ↓	
Consider Diagnosis	**Suggestive Features**	**Ancillary Evaluation**
Hemolytic uremic syndrome	Prodrome of colitis, pallor and fatigue, oliguria, petechiae	CBC, blood smear for schistocytes, reticulocyte count, lactate dehydrogenase, stool culture
Henoch-Schönlein purpura	Purpuric rash distal to buttocks, arthralgias, abdominal colic/diarrhea, hematochezia, hematuria, proteinuria	BMP, CBC, urine protein/Cr
IgA nephropathy	Recurrent macroscopic hematuria	Urine protein/Cr
Alport syndrome	Hearing deficit; family history of hearing loss; renal failure	BMP, CBC, hearing screen, slit eye examination
Benign familial hematuria	Family history of hematuria	BMP, CBC, urinalysis from family

Figure 7-4., continued

Evaluation of symptomatic microscopic hematuria. Cr indicates creatinine; CBC, complete blood count; UT, urinary tract; Ca, calcium; BMP, basic metabolic profile; HT, hypertension; RBC, red blood cell; ASO, antistreptolysin-O; ANA, antinuclear antibody; ESR, erythrocyte sedimentation rate; IgA, immunoglobulin A.

References

1. Crompton CH, Ward PB, Hewitt IK. The use of urinary red cell morphology to determine the source of hematuria in children. *Clin Nephrol.* 1993;39:44–49

2. Stapleton FB. Idiopathic hypercalciuria: association with isolated hematuria and risk for urolithiasis in children. The Southwest Pediatric Nephrology Study Group. *Kidney Int.* 1990;73:807–811

3. Bergstein J, Leiser J, Andreoli S. The clinical significance of asymptomatic gross and microscopic hematuria in children. *Arch Pediatr Adolesc Med.* 2005;159:353–355

4. Wilson PD. Polycystic kidney disease. *New Engl J Med.* 2004;350:151–164

5. Rakowski SK, Winterkorn EB, Paul E, Steele DJ, Halpern EF, Thiele EA. Renal manifestations of tuberous sclerosis complex: incidence, prognosis, and predictive factors. *Kidney Int.* 2006;70:1777–1782

6. Davis CJ, Mostofi FK, Sesterhenn IA. Renal medullary carcinoma. The seventh sickle cell nephropathy. *Am J Surg Pathol.* 1995;19:1–11

7. Ten RM, Torres VE, Milliner DS, Schwab TR, Holley KE, Gleich GJ. Acute interstitial nephritis: immunologic and clinical aspects. *Mayo Clin Proc.* 1988;63:921–930

8. Lau KK, Wyatt RJ. Glomerulonephritis. *Adolesc Med Clin.* 2005;16:67–85

9. Falk RJ, Nachman RP, Hogan SL, Jennette JC. ANCA glomerulonephritis and vasculitis: a Chapel Hill Perspective. *Semin Nephrol.* 2000;20:233–243

10. Delos Santos NM, Wyatt RJ. Pediatric IgA nephropathies: clinical aspects and therapeutic approaches. *Semin Nephrol.* 2004;24:269–286

11. Petri M. Review of classification criteria for systemic lupus erythematosus. *Rheum Dis Clin North Am.* 2005;31:245–254

12. Kalluri R, Wilson CB, Weber M, et al. Identification of the alpha 3 chain of type IV collagen as the common autoantigen in antibasement membrane disease and Goodpasture syndrome. *J Am Soc Nephrol.* 1995;6:1178–1185

13. Kaplan BS, Meyers KE, Schulman SL. The pathogenesis and treatment of hemolytic uremic syndrome. *J Am Soc Nephrol.* 1998;9:1126–1133

14. American Academy of Pediatrics Committee on Practice and Ambulatory Medicine. Recommendations for preventive pediatric health care. *Pediatrics.* 1995;96:373–374

15. Dodge WF, West EF, Smith EH, Bunce H. Proteinuria and hematuria in school children: epidemiology and early natural history. *J Pediatr.* 1976;88:327–347

16. Vehaskari VM, Rapola J, Koskimies O, Savilahti E, Vilska J, Hallman N. Microscopic hematuria in school children: epidemiology and clinicopathologic evaluation. *J Pediatr.* 1979;95:676–684

17. Ingelfinger JR, Davis AE, Grupe WE. Frequency and etiology of gross hematuria in a general pediatric setting. *Pediatrics.* 1977;59:557–561

18. Diven SC, Travis LB. A practical primary care approach to hematuria in children. *Pediatr Nephrol.* 2000;14:65–72

Chapter 8

Proteinuria

Victoria F. Norwood

Introduction	Abbreviations	
"Normal" Urinary Protein Excretion	AAP	American Academy of Pediatrics
Etiology	ATN	Acute tubular necrosis
Measurement of Proteinuria	GN	Glomerulonephritis
Causes of Proteinuria	MW	Molecular weight
Workup of Proteinuria	kDa	Kilodalton
Treatment of Proteinuria	UTI	Urinary tract infection
Summary		

Introduction

Abnormal urinary protein excretion is a highly sensitive marker of significant renal disease, albeit often a silent one. The AAP currently recommends screening urinalysis for all children as they enter kindergarten.[1] The urinalysis is a routine part of most preparticipation physical examinations for athletics, and many pediatricians screen more frequently.[2] Given the reasonable frequency with which proteinuria can be detected in these settings and in the setting of illness, pediatric practitioners should clearly understand the laboratory methods for evaluation of urinary protein and the potential diagnostic outcomes of these evaluations (Chapter 3). Subsequently, decisions regarding management, follow-up, and referral to nephrology colleagues become straightforward and efficient. For additional recommendations, especially for patients with nephrotic syndrome, refer to Chapter 9 and a review by Hogg et al.[3]

A pediatric practitioner will detect proteinuria in 3 circumstances: routine screening as outlined by AAP guidelines, incidentally as a part of an evaluation for another disorder for which urine studies were sent (ie, presurgical evaluation), and during the investigation of suspected renal or urinary tract disease. Signs and symptoms such as edema, hematuria, hypertension, failure to thrive, growth delay, suspicion of vasculitis, UTI, recurrent abdominal pain, or a history of past renal disease are all indications for the evaluation for possible proteinuria.

ஃ *Pearl*

Low-level proteinuria discovered on routine dipstick evaluation will most likely prove transient.

The circumstances of diagnosis along with the severity of proteinuria should be the primary guide for further evaluation. In otherwise healthy patients, low-level positive dipstick evaluations discovered at screening will most likely prove transient or false-positive on repeat studies. Patients with medical illness and moderate-to high-level proteinuria should be thoroughly evaluated because they are most likely to have clinically important renal disease.

"Normal" Urinary Protein Excretion

Although final daily urinary losses of protein are low, the normal nephron filters, reabsorbs, secretes, and catabolizes proteins. The glomerular filtration mechanism, which comprises the fenestrated glomerular endothelium, the acellular glomerular basement membrane complex, and the specialized epithelial podocyte, provides an effective barrier against loss of plasma proteins (Figure 8-1).

Permeability of proteins across the glomerulus varies in normal physiology depending on MW and electrical charge. Small plasma proteins and peptides (<40 kDa) are effectively filtered, whereas those of high MW and electronegativity (ie, albumin, MW 67 kDa; or immunoglobulin G, MW 150 kDa) are restricted from crossing the barrier. Most filtered small proteins and peptides are reabsorbed and catabolized quickly in the proximal tubule, whereas the scant filtration of albumin and other large proteins is also normally corrected in the proximal tubule through the reabsorptive capabilities of megalin, a proximal tubular receptor that mediates endocytosis of albumin. In normal individuals, the major component of urinary protein is Tamm-Horsfall protein (also known as uromodulin). Although its physiologic importance remains unknown, this large-MW protein (95 kDa) is actively secreted by the proximal tubule. Other small-MW proteins that are normally found in urine include ß2- and α1-microglobulins.

ஃ *Pearl*

Normal urinary protein excretion is less than 4 mg/m^2/h.

Given that glomerular filtration characteristics and proximal tubular function determine final normal urinary protein levels, it is not unexpected that the final total daily urinary protein quantity varies with body mass and

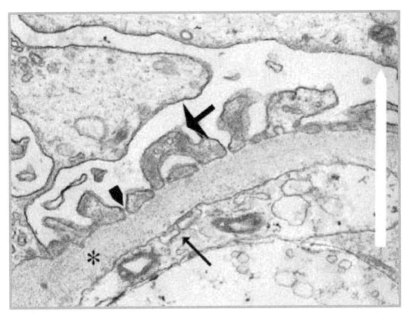

Figure 8-1.

High-power electron microscopy view of the glomerular filtration barrier. Small black arrow indicates fenestrated endothelial cell; *, glomerular basement membrane; large black arrow, podocyte foot process; arrowhead, podocyte slit membrane; white arrow, direction of filtration.

renal maturity. When corrected for urinary creatinine excretion (discussed later), normal urinary protein excretion ranges from a protein/creatinine ratio of 0.7 in the immature newborn to 0.2 or less in the mature individual (Table 8-1). When expressed quantitatively by timed urine collections, normal urinary protein excretion is less than 4 mg/m^2/h (100 mg/m^2/d) (see Table 8-1).

Etiology

Clinically important urinary protein excretion comes from 3 possible sources: a breakdown in the glomerular barrier, tubular dysfunction, or excessive plasma protein concentrations that overwhelm the normal reabsorptive process. The most common clinical scenario involves a loss of glomerular integrity and excretion of high-MW proteins such as albumin. Whether caused by congenital podocyte disorders (such as Finnish-type

Table 8-1. Normal Urinary Protein Excretion		
Age	mg/m²/d (mean, [range])[a]	Protein/Creatinine Ratio (mg/mg)[b]
Premature infant (<30 wks)	182, [8–377]	0.7
Term infant (>30 wks)	145, [68–309]	0.7
2 months–4 y	100, [37–244]	0.55–0.7 (up to 1 y) 0.4 (1–2 y) 0.3 (2–3 y)
5–10 y	85, [21–234]	0.2
>10 y	63, [22–181]	0.15–0.2

[a]Data from Miltenyi M. Urinary protein excretion in healthy children. *Clin Nephrol.* 1979;12:216–221.

[b]Adapted from Guignard J-P, Santos F. Laboratory investigations (Chapter 21). In: *Pediatric Nephrology.* 5th ed. Philadelphia, PA: Lippincott, Williams & Wilkins; 2004.

congenital nephrosis) or acquired disorders (such as minimal change disease, poststreptococcal GN, renal scarring, or long-standing diabetes), the structure and function of the glomerulus is altered so that the size and charge selectivity of endothelial cells, the basement membrane, and/or podocytes are disrupted, resulting in leakage of high-MW plasma proteins into Bowman space and ultimately into the final urine. These are the disorders that result in the highest urine protein contents and features of the nephrotic syndrome, often with progressive loss of overall renal function.

Tubular proteinuria is characterized by abnormal excretion of the low-MW proteins normally reabsorbed by the proximal tubule. Tubular proteinuria is most commonly seen with ATN, as a side effect of chemotherapy or aminoglycoside use, or from the inherited tubulopathies such as Fanconi syndrome.

In the pediatric population, disorders resulting in excessive plasma protein concentrations leading to overflow proteinuria are rare. However, hemoglobinuria from hemolytic crises, myoglobinuria from rhabdomyolysis, and hypergammaglobulinemic states may all be associated with elevated urine protein.

Measurement of Proteinuria

Screening urine studies are routinely performed using dipstick technologies such as Multitstix or Albustix (Bayer Inc.). These reagent strips contain a color indicator dye that changes from yellow to green on binding with protein, and the color change can be semiquantitated in ranges from negative through greater than 4+. False-negative results can occur using this technique in very dilute urine samples and in cases of purely low-MW proteinuria (which bind poorly to the indicator), whereas false-positives can occur in very alkaline urine, very concentrated samples, or those contaminated with chlorhexidine. False results can also be obtained with reagent strips that have been inappropriately stored or if appropriate timing between exposure and reading is not accomplished. Consistent positive results using dipstick techniques should be more definitively quantitated.

Quantitative urine protein determinations are performed using timed urine collections, most commonly for 24 hours, although shorter, well-documented intervals are effective as well. These studies are commonly error prone and can be difficult to accomplish in smaller children. Patients and families should be given specific instructions to begin and end the collection with an empty bladder to measure only the urine produced during the interval of investigation. Even in highly controlled circumstances, up to 15% of collections will be deemed inaccurate.[4] It is mandatory that urine creatinine content be assessed in any timed collection as an internal standard; daily creatinine excretion is normally 15 to 20 mg/kg/24 hours in patients of normal muscle mass. A collection containing more or less than this amount of creatinine should be considered of suspect quality, although extrapolation of the protein content to "normal" creatinine content may be considered. Patients with unusually high or low muscle mass or those who are obese may be difficult to assess, but in most instances, progress over time can be followed using this technique and using the patient as the control.

In recent years the use of a protein/creatinine ratio in spot urine samples has gained wide acceptance as a middle ground between the screening dipstick tests and the more involved timed collections. In samples taken from normal adults and patients with varying degrees of proteinuria defined by quantitative studies, the protein/creatinine ratio in approximately 80% of random samples correlated numerically with 24-hour excretion rates.[4] The ease of collection of a spot sample for pediatric patients and the availability of age-dependent normative values make this technique quite popular despite an approximately 20% error rate. The practitioner is warned to carefully assess the units reported for both creatinine and protein to ensure that the ratios are appropriately calculated.

The discovery that low-level urinary albumin excretion marks the earliest phase of diabetic nephropathy has led to the development of a test for microalbumin. In contrast to the routine urinary protein assays, which use turbidimetric methods following ammonium salts and therefore detect all forms of urinary protein, the microalbumin assay is specific for albumin alone and is highly sensitive to detect very low levels of urinary albumin. Its utility is in these very low ranges of albuminuria, and the cost is high compared with the routine assay. This test is not routinely used for the assessment of nondiabetic proteinuria or for established diabetic nephropathy.

Causes of Proteinuria

The differential diagnosis of proteinuria is listed in Box 8-1. Although a complete description and discussion of this large list is beyond the scope of this review, those diagnoses most commonly encountered by pediatricians and those of most concern will be addressed. Nephrotic syndrome and GN are discussed in Chapter 9.

Proteinuria may be best categorized as transient, orthostatic, or fixed. Transient proteinuria is defined by the disappearance of urinary protein following one or more positive tests. Transient proteinuria accounts for

---

Box 8-1. Causes of Proteinuria

Transient
- Exercise
- Fever
- Stress/illness

Orthostatic

Drugs
- Chemotherapy
- Aminoglycosides
- Heavy metal intoxication

Tubular disease
- Acute tubular necrosis
- Interstitial nephritis
- Cystic kidney diseases
- Fanconi syndrome
- Graft-versus-host disease

Reflux nephropathy

Glomerulonephritis
- All forms, including minimal change nephrotic syndrome

Other chronic renal disease
- Obstructive uropathy
- Congenital renal dysplasia
- Permanent residual dysfunction from acute disease (ie, cortical necrosis, hemolytic uremic syndrome, glomerulonephritis)

Diabetes mellitus

Protein overload syndromes
- Hemolysis
- Rhabdomyolysis
- Hypergammaglobulinemia

most cases of isolated proteinuria without a history of significant illness or concerning symptoms and results from heavy exercise, fever, and significant heat or cold stress. It is commonly seen in the settings of evaluations for sports participation physical examinations, especially those occurring directly following practice or in highly active or athletic teens. The degree of proteinuria is mild to moderate in these circumstances (<1 g/24 hours, protein/creatinine <1.0), and repeated assessments should be made in the absence of the probable stressor prior to more involved evaluation.

Orthostatic proteinuria is the next most frequently diagnosed form of isolated proteinuria and is most commonly seen in otherwise healthy adolescents. By definition, orthostatic proteinuria is that which is present only in the upright position and is not associated with abnormal renal function or hypertension. Its cause is unknown, and it is usually present for some time, at least years, although it may eventually resolve or may be permanent.[5] Recumbent collections or samples will be negative by dipstick, with protein levels less than 100 mg/8 to 12 hours (or protein/creatinine <0.2); whereas upright collections will be positive by dipstick, with protein levels 300 to 900 mg/12 to 16 hours. Orthostatic proteinuria becomes a less likely diagnosis than other forms of renal disease if the total daily urinary protein content exceeds 1 g/d or if there is any degree of associated hematuria.

Persistent nonorthostatic proteinuria of any degree is indicative of some form of underlying renal disease (see Box 8-1) and should be more thoroughly evaluated. Nephrotic range proteinuria, defined as greater than 40 mg/m^2/h or 3 g/24 hours, may be due to minimal change disease or any other form of potentially aggressive GN but is uncommon with congenital dysplasia, reflux nephropathy, obstructive uropathy, or tubular disorders. In these conditions, the proteinuria is usually mild to moderate (500–1,000 mg/d).

❧ Pearl

Orthostatic proteinuria is present only in the upright position and is not associated with abnormal renal function or hypertension.

Workup of Proteinuria

The evaluation of proteinuria is outlined in algorithmic form in Figure 8-2. In the cases of otherwise healthy normotensive patients and isolated proteinuria detected by routine screening, repeated assessments should be

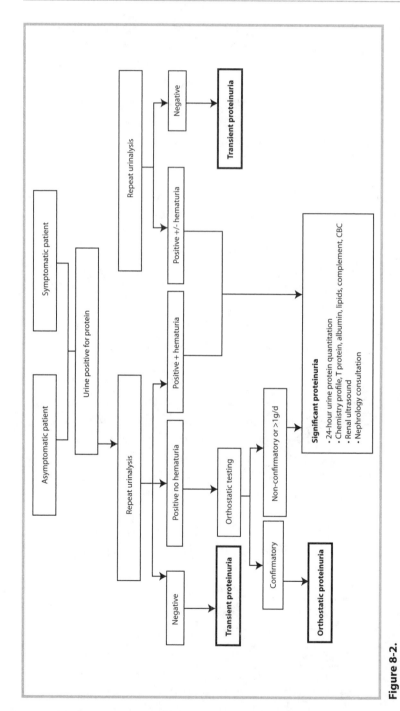

Figure 8-2.

Evaluation of children with proteinuria. CBC indicates complete blood count.

performed in the absence of heavy exercise or other causes of transient proteinuria. More accurate assessments with spot protein/creatinine ratios will also clarify false-positive dipstick results in patients with highly concentrated urine samples. Should these values be normal, no further evaluation is necessary and families may be reassured. Although hematuria occasionally occurs in association with the identical stressors known to cause transient proteinuria, the finding of proteinuria and hematuria should lead to further consideration of more significant renal disease unless all issues resolve completely.

In the cases of otherwise healthy normotensive patients whose isolated proteinuria is confirmed on repeated sampling, evaluation for orthostatic proteinuria should be undertaken. The gold standard for confirmation of orthostatic proteinuria is the "split" 24-hour urine collection (Box 8-2). As mentioned earlier, a normal nighttime collection associated with an abnormal daytime collection (with the total protein excretion <1 g/d) is diagnostic of orthostatic proteinuria. A more practical alternative to timed collections, first morning spot samples, and midday samples can be assessed using protein/creatinine ratios to confirm orthostasis, with the caveat that the first morning sample should not contain urine generated during waking hours the evening prior. A concentrated first morning sample that is negative by dipstick may also be considered strong evidence of orthostatic proteinuria, but many nephrologists still prefer more accurate determinations before confirming this benign condition. Similarly, although scant data suggest that orthostatic proteinuria is indeed benign even if persistent, many specialists still suggest follow-up testing at least 1 year after the diagnosis to confirm the lack of any progression.

Pediatricians are occasionally confronted with patients in whom no renal disease is suspected or known, but who are found to have proteinu-

---

Box 8-2. Split 24-Hour Urine Collection for Evaluation of Possible Orthostatic Proteinuria

- Use 2 clean containers (no detergents remaining).
- First morning: first void is discarded (empty bladder).
- Collect all urine until sleep in container 1 (day), including a final void before sleep.
- Next morning (including any nighttime voids): void into container 2 (night).
- Submit both samples for protein and creatinine quantitation.

ria during an intercurrent illness or screening for an invasive procedure. In these circumstances, it is prudent to take a thorough look at the history and physical examination with an eye toward possible renal disease. Low to moderate levels of proteinuria; normal blood pressure; and the absence of hematuria, edema, or vasculitis are all reassuring. Evaluation of serum creatinine is often prudent in these circumstances as reassurance of the absence of a significant renal process. Transient proteinuria is the most likely cause as a result of the stress of the underlying issue that brought the child to attention. Even if the proteinuria is reflective of previously unknown renal disease, in the absence of significantly elevated creatinine or hypertension, it is unlikely to affect the outcome of the intercurrent event. Should high-level proteinuria be detected on screening, accurate quantitation should be performed along with evaluation of serum creatinine.

In settings where renal disease is suspected from history and examination, pediatric practitioners may undertake a variety of evaluations, often dependent on the suspected diagnosis. When tubular dysfunction is possible, accurate quantitation of urinary protein and serum creatinine and electrolytes (including calcium and phosphorus) may be sufficient for baseline measurements. Quality renal ultrasonography will assess anatomy, size, and echogenicity with comparison to normal children, although it is often normal or minimally nonspecific in tubular disorders. Aminoglycoside toxicity and interstitial nephritis usually resolve in days to a few weeks, whereas chemotherapeutic agents such as platinum may result in permanent damage. Inherited disorders such as Fanconi syndrome are often associated with growth failure and rickets, which may be further evaluated by routine x-ray. In these circumstances, evaluation need not be emergent and is often best managed in consultation with a nephrologist.

The presence of associated edema, hypertension, and/or hematuria makes glomerular disease the most likely cause of proteinuria. Urinary protein should be accurately quantitated, and serum creatinine, electrolytes, total protein and albumin, and C3 complement and streptococcal titers (for consideration of postinfectious GN) measurements would be considered baseline requirements. Quality renal ultrasonography is appropriate, and consultation with a nephrologist is reasonable. Many pediatricians are comfortable with the management of mild acute poststreptococcal glomerulonephritis and minimal change nephrotic syndrome, especially with the assistance of nephrology consultation as needed. In situations where the presentation or course is atypical or more severe, prompt evaluation by a nephrologist should be organized.

Special mention should be made regarding the presentation and evaluation of proteinuria from reflux nephropathy. When associated with known urologic disorders of repeated UTIs in early childhood, the proteinuria and hypertension that accompany nephropathy from vesicoureteral reflux are not unexpected. However, reflux nephropathy may go undiagnosed for years and may present as asymptomatic proteinuria (commonly <1 g/d) with or without hypertension in the older child or adolescent. A careful history inquiring for past UTIs or recurrent antibiotic use for fevers without urine testing during early childhood may point to this diagnosis. Renal ultrasonography may be suggestive if renal asymmetry or parenchymal defects are seen, but this modality is poorly sensitive in situations where the scarred areas are small. Nuclear imaging with a cortical agent such as dimercaptosuccinic acid is the most sensitive for diagnosis. Voiding cystourethrography will be negative in a child whose reflux has resolved spontaneously and can be reserved for those in whom cortical imaging has confirmed scarring.

Timing of referral of a patient with proteinuria to a pediatric nephrologist is dependent on the likely severity of the underlying process, the comfort level of the treating physician, and the practical availability of nephrology services. Evaluation of asymptomatic proteinuria and the diagnosis of transient and orthostatic proteinuria are easily managed in the primary care setting. The additional evaluations provided by a nephrologist will be dependent on the suspected underlying process but may be expected to include more extensive biochemical testing, such as complement assays and serologic studies for immune-mediated diseases, repeat quantitative urine studies for confirmation and trending, and specialized imaging. Percutaneous renal biopsy is usually needed for specific diagnosis and/or prognosis in cases of progressive or persistent GN.

₰ *Pearl*

Presence of associated edema, hypertension, and/or hematuria makes glomerular disease the most likely cause of proteinuria.

Treatment of Proteinuria

Transient proteinuria and orthostatic proteinuria, by virtue of their benign natures, do not require therapy. In acute or self-limited processes such as ATN, postinfectious GN, or mild hemolytic uremic syndrome, proteinuria may persist for months following resolution of the primary disorder. In these circumstances, protein quantitation is usually of relatively low degree (<1 g/24 hours or protein/creatinine ratio <1.0) and does not require specific therapy. With time, the level of proteinuria should decline in these disorders, making worsening proteinuria an indication for more detailed investigation.

In most circumstances of clinically important proteinuria, the treatment is directed toward cure or management of treatment of the primary disease, and changes in urinary protein excretion are often used as a marker of the success of treatment. Most acquired glomerular diseases are treated with immunomodulatory therapies such as corticosteroids, calcineurin inhibitors, cytotoxic drugs, or antibody therapies, with varying degrees of success. Because cure of many of these disorders is not always accomplished or permanent glomerular damage often remains after successful treatment of the primary disease, the treatment of persistent proteinuria has become an additional option. Led by discoveries that showed benefits in renal life span in patients with nephropathy from type 1 diabetes mellitus,[6] it is now routine practice to use angiotensin-converting enzyme inhibitors and/or angiotensin receptor antagonists to decrease urinary protein excretion in patients with persistent high-grade glomerular proteinuria (>1 g/24 hours). Although not specifically proven effective to improve long-term renal outcomes in all forms of glomerular disease, especially in children, these agents clearly decrease urinary protein excretion by their hemodynamic effects of decreasing glomerular filtration pressure. Whether the long-term benefits are directly due to decreasing tubular protein or secondary to reduction in the effects of hypertension so commonly associated with these disorders remains an area of debate. Likewise, the need for and efficacy of these agents in chronic low-grade proteinuria or purely tubular proteinuria remains unclear.

❧ Pearl

Transient and orthostatic proteinuria do not require therapy.

Summary

The detection of proteinuria in pediatric patients is most commonly diagnosed as a transient or benign process. A thorough evaluation by a primary care pediatrician will usually separate these processes from those in which proteinuria is associated with more serious underlying renal disease. The relatively simple steps of a complete history and physical examination and quantitation of urine protein and creatinine can reassure many patients and families and also speed the evaluation by a nephrologist for those patients with concerning processes.

References

1. American Academy of Pediatrics Committee on Practice and Ambulatory Medicine. Recommendations for preventive pediatric health care. *Pediatrics*. 2000;105(3):645–646

2. Sox CM, Christakis DA. Pediatricians' screening urinalysis practices. *J Pediatr*. 2005; 147(3):362–365

3. Hogg RJ, Portman RJ, Milliner D, Lemley KV, Eddy A, Ingelfinger J. Evaluation and management of proteinuria and nephrotic syndrome in children: recommendations from a pediatric nephrology panel established at the National Kidney Foundation conference on proteinuria, albuminuria, risk, assessment, detection, and elimination (PARADE). *Pediatrics*. 2000;105(6):1242–1249

4. Shaw AB, Risdon P, Lewis-Jackson JD. Protein creatinine index and Albustix in assessment of proteinuria. *Br Med J*. 1983;287:929–932

5. Springberg PD, Garrett LE, Thompson AL Jr, Collins NF, Lordon RE, Robinson RR. Fixed and reproducible orthostatic proteinuria: results of a 2-year follow-up study. *Ann Intern Med*. 1982;97:516–519

6. Cook J, Daneman D, Spino M, Sochett E, Perlman K, Balfe JW. Angiotensin converting enzyme inhibitor therapy to decrease microalbuminuria in normotensive children with insulin-dependent diabetes mellitus. *J Pediatr*. 1990;117:39–45

Chapter 9

Glomerular Disease

M. Colleen Hastings and Robert J. Wyatt

Abbreviations

ANCA	Antineutrophil cytoplasmic antibody
APSGN	Acute poststreptococcal glomerulonephritis
ARBs	Angiotensin receptor blocker
ASO	Antistreptolysin-O
C1qN	C1q nephropathy
C3NeF	C3 nephritic factor
ESRD	End-stage renal disease
FSGS	Focal segmental glomerulosclerosis
GBM	Glomerular basement membrane
GN	Glomerulonephritis
HIV	Human immunodeficiency virus
HSP	Henoch-Schönlein purpura
IgA	Immunoglobulin A
IgG	Immunoglobulin G
IgM	Immunoglobulin M
IgAN	Immunoglobulin A nephropathy
ISKDC	International Study of Kidney Disease in Childhood
MLNS	Minimal lesion nephritic syndrome
MMF	Mycophenolate mofetil
MPGN	Membranoproliferative glomerulonephritis
NS	Nephrotic syndrome
RBC	Red blood cell
RPGN	Rapidly progressive glomerulonephritis
SLE	Systemic lupus erythematosus
SRINS	Steroid-responsive idiopathic nephrotic syndrome

Introduction

Glomerular diseases in children may be associated with serious morbidities, and in some instances the potential for progression to ESRD (ie, the need for dialysis or renal transplantation). Although glomerular diseases occur less frequently in children and adolescents than in adults, these diseases remain a common cause of ESRD in the pediatric population. Many patients with onset of glomerular disease in childhood or adolescence will progress to ESRD after reaching adulthood.

Pediatricians should recognize the clinical and diagnostic features of (1) NS, (2) acute GN, and (3) chronic GN. Classic features at presentation for each of these diagnostic groups are shown in Table 9-1. Although some overlap for clinical features may occur for specific disorders, the typical features for each of the 3 groups will be discussed in this chapter.

Table 9-1. Clinical Features of Pediatric Glomerular Syndromes			
Feature	**Nephrotic Syndrome**	**Acute Nephritis**	**Chronic (Primary) GN**
Hematuria	Minimal or none	Macroscopic or microscopic	Microscopic or episodic macroscopic
Proteinuria	Heavy	Mild to moderate	None to moderate
Serum albumin	Severely depressed	Normal or mildly depressed	Normal or mildly depressed[a]
Edema	Moderate to severe	Mild to moderate	None to mild[a]
Hypertension	Mild or none	Severe to none	None to moderate
Urinary sediment	Hyaline (fatty casts), oval fat bodies	RBC casts, WBC, dysmorphic RBCs	Dysmorphic RBCs, RBC casts +/–
Intravascular volume	Normal or decreased	Increased	Usually normal
Chest x-ray	Pleural effusion	Cardiomegaly +/–, pulmonary edema +/–	Normal

Abbreviations: GN, glomerulonephritis; RBC, red blood cell; WBC, white blood cell.
[a]Unless the patient has a mixed nephritic or nephrotic syndrome.

Nephrotic Syndrome

Nephrotic syndrome is defined by massive proteinuria, hypoalbuminemia, edema, and hypercholesterolemia. Edema may be the only initial symptom. Urinalysis shows concentrated urine with 3+ to 4+ protein on the dipstick. Hyaline or fatty casts and oval fat bodies may be seen in the spun urinary sediment.

Nephrotic-range proteinuria is defined as protein excretion greater than 40 mg/m²/h using a timed urine collection. Random urine specimens with protein/creatinine ratios above 2.0 suggest nephrotic-range proteinuria. Nephrotic-range proteinuria is not synonymous with NS because some individuals with nephrotic-range proteinuria do not have depressed serum albumin levels.

The incidence for primary NS in the United States in 1968 was about 2 cases per 100,000 children per year.[1] Proteinuria is believed to result from disruption of the glomerular filtration barrier that normally restricts passage of proteins based on both size and negative charge. Although the precise etiology of NS remains elusive, a soluble permeability factor has been postulated as a cause for the proteinuria for MLNS and focal segmental FSGS.[2]

✌ Pearl

Nephrotic range proteinuria is defined as protein excretion greater than 40 mg/m²/h.

Minimal Lesion Nephrotic Syndrome

Minimal lesion nephrotic syndrome (minimal change disease) is also known as SRINS because most patients with MLNS have complete resolution of proteinuria and normalization of serum albumin within the first month of treatment with corticosteroids. Minimal lesion nephrotic syndrome has a peak incidence in children between 2 and 6 years of age. The incidence of SRINS in the 1970s for eastern and central Kentucky was 1.8 cases per 100,000 per year for children younger than 10 years.[3]

Patients with MLNS typically have periorbital and dependent edema. Mild periorbital edema may be mistakenly diagnosed as an allergic symptom until urinalysis is performed. Ascites, pleural effusions, and scrotal or labial edema may also occur. Children with MLNS are typically not hypertensive and only rarely have hematuria.[4] Because the probability of MLNS is greater than 90% for a young child who presents with NS, renal biopsy is not performed unless there is no response to treatment. Response or remission is defined by complete resolution of proteinuria. Renal biopsy shows normal light microscopy (Figure 9-1) with the diffuse effacement of podocyte foot processes demonstrable only by electron microscopy.

Treatment is started with prednisolone or prednisone at a dose of 60 mg/m² divided twice daily, with a maximum dose of 80 mg/d. Although the original recommendation of the ISKDC was for 4 weeks of daily treatment for the first episode before tapering, the use of 6 weeks of daily corticosteroids followed by 6 weeks of alternate day therapy for treatment of initial presentation was shown in at least one study to decrease the incidence of relapse after 1 year of follow-up versus shorter steroid courses.[5] Proteinuria will resolve within 10 days for nearly half of affected children and by 4 weeks for 94%.[6]

Parents and children should be counseled on the maintenance of a low-sodium diet to minimize edema while proteinuria is present. Families should also be taught how to monitor children for relapse by frequent testing of urine for protein with Albustix.

Approximately 15% of children with MLNS will have only one episode of NS, and rarely a child will have a spontaneous remission before institution of treatment. Relapses are common until the onset of puberty but may continue in adulthood. Relapse most frequently occurs after other illnesses, particu-

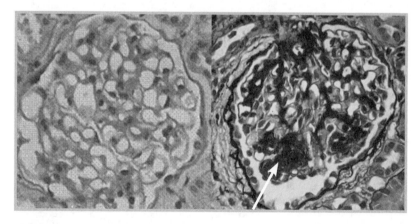

Figure 9-1.
Left (LM) Normal glomerulus (minimal lesion). Right (LM) PAS stain with focal segmental glomerulosclerosis (arrow).

larly viral upper respiratory tract infections. Treatment of relapses typically requires daily steroid therapy only until the proteinuria resolves, and then an alternate-day steroid taper is started. The usual course is for a child to have problems with relapses for 2 to 5 years followed by prolonged, often permanent, remission off all medications.

Complications of this disease are mostly related to the low serum levels of immunoglobulins and anticoagulant proteins, presumably owing to urinary loss. Bacteremia and peritonitis resulting from encapsulated organisms, especially *Streptococcus pneumoniae,* are related to low serum IgG levels, abnormal alternative complement pathway function, and lymphocyte dysfunction.[7] A febrile child with active NS should be immediately referred to the hospital for septic workup because of the risk for peritonitis. Parenteral antibiotic coverage for *S pneumoniae* should be instituted pending culture results. Thrombotic events involving the cerebral, pulmonary, and renal vasculature can occur because of the hypercoagulable state resulting from increased platelet aggregability, increased fibrinogen, and loss of proteins involved in the coagulation cascade.[7]

Steroid sensitivity is the most important prognostic indicator. Even in children who relapse, renal function should be preserved in children who respond to treatment with steroids. In children who do not respond to treatment within 4 to 6 weeks, a renal biopsy is indicated to search for other diagnoses such as FSGS, diffuse mesangial proliferation, or membranous nephropathy. Children younger than 1 year or older than 10 years should be biopsied at the time of presentation because they are less likely to have MLNS as the etiology.[7]

> ## ₴➤ Pearl
>
> Steroid sensitivity is the most important prognostic indicator in NS.

Focal Segmental Glomerulosclerosis

Approximately 75% of pediatric patients with FSGS have NS at presentation. Focal segmental glomerulosclerosis is usually characterized by resistance to sufficient corticosteroid therapy and high risk for eventual progression to ESRD.

Focal segmental glomerulosclerosis may be due to primary or secondary causes. Secondary causes of FSGS may result from hyperfiltration injury to glomeruli, often in the setting of decreased nephron mass. Some condi-

tions that can result in secondary FSGS include renal dysplasia, reflux nephropathy, morbid obesity, and sickle cell disease.[8] Secondary FSGS may also
occur in association with HIV infection and heroin abuse.[9] Genetic forms
of FSGS have been observed, so it is important to elicit any family history
of kidney disease.

Recent studies raise the concern that the incidence of primary FSGS is
increasing.[10] In the midwestern United States, 55% of cases of primary NS
were due to MLNS, and 25% were due to FSGS.[11] Another study showed that
FSGS had increased from 38% to 69% in biopsies performed before and after
1990.[12] Inference regarding disease incidence based on renal biopsy series
is clearly confounded by the practice of not performing biopsies in children
who are presumed to have steroid-responsive MLNS.

The initial clinical presentation of primary FSGS may be similar to
MLNS, with high-grade proteinuria and hypoalbuminemia. Children with
FSGS are more likely to have hematuria, hypertension, and/or renal insufficiency at the time of presentation than children with MLNS. Focal segmental glomerulosclerosis may also present with isolated proteinuria and a
normal serum albumin.[8]

Renal biopsy shows segmental scarring involving some but not all of
the sampled glomeruli. These glomerular scars are composed of collapsed
glomerular capillaries, adhesions between the tuft and Bowman capsule,
and hyaline deposits (see Figure 9-1). Uninvolved areas of the glomerulus
appear normal.[9]

Initial treatment is identical to that for patients with minimal change
disease: prednisone doses at 60 mg/m^2/d with a maximal dose of 80 mg/d.
After 4 weeks of daily therapy, the ISKDC protocol tapers the dose to
40 mg/m^2 given on alternate days for 4 weeks, then finally tapers the steroids
off over 4 weeks. Response rates of approximately 30% have been reported.
Genetic forms of FSGS caused by mutations in nephrin (congenital NS),
podocin (autosomal recessive FSGS), or alpha-actinin 4 (autosomal dominant FSGS) are steroid resistant.[8]

Angiotensin-converting enzyme inhibitors or ARBs are often used for
treatment of proteinuria in both hypertensive and normotensive patients
with proteinuria. Cytotoxic agents such as cyclophosphamide and chlorambucil have not been shown to be efficacious for treatment of FSGS in randomized controlled trials. Mendoza et al[13] achieved complete remission in

52% of 23 children by using methylprednisolone infusions, oral prednisone, and either cyclophosphamide or chlorambucil. Calcineurin inhibitors such as cyclosporine A or tacrolimus have been used to induce partial or complete remission and/or to reduce the amount of steroid exposure. Because calcineurin inhibitors, particularly at higher doses, are nephrotoxic, some centers are now using MMF. The National Institutes of Health currently supports a randomized controlled trial comparing treatment regimens using either cyclosporine A or pulsed oral dexamethasone and MMF. Plasmapheresis is used primarily in the setting of recurrent disease after renal transplantation. Hyperlipidemia may require treatment with 3-hydroxy-3-methyl-glutaryl coenzyme A reductase inhibitors (statins).

Children may progress to ESRD within 5 to 10 years of diagnosis if untreated.[8] Severity of proteinuria is the clinical feature most predictive of outcome, with persistence of nephrotic range proteinuria most often leading to ESRD. If proteinuria remits, the prognosis is markedly improved. Elevated serum creatinine at presentation is also a poor prognostic factor. Disease progression has not been correlated with age, gender, hematuria, or hypertension. Interstitial fibrosis, but not the number of affected glomeruli or percentage with global sclerosis, is the biopsy finding associated with increased likelihood of progression to renal failure.[9]

Focal segmental glomerulosclerosis is the most common cause of renal failure and need for transplantation among acquired renal diseases in children.[14] Focal segmental glomerulosclerosis may be more common and more aggressive in black children than in white children. Recurrence of the disease after renal transplantation is common and may result in allograft loss.

ᴬᵎ *Pearl*

Children with FSGS are more likely to have hematuria, resistance to corticosteroids, and eventual progression to ESRD.

Diffuse Mesangial Proliferation

This is a rare cause of NS with mesangial proliferation as the dominant feature on renal biopsy. Immunofluorescence and electron microscopy show no deposits typical for immune complexes. The outcome and response to treatment is variable. In some instances diffuse mesangial proliferation may be a precursor to the development of FSGS.

Membranous Nephropathy

Membranous nephropathy is the most common cause of NS in adults, yet it is very rare in children.[15] The ISKDC calculated an incidence of only 0.8% when 400 nephrotic children from 21 centers in 11 countries underwent renal biopsy.[16]

Membranous nephropathy may be either primary (idiopathic) or secondary. Secondary causes are seen in 23% to 43% of cases, with the most common secondary cause being hepatitis B infection. Other secondary causes include autoimmune disease (especially SLE), sickle cell disease, syphilis, complement deficiencies (particularly C2), malignancy, and drugs (eg, penicillamine, rarely captopril).[16]

Most children with membranous nephropathy have heavy proteinuria, hypoalbuminemia, and hyperlipidemia. Children may have asymptomatic proteinuria. Hematuria, usually microscopic as opposed to macroscopic, is more common in children than adults. Hypertension may be present.[16] Serum complement CH_{50}, C3, and C4 levels are typically normal.

Renal biopsy shows normal or slightly enlarged glomeruli with subepithelial immune deposits but without an inflammatory response or proliferation. Electron microscopy shows the hallmark electron-dense deposits located exclusively in the subepithelial position.[17] The severity of the basement membrane involvement may progress from small subepithelial deposits with a normal-appearing basement membrane (stage I); to larger, more numerous, and uniform deposits creating spikes projecting from the basement membrane toward the urinary space (stage II); and, finally, to a thickened basement membrane with fewer apparent deposits (stage IV). It is unclear whether the histologic stage is associated with prognosis.[15] Immunofluorescence studies in idiopathic membranous nephropathy show fine granular staining with IgG and C3 along the glomerular capillary wall. Mesangial IgG staining suggests that the membranous lesion may be secondary to SLE.[17]

The pathogenesis of idiopathic membranous nephropathy is uncertain, but it is most likely immune mediated. In contrast to other types of GN in which the immune complexes initially form in the circulation, the immune deposits in membranous nephropathy are believed to form in situ from binding of an autoantibody to a glycoprotein antigen expressed on the podocyte cell membrane.[17]

There are no evidence-based treatment guidelines for pediatric cases because of the rarity of this disease. In adults, treatment regimens using corticosteroids with or without alkylating agents (chlorambucil or cyclophosphamide) have resulted in equivocal outcomes.[16] The factors associated with loss of renal function in adults include abnormal creatinine at presentation, persistent heavy proteinuria, and tubulointerstitial injury on renal biopsy.[16]

> **ᵊᵥ Pearl**
>
> Membranous nephropathy is very rare in children.

C1q Nephropathy

C1q nephropathy may present as NS with minimal or no hematuria or with isolated proteinuria.

Acute Glomerulonephritis

A child with acute GN often has hematuria (microscopic or macroscopic), proteinuria, and intravascular volume expansion. Hypertension may be associated with headaches or, rarely, result in seizures. Volume overload may necessitate hospitalization for treatment of severe hypertension or congestive heart failure and pulmonary edema.

Acute Poststreptococcal Glomerulonephritis

Acute poststreptococcal glomerulonephritis, the most common type of postinfectious GN, occurs at a peak age of 4 to 5 years. A latent period occurs between infection, with a nephritogenic subtype of group A β-hemolytic streptococci and the onset of nephritis. Approximately 1 to 2 weeks after pharyngitis or 3 to 6 weeks after onset of pyoderma, the now afebrile child has hematuria. Hypertension and edema secondary to avid sodium retention are often found at the time of presentation. Hypertensive encephalopathy and pulmonary edema are potential complications. Antibiotic therapy for *Streptococcus pyogenes* does not prevent the development of GN.

In addition to dysmorphic RBCs, examination of the urine may reveal cellular casts composed of both RBCs and white blood cells. Laboratory studies show increased ASO levels if the GN was preceded by pharyngitis or elevated anti-deoxyribonuclease-B titers if the disease was preceded by a skin infection. The C3 level is depressed at time of presentation, but should return to normal within 6 weeks after onset of the disease. In children who present with gross hematuria, the urine usually becomes yellow approximately 2 weeks after disease onset.

Oliguria may occur but is transient, and rarely is it severe enough to require dialysis. Treatment is supportive with antihypertensive therapy, typically using a calcium channel blocker such as amlodipine, dietary sodium restriction, and administration of a loop diuretic such as furosemide. Patients may require hospitalization for control of hypertension.

Renal biopsy is not required in typical cases but should be performed to rule out MPGN if C3 levels are decreased for longer than 6 to 8 weeks, recurrent episodes of gross hematuria occur, proteinuria persists, or there is progressive decline in renal function. The classic finding on renal biopsy is a large electron-dense "hump" in a subepithelial location visualized with electron microscopy. Light microscopy reveals numerous neutrophils and enlarged glomeruli with narrowed capillary lumens (Figure 9-2A). Granular deposits of IgG, C3, properdin and, occasionally, IgM and IgA are seen in a capillary loop pattern with immunofluorescent stains (Figure 9-2).[18]

⪼ Pearl

Antibiotic therapy for *S pyogenes* does not prevent development of GN.

Prognosis is excellent in children with APSGN. Antihypertensive therapy is usually required for only a few weeks. The urinalysis is usually normal by 1 year after onset. Progression to ESRD is rare, and when it does occur the patient likely had atypical features such as crescent formation in a high percentage of the glomeruli.

Other Types of Postinfectious Acute Glomerulonephritis

A number of other bacterial and viral infections are reported as etiologies of acute proliferative GN. Staphylococci, pneumococci, and meningococci have been reported as underlying causes. Viruses such as varicella, influenza, adenovirus, and parvovirus have also been associated with this condition.[19]

Nephritis of Chronic Bacteremia

Postinfectious GN owing to atrioventricular shunt infection or subacute bacterial endocarditis may have either an acute or chronic presentation (Chapter 20). In these conditions the individual generally has an unsus-

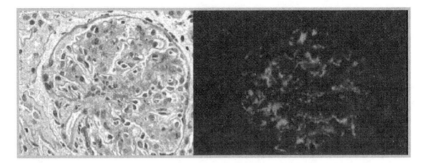

Figure 9-2.
Acute poststreptococcal glomerulonephritis. Left (LM), endocapillary proliferation.
Right (IF), IgG in capillary loop pattern.

pected chronic bacteremia with an organism of low virulence, such as
Staphylococcus epidermidis for shunt nephritis or viridans streptococci.
Over time these organisms induce the production of specific antibodies
that form circulating immune complexes and deposit in the glomerulus,
producing a chronic GN resembling MPGN. Treatment is directed at
eradication of the underlying infection.[20]

Chronic (Primary) Glomerulonephritis

Early detection of chronic GN offers the best opportunity for therapeutic
intervention directed at prevention or attenuation of glomerular injury.
The only presenting sign may be an abnormal urinalysis. Initial evaluation
should include urinalysis with microscopy (looking for dysmorphic RBCs
and RBC casts), serum creatinine and electrolytes, serum albumin, a complete blood count, total cholesterol, and complement levels (particularly C3
and C4). Proteinuria should be quantified using either a timed urine collection or, more easily, with a ratio of urine protein/creatinine measured from a
random urine specimen. A normal urine protein/creatinine ratio is less than
0.2; a ratio greater than 2 signifies nephrotic range proteinuria. Depending
on the presentation of the patient, it may also be necessary to include ASO,
fluorescent antinuclear antibodies, hepatitis serology, HIV testing, and antineutrophil antibodies (antimyeloperoxidase and antiproteinase 3 antibod-

ies).[18] Children with suspected glomerular disease should be referred to a pediatric nephrologist for evaluation, with the time frame for referral dependent on the severity of the child's symptoms.

Although comorbid symptoms may also suggest an etiology, renal biopsy is usually necessary to provide the definitive diagnosis and to direct clinical management. Unexplained fevers, arthralgias, rashes, hemoptysis, cough, or sinus disease suggests an underlying vasculitic etiology. Prior episodes of painless gross hematuria associated with upper respiratory infections are commonly seen in IgAN. Family history may also be useful in determining the etiology of the glomerular disease, particularly a history of dialysis and/or renal transplantation.

> **ᘒ Pearl**
>
> Abnormal urinalysis may be the only presenting sign of chronic GN.

IgA Nephropathy

IgAN is the most commonly occurring type of chronic GN in children and adults.[21] Berger and Hinglais[22] initially described IgAN in 1968 by reporting mesangial deposition of IgA in renal tissue obtained from children and young adults with episodic gross hematuria occurring concurrent with upper respiratory infections. The only US study estimating the incidence of this disorder in a pediatric population was performed in eastern Kentucky, showing an incidence of 5.6 and 10.2 per 1 million population per year for children 1 to 9 years of age and 10 to 19 years of age, respectively.[23] Most pediatric series show a male/female predominance of about 2:1.[24]

Children with IgAN in the United States tend to have gross hematuria.[25] In countries such as Japan, where screening is common, a much higher percentage of children have microscopic hematuria with or without proteinuria. Less than 10% of children have nephrotic range proteinuria.[26] Some children may be hypertensive at presentation, though severely elevated blood pressure is unusual.[27] Children are less likely than adults to have impaired renal function.[24] Numerous reports of familial IgAN affecting first-, second-, or third-degree relatives and the identification of the IgAN1 locus in some families strongly suggests a genetic basis for the disease.[28]

The pathogenesis of IgAN appears to be related to aberrant glycosylation of O-linked glycans in the hinge region of IgA1. Rather than terminating with galactose, these glycans terminate with N-acetylgalactosamine and are recognized by IgG or IgA1 antibodies. Circulating immune complexes are formed and deposit in the mesangium.[29]

At the present time there is no diagnostic test for IgAN other than the renal biopsy. An assay measuring levels of galactose-deficient IgA appears to have potential for development as a diagnostic test for IgAN.[30] When a noninvasive diagnostic test becomes available and is used in the evaluation of hematuria, more mild cases of IgAN will likely be detected.

Immunofluorescent studies on renal biopsy tissue show dominant or co-dominant deposition of IgA, primarily in a mesangial distribution. IgG, IgM, and C3 deposition may also be seen in the same pattern (Figure 9-3). Severity of involvement based on light microscopy examination may be graded, with histologically normal tissue designated as type I, mesangial hypercellularity as type 2, and proliferative changes associated with scarring as type 3.[31] When there is renal involvement in HSP, the renal biopsy findings are identical to IgAN.

Angiotensin-converting enzyme inhibitors and/or ARBs are the mainstays of medical therapy owing to renoprotective effects. These medications are used when the urine protein/creatinine ratio is greater than 1.0, even if the child is normotensive. Despite lack of evidence from randomized controlled trials, oral or intravenous corticosteroids are recommended for severe

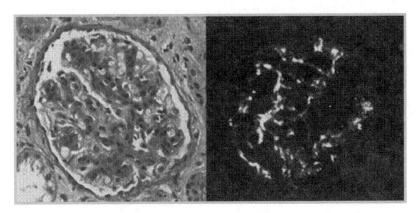

Figure 9-3.
Renal biopsy in immunoglobulin A (IgA) nephropathy: Left (LM), mesangial matrix and cellular proliferation. Right (IF), typical mesangial pattern of IgA.

or rapidly progressive disease.[32] Therapy with omega-3 fatty acid in the form of fish oil supplements, azathioprine, and vitamin E has been tried.[24] Tonsillectomy is advocated as an adjunct therapy in countries such as France and Japan, but its efficacy is not supported by well-designed randomized controlled trials.

Pediatric patients with IgAN often do not progress to ESRD until adulthood.[25] In 1995 kidney survival from the time of biopsy was 94% at 5 years, 87% at 10 years, and 70% at 20 years.[26] Ronkainen et al[33] recently reported renal survival in a Finnish pediatric cohort from the time of presentation as 93% at 10 years and 87% at 20 years. Race does not appear to be a risk factor for progression to ESRD.[27]

> **≈► Pearl**
>
> IgA nephropathy is the most commonly occurring type of chronic GN in children and adults.

Membranoproliferative Glomerulonephritis

Membranoproliferative glomerulonephritis is a relatively rare form of chronic GN, with an estimated incidence in pediatric patients of 1 to 2 cases per million per year.[34] Membranoproliferative glomerulonephritis is also known as mesangiocapillary GN and is typically characterized by persistent hypocomplementemia or low serum C3 concentration. Proliferation of the mesangial and endothelial cells is of such severity that the glomerulus is enlarged and glomerular tufts may appear lobulated. The failure of the C3 level to return to normal within 6 weeks after onset of APSGN should lead to referral to a pediatric nephrologist for renal biopsy.

Membranoproliferative glomerulonephritis is subdivided into types I, II, and III based on location of the immune deposits and GBM appearance on electron microscopy. In type I, the GBM structure is normal, and the large electron-dense deposits occur in a subendothelial location. Deposits, felt by some to be dense "alterations" rather than immune complexes, are within the GBM and Bruch membrane of the eye in type II MPGN. In type III MPGN, the GBM may be frayed and disrupted and dense deposits may be subendothelial, intramembranous, and subepithelial.

Membranoproliferative glomerulonephritis presents with NS in approximately 33% of patients, acute nephritis in 25%, and asymptomatic hematuria and proteinuria in the rest. Constitutional symptoms, mild anemia, and hypertension are more common in patients with MPGN type I.[34] C3 levels are low in 80% of patients with all types of MPGN. In patients with type I disease who have low C3 levels, 40% will have significant depression of C4 levels. Secondary type I MPGN may occur in association with viral infection from agents such as hepatitis C, autoimmune diseases such as SLE, or neoplasia.

Type II MPGN, or dense deposit disease, constitutes less than 20% of pediatric MPGN. In most patients with type II disease, the alternative complement pathway is activated by C3NeF, an autoantibody to the C3 convertase C3bBb, resulting in continuous consumption of C3. Presumably this complement abnormality precedes the development of GN. C3 nephritic factor is also associated with another rare condition, partial lipodystrophy, that may also be a precursor to type II MPGN.

Children with type III MPGN are more likely than those with types I and II to have abnormal urinalyses in the absence of other symptoms.[35] Patients with type III MPGN and depressed serum C3 levels often have normal C4 levels, but depression of terminal complement component levels. This appears because of a C3NeF that consumes C3 slower than the C3NeF associated with type II MPGN.[34]

The pathogenetic mechanisms for all types of MPGN are not well understood. Association with an extended human leukocyte antigen haplotype and inherited deficiencies of individual complement proteins suggest a genetic susceptibility.[35] Type III MPGN was linked to chromosome 1q31–32 in an Irish pedigree.[36]

A few patients have rapid progression to ESRD, but most lose renal function over a period of years. In the 1970s the 10-year kidney survival rate for all types of MPGN was 50%. A more recent study showed a 10-year kidney survival rate of approximately 80% for type I and 70% for type III MPGN.[37] Membranoproliferative glomerulonephritis types I and II frequently recur in renal transplants and pose a significant risk for graft loss over time.

ᴥ *Pearl*

Membranoproliferative glomerulonephritis presents with NS in 33% of patients, acute nephritis in 25%, and asymptomatic hematuria and proteinuria in the rest.

An ISKDC trial compared alternate-day prednisone with placebo and showed better kidney survival for the prednisone group for types I and III but not for type II MPGN.[38] Angiotensin-converting enzyme inhibitors and/or ARBs should be used to control hypertension and reduce proteinuria. Statins are generally recommended for older children with NS.

C1q Nephropathy

Jennette and Hipp[39] used the term *C1qN* in 1985 to describe a pathologic renal lesion closely resembling lupus nephritis in a set of patients who had no evidence of that disease. Immunofluorescent studies showed extensive C1q deposits in a predominantly mesangial distribution along with C3 and immunoglobulins. Electron microscopy revealed mesangial dense deposits in 100% and capillary wall dense deposits in 20% of patients. The patients were 53% male and 60% black and they had a mean age of 17.8 years. All patients had proteinuria, with more than 50% described as steroid resistant. Hematuria was present in 40%. All patients had normal serum levels for complement components, and none were positive for antinuclear antibodies.[39]

In a cohort of 20 pediatric patients (mean age 11.2 years, 60 % black, 55% male) with C1qN, Lau et al[40] reported 40% had NS, whereas 30% had normal serum albumin despite nephrotic range proteinuria. In patients with NS, renal survival was 88% and 49% at 1 and 5 years, respectively.

Rapidly Progressive Glomerulonephritis

Rapidly progressive glomerulonephritis, or crescentic GN, is a clinical term used to describe deterioration in renal function occurring over days to weeks[41] (see also Chapter 20). The presence of large epithelial crescents within Bowman space (with percentages varying from 20%–75%) is used as the histologic criterion for crescentic GN.[42] These crescents may result in complete and irreversible destruction of the glomerular tuft. A wide variety of glomerular disorders may have crescent formation with rapid progression including APSGN, SLE, MPGN type II, IgAN, HSP nephritis, anti-GBM disease, and ANCA-associated pauci-immune GN.[43]

At presentation, patients with RPGN may have hematuria (73%), moderate to severe proteinuria (78%), and decreased glomerular filtration rate (86%).[43] Oliguria and edema may also be present. Patients with anti-GBM disease may also have pulmonary involvement with hemoptysis because of pulmonary hemorrhage.[44] Children with ANCA-associated GN, such as Wegener granulomatosis or polyarteritis nodosa, may present with constitutional symptoms along with multisystem disease.

Diagnosis of RPGN must be made promptly because urgent treatment is needed to preserve renal function. Differing patterns of immunofluorescence on renal biopsy may be helpful in determining the underlying cause. Linear IgG staining along the capillary walls occurs in anti-GBM disease. Immune complex GN shows granular glomerular deposition of immunoglobulins and complement. *Pauci-immune* refers to negative or scanty immunoglobulin deposition often seen in ANCA-associated disease.[44]

Treatment is directed by suspected etiology. Anti-GBM disease is often treated by plasma exchange with albumin, corticosteroids, and cyclophosphamide. Antineutrophil cytoplasmic antibody–associated disease is treated with corticosteroids and cyclophosphamide, with the addition of plasma exchange for pulmonary involvement. Treatment of pauci-immune disease is more controversial, with no clear benefit for plasma exchange in adult randomized controlled trials. These studies also used steroids, cytotoxic agents, azathioprine, and heparin.[44] Treatment of immune complex–mediated disease such as IgAN and MPGN was discussed previously. Despite aggressive therapy, at least half of pediatric patients with RPGN will progress to ESRD.[43]

> ⋧ *Pearl*
>
> Rapidly progressive glomerulonephritis, or crescentic GN, is a clinical definition used to describe deterioration in renal function occurring over days to weeks.

References

1. Schlesinger ER, Sultz HA, Mosher WE, Feldman JG. The nephrotic syndrome. Its incidence and implications for the community. *Am J Dis Child.* 1968;116:623–632

2. Trachtman H, Greenbaum LA, McCarthy ET, Sharma M, Gauthier BG, Frank R, Glomerular permeability activity: prevalence and prognostic value in pediatric patients with idiopathic nephrotic syndrome. *Am J Kidney Dis.* 2004;44:604–610

3. Wyatt RJ, Marx MB, Kazee M, Holland NH. Current estimates of the incidence of steroid responsive idiopathic nephrosis in Kentucky children 1–9 years of age. *Int J Pediatr Nephrol.* 1982;3:63–65

4. Tune BM, Mendoza SA. Treatment of the idiopathic nephrotic syndrome: regimens and outcomes in children and adults. *J Am Soc Nephrol.* 1997;8:824–832

5. Brodehl J. The treatment of minimal change nephrotic syndrome: lessons learned from multicentre co-operative studies. *Eur J Pediatr.* 1991;150:380–387

6. A report of the International Study of Kidney Disease in Children. The primary nephrotic syndrome in children. Identification of patients with minimal change nephrotic syndrome from initial response to prednisone. *J Pediatr.* 1981;98:561–564

7. Niaudet P. Steroid-sensitive idiopathic nephrotic syndrome in children. In: Avner ED, Harmon WE, Niaudet P, eds. *Pediatric Nephrology.* 5th ed. Philadelphia, PA: Lippincott, Williams & Wilkins; 2004:543–556

8. Benchimol C. Focal segmental glomerulosclerosis: pathogenesis and treatment. *Curr Opin Pediatr.* 2003;15:171–180

9. Korbet SM. Primary focal segmental glomerulosclerosis. *J Am Soc Nephrol.* 1998;9: 1333–1340

10. Chesney R. The changing face of childhood nephrotic syndrome. *Kidney Int.* 2004;66: 1294–1302

11. Srivastava T, Simon SD, Alon US. High incidence of focal segmental glomerulosclerosis in nephrotic syndrome of childhood. *Pediatr Nephrol.* 1999;13:13–18

12. Bonilla-Felix M, Parra C, Dajani T, Ferris M, Swinford RD, Portman RJ. Changing patterns in the histopathology of idiopathic nephrotic syndrome in children. *Kidney Int.* 1999;55:1885–1890

13. Mendoza SA, Reznik VM, Griswold WR, Krensky AM, Yorgin PD, Tune BM. Treatment of steroid-resistant focal segmental glomerulosclerosis with pulse methylprednisolone and alkylating agents. *Pediatr Nephrol.* 1990;4:303–307

14. Benfield MR, McDonald R, Sullivan EK, Stablein DM, Tejani A. The 1997 Annual Renal Transplantation in Children Report of the North American Pediatric Renal Transplant Cooperative Study (NAPRTCS). *Pediatr Transplant.* 1999;3:152–167

15. Reichert LJ, Koene RA, Wetzels JF. Prognostic factors in idiopathic membranous neph-ropathy. *Am J Kidney Dis.* 1998;31:1–11

16. Cameron JS. Membranous nephropathy in childhood and its treatment. *Pediatr Nephrol.* 1990;4:193–198

17. Makker SP. Membranous nephropathy. In: Avner ED, Harmon WE, Niaudet P, eds. *Pediatric Nephrology.* 5th ed. Philadelphia, PA: Lippincott, Williams & Wilkins; 2004: 641–654

18. Lau KK, Wyatt RJ. Glomerulonephritis. *Adolesc Med Clin.* 2005;16:67–85

19. Nadasdy T, Silva FG. Chapter 8: Acute post-infectious glomerulonephritis and glomerulo-nephritis caused by persistent bacterial infection. In: Jennette JC, Olson JL, Schwartz MM, Silva FG, eds. *Heptinstall's Pathology of the Kidney.* Vol 1. 6th ed. Philadelphia, PA: Lippin-cott, Williams & Wilkins; 2007:321–396

20. Wyatt RJ, Walsh JW, Holland NH. Shunt nephritis. Role of the complement system in its pathogenesis and management. *J Neurosurg.* 1981;55:99–107

21. D'Amico G. The commonest glomerulonephritis in the world: IgA nephropathy. *Q J Med.* 1987;64:709–727

22. Berger J, Hinglais N. [Intercapillary deposits of IgA-IgG]. *J Urol Nephrol (Paris)*. 1968;74:694–695

23. Wyatt RJ, Julian BA, Baehler RW, Stafford CC, McMorrow RG, Ferguson T, et al. Epidemiology of IgA nephropathy in central and eastern Kentucky for the period 1975 through 1994. Central Kentucky Region of the Southeastern United States IgA Nephropathy DATABANK Project. *J Am Soc Nephrol*. 1998;9:853–858

24. Delos Santos NM, Wyatt RJ. Pediatric IgA nephropathies: clinical aspects and therapeutic approaches. *Semin Nephrol*. 2004;24:269–286

25. Wyatt RJ, Julian BA, Bhathena DB, Mitchell BL, Holland NH, Malluche HH. IgA nephropathy: presentation, clinical course, and prognosis in children and adults. *Am J Kidney Dis*. 1984;4:192–200

26. Wyatt RJ, Kritchevsky SB, Woodford SY, Miller PM, Roy S III, Holland NH, et al. IgA nephropathy: long-term prognosis for pediatric patients. *J Pediatr*. 1995;127:913–919

27. Lau KK, Gaber LW, Delos Santos NM, Fisher KA, Grimes SJ, Wyatt RJ. Pediatric IgA nephropathy: clinical features at presentation and outcome for African-Americans and Caucasians. *Clin Nephrol*. 2004;62:167–172

28. Beerman I, Novak J, Wyatt RJ, Julian BA, Gharavi AG. The genetics of IgA nephropathy. *Nature Clin Pract Nephrol*. 2007;3:325–338

29. Tomana M, Novak J, Julian BA, Matousovic K, Konecny K, Mestecky J. Circulating immune complexes in IgA nephropathy consist of IgA1 with galactose-deficient hinge region and antiglycan antibodies. *J Clin Invest*. 1999;104:73–81

30. Moldoveanu Z, Wyatt RJ, Lee JY, Tomana M, Julian BA, Mestecky J, et al. Patients with IgA nephropathy have increased serum galactose-deficient IgA1 levels. *Kidney Int*. 2007;71:1148–1154

31. Hogg RJ, Silva FG, Wyatt RJ, Reisch JS, Argyle JC, Savino DA. Prognostic indicators in children with IgA nephropathy—report of the Southwest Pediatric Nephrology Study Group. *Pediatr Nephrol*. 1994;8:15–20

32. Wyatt RJ, Hogg RJ. Evidence-based assessment of treatment options for children with IgA nephropathies. *Pediatr Nephrol*. 2001;16:156–167

33. Ronkainen J, Ala-Houhala M, Autio-Harmainen H, et al. Long-term outcome 19 years after childhood IgA nephritis: a retrospective cohort study. *Pediatr Nephrol*. 2006;21:1266–1273

34. Strife CF, Braun MC, West CD. Membranoproliferative glomerulonephritis. In: Avner ED, Harmon WE, Niaudet P, eds. *Pediatric Nephrology*. 5th ed. Philadelphia, PA: Lippincott, Williams & Wilkins; 2004:629–637

35. West CD. Idiopathic membranoproliferative glomerulonephritis in childhood. *Pediatr Nephrol*. 1992;6:96–103

36. Neary JJ, Conlon PJ, Croke D, et al. Linkage of a gene causing familial membranoproliferative glomerulonephritis type III to chromosome 1. *J Am Soc Nephrol*. 2002;13:2052–2057

37. Braun MC, West CD, Strife CF. Differences between membranoproliferative glomerulonephritis types I and III in long-term response to an alternate-day prednisone regimen. *Am J Kidney Dis*. 1999;34:1022–1032

38. Tarshish P, Bernstein J, Tobin JN, Edelmann CM Jr. Treatment of mesangiocapillary glomerulonephritis with alternate-day prednisone—a report of the International Study of Kidney Disease in Children. *Pediatr Nephrol.* 1992;6:123–130

39. Jennette JC, Hipp CG. C1q nephropathy: a distinct pathologic entity usually causing nephrotic syndrome. *Am J Kidney Dis.* 1985;6:103–110

40. Lau KK, Gaber LW, Delos Santos NM, Wyatt RJ. C1q nephropathy: features at presentation and outcome. *Pediatr Nephrol.* 2005;20:744–749

41. Couser WG. Glomerulonephritis. *Lancet.* 1999;353:1509–1515

42. Dillon MJ. Crescentic glomerulonephritis. In: Avner ED, Harmon WE, Niaudet P, eds. *Pediatric Nephrology.* 5th ed. Philadelphia, PA: Lippincott, Williams & Wilkins; 2004: 655–662

43. Southwest Pediatric Nephrology Study Group. A clinico-pathologic study of crescentic glomerulonephritis in 50 children. A report of the Southwest Pediatric Nephrology Study Group. *Kidney Int.* 1985;27:450–458

44. Jindal KK. Management of idiopathic crescentic and diffuse proliferative glomerulonephritis: evidence-based recommendations. *Kidney Int Suppl.* 1999;70:S33–S40

Chapter 10

▌ *Renal Tubular Disease*

Russell W. Chesney

Introduction

The renal tubule consists of an epithelium that acts as the principal site of transport of ions, organic solutes, drugs and toxins, and water (Box 10-1). These transport processes can include reabsorption and/or secretion.[1-7] Different segments of the nephron are responsible for both quantitative and qualitative transport, with bulk reabsorption occurring in proximal tubular segments and fine-tuning in distal tubular sites. Disorders can involve a single solute, water, or a class of solutes. With generalized damage to the renal tubular epithelium, many solutes will be lost in the urine, which is a condition termed *Fanconi syndrome*.[1-6] The syndrome occurs whenever an agent, toxin, or mutation disrupts oxidative phosphorylation and energy production and a more global wasting of ions and solutes occurs.

Box 10-1. Nephron Locations of Ion or Solute Reabsorption and/or Secretion

Proximal tubule

Sodium, chloride, glucose, amino acids, ketoacids, low-molecular-weight proteins (<50,000 daltons), phosphate, water

Loop of Henle

Sodium, chloride, calcium, potassium

Distal convoluted tubule

Sodium, chloride

Collecting ducts

Sodium, chloride, potassium, hydrogen ions (protons)

Renal tubular disorders are largely a result of abnormal transport function. Because many of the tubule transporter systems are ion channels, water channels, or solute transporters (eg, sodium-glucose co-transporter), disorders resulting in mutation of the transporter DNA can result in defective transporter protein with a loss or diminution of transport function. Hence, when these transport systems are abnormal, excessive amounts of ions or solute will be excreted into the urine.

These transport processes represent both active and passive (diffusional) transport. Essentially all active transport systems require energy derived from ATP hydrolysis. Accordingly, the renal tubule is a site of oxidative phosphorylation that produces the ATP necessary for transport processes. Function follows form in that the proximal tubule, where bulk reabsorption takes place, has a far greater density of, and number of, mitochondria than do distal tubule segments. Renal tubular disorders usually have universal characteristics.[1-7]

1. These disorders are usually inherited.
2. Affected children frequently have growth failure.
3. Some of these disorders are benign and require no therapy, thus it is important to make the correct diagnosis.
4. These disorders may be treated with replacement of the substance being lost in the urine or removal of an offending substance or metabolite.

A primary care physician will probably need the help of a pediatric nephrologist in the diagnosis and management of major renal tubular disorders. The more common renal tubular disorders are presented in Table 10-1. Tests performed to evaluate these disorders are presented in Table 10-2.

Table 10-1. Renal Tubular Disorders				
Disorder	Inheritance	Prevalence	Tubular Abnormality	Clinical Consequence
Renal glucosuria	AR	1/20,000	Glucose transport affected; benign	Glucosuria at normal blood glucose
Cystinuria	AR	1/7,000–12,000	Transport system for cystine and dibasic AAs affected in kidney and intestine	Cystinuria results in stones and obstruction; gut defect benign
Hartnup disease	AR	1/16,000–130,000	Transport system for neutral AAs defective in kidney and intestine	Loss of tryptophan causes nicotinamide deficiency and symptoms of pellagra
RTA, type I		Uncommon	Defect in acidification mechanism of distal tubule	Metabolic acidosis with or without hypercalciuria
Fanconi syndrome	AR, AD, acquired	1/40,000 for cystinosis, others unknown	Generalized proximal tubular defect	Disease dependent
X-linked hypophosphatemic rickets (vitamin D–resistant rickets)	XLD, rarely; AR, AD	1/20,000	Renal defect in phosphate reabsorption and vitamin D metabolism	Bowing of lower extremities, short stature
Nephrogenic diabetes insipidus	XLR	Uncommon	Unknown	Renal tubular cells insensitive to vasopressin; polyuria
Bartter syndrome	AR?	Rare	Impaired chloride reabsorption, potassium wasting	Hypokalemic alkalosis

Abbreviations: AR, autosomal recessive; AA, amino acid; AD, autosomal dominant; XLD, X-linked dominant; XLR, X-linked recessive.

Table 10-2. Evaluation of Renal Tubular Disorders		
Test	**Abnormality**	**Suspected Diagnosis**
Urinalysis	Concentration defect	Bartter, Fanconi syndromes
	Glucosuria	Glucosuria, Fanconi syndrome
	Ketonuria	Fanconi syndrome
	Proteinuria	Fanconi syndrome
	Cystine crystals	Cystinuria
	Alkaline pH	Renal tubular acidosis, Fanconi syndrome
Serum electrolytes	Hypokalemia	Fanconi, Bartter syndromes
	Reduced bicarbonate	Renal tubular acidosis, Fanconi syndrome
	Elevated bicarbonate	Bartter syndrome
Serum chemistries	Reduced phosphate	Phosphaturias
	Reduced calcium	Vitamin D abnormality
	Elevated alkaline phosphatase	Phosphaturias, vitamin D abnormality
	Elevated phosphate	Renal failure, hypoparathyroidism or pseudohypoparathyroidism
	Hypercalcemia	Primary hyperparathyroidism
	Hypomagnesemia	Renal leak, drug-induced magnesium deficiency
Urine metabolic screen	Amino acids	Aminoaciduria, vitamin D deficiency, Fanconi syndrome
	Cyanide-nitroprusside	Cystinuria
	Organic acids	Fanconi syndrome
	Excessive phosphaturia (tubular reabsorption of phosphate <85%)	Phosphaturia, Fanconi syndrome, hyperparathyroidism
	Excessive phosphate retention (tubular reabsorption of retention >85%, with hyperphosphatemia)	Hypoparathyroidism or pseudohypoparathyroidism

Proximal Tubulopathies

Familial Glucosuria

An uncommon condition (about 1 in 20,000 individuals), familial glucosuria is the result of mutations in 1 of 2 sodium-dependent glucose transporters.[6] Affected patients spill glucose in the urine at normal or low-normal plasma glucose concentrations. A urinalysis will reveal glucose in the urine, which often results in a misdiagnosis of diabetes mellitus. No treatment is necessary for familial glucosuria, but a physician may be required to inform insurance companies of this benign condition when a patient applies for life insurance or health insurance. When the sodium-dependent glucose-galactose transporter malfunctions, both glucose and galactose are hyperexcreted. These 2 hexoses are also malabsorbed by the gut because this transporter is expressed at both epithelial surfaces.

ᗌ Pearl

Familial glucosuria is a benign condition that needs no treatment.

Aminoacidurias

Aminoacidurias generally represent the effect of mutations in transporter proteins responsible for the reabsorption of α-amino acids from proximal tubular ultrafiltrate.[4-6] These can be amino acid–specific or group-specific. Based on their structure and charge, amino acids are divided into several groups: neutral monoamino acids, dibasic amino acids, imino acids, and dicarboxylic amino acids. Several of these aminoacidurias, including iminoaciduria and dicarboxylic aminoaciduria, and the loss of α-amino acids are benign and will not be discussed further.

The main aminoaciduria of pathologic significance is cystinuria, an autosomal recessive disorder that occurs in 1 in 9,000 to 12,000 individuals. Cystinuria can be isolated or represent a defect in the dibasic amino acid system that includes cystine. In this case, the amino acids lost are cystine, ornithine, arginine, and lysine (COAL), but the key is the loss of cystine. Cystine, a dimer of cysteine, is highly insoluble in aqueous fluid and, hence, precipitates to form hexagonal crystals. These crystals coalesce to form cystine stones. Thus the direct pathogenesis of cystinuria is a result of the physical-chemical insolubility of cystine. Increased cystine excretion can lead to staghorn calculi, stasis, infection, bleeding, and pain.

Therapy is aimed at increasing the solubility of cystine, which includes forced hydration, alkalinization of the urine, and the use of agents that cause the formation of mixed disulfides, which are far more soluble than cystine. The major agent used is tiopronin, or 2-mercaptopropionylglycine, which has fewer side effects than other agents.

Hartnup disease is a rare autosomal recessive disorder of the neutral monocarboxylic amino acid transport system.[4-6] In patients with the disease, 12 amino acids are lost as a result of a defective transporter, but the pathogenesis of the disorder results from the loss of tryptophan in the urine and its failure to be absorbed by the gut. Tryptophan is important in the formation of nicotinamide, and patients manifest niacin deficiency or pellagra-like features. Patients exhibit the triad of a red rash in sun-exposed sites, dementia, and chelosis (cracks at the corners of the mouth). Therapy, which reverses clinical characteristics, is the provision of nicotinamide, but aminoaciduria and tryptophan loss persists for life. Ataxia found may also persist.

❧ Pearl

Increased cystine excretion in cystinuria can lead to staghorn calculi, stasis, infection, bleeding, and pain.

Phosphaturia

Hereditary phosphaturias are important because they result in hypophosphatemia and diminished mineralization of bone osteoid, especially at the growth plate. Because undermineralization of the growth plate results in soft bone (termed *osteomalacia*), which will bend on weight bearing, these conditions are frequently termed *hypophosphatemic rickets*. Moreover, despite the cause of phosphaturia, the clinical features are similar. Biochemical features include normocalcemia or hypercalcemia, hypophosphatemia, elevation of serum alkaline phosphatase and other markers of rapid bone turnover (raised osteocalcin levels, etc), and a normal or subnormal circulating parathyroid hormone level.[2-6]

Hypophosphatemic rickets can be hereditary, either the result of a mesenchymal tumor (which produces a phosphaturic substance) or the result of Fanconi syndrome from any of its causes. The hereditary forms of hypophosphatemic rickets are usually X-linked dominant in transmission, but autosomal dominant and recessive inheritance modes may occur. X-linked hypophosphatemic rickets is the most common form of rickets other than nutritional rickets, and it usually appears after a child bears weight with lower limb bowing, metaphyseal widening, fraying at the ends of bones, and osteopenia on x-ray with short stature (Figure 10-1). Because males have a single X chromosome, they are hemizygous for the mutation causing this condition; thus, the disease is more marked in males than in females. Although the mutation is found on the X chromosome, it also influences a protein termed *PHEX* that regulates FGF-23, which in turn regulates the function of the sodium-dependent phosphate transporter located in the apical membrane of the proximal tubule. Because most phosphate is reclaimed by the epithelial surface of the proximal tubule, it is this transport system that is affected in X-linked hypophosphatemia and, accordingly, renal phosphate wasting is massive.

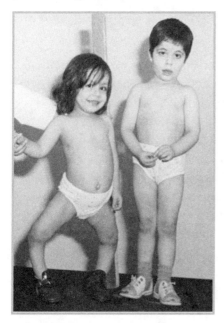

Figure 10-1.
A girl with hypophosphatemic rickets with her normal twin sister. (Courtesy of Dr S.S. Najjar.) (Reprinted with permission from Barakat AY, et al. *The Kidney in Genetic Disease.* Edinburgh, UK: Churchhill Livingstone; 1986:97.)

Oncogenous, or tumoral, rickets is found whenever a mesenchymal (bone or soft tissue) tumor develops that elaborates a phosphaturic substance and alters the interaction of FGF-23 and the sodium-dependent phosphate transporter. The biochemical features are similar to hereditary hypophosphatemic rickets except that the circulating values of 1,25-dihydroxyvitamin D are extremely low.[1] Patients with this disorder develop bone pain, osteomalacia, and hypophosphatemia. Careful evaluation for the presence of a tumor, including a skeletal x-ray survey or bone scan, will often reveal a small lesion. Whenever this tumor is completely removed, the hypophosphatemia and other biochemical features reverse. The tumor, depending on its size and location, may not be completely removable, and therapy with oral phosphate and calcitriol is essential.[1,3,4]

The phosphaturia and hypophosphatemic osteomalacia resulting from Fanconi syndrome is discussed in relation to the entire syndrome later in this chapter.

ટ Pearl

Other than nutritional rickets, X-linked hypophosphatemic rickets is the most common form of rickets.

In general, treatment of the phosphaturic syndrome is the provision of oral phosphate and calcitrol. Because phosphaturia is continuous, oral phosphate must be given around the clock, usually as a neutral phosphate solution given 3 to 5 times daily. Because oral phosphate solutions reduce calcium absorption from the intestine, calcium absorption can be enhanced by calcitriol therapy.[2-5]

Bicarbonaturia

Proximal RTA results in massive loss of sodium and potassium bicarbonate into the urine. Because the bulk of HCO_3^- reabsorption occurs in the

ટ Pearl

Type II proximal RTA is usually a component of Fanconi syndrome.

proximal tubule, it is necessary to replace between 10 to 15 mEq of HCO_3^-/kg/d as therapy. Proximal RTA is usually termed *type II* (versus distal RTA, which is *type I*), and as an isolated disorder is rare. Forms of type II may be hereditary (autosomal dominant or recessive) and include ocular abnormalities. Most patients with type II RTA have this condition as a component of Fanconi syndrome.[1-6]

Fanconi Syndrome

Fanconi syndrome is a global proximal tubule dysfunction abnormality that is characterized by glucosuria, generalized aminoaciduria, phosphaturia, proximal RTA, low-molecular-weight proteinuria, hypokalemia and, often, hypomagnesemia.[1-4,6] This syndrome may be primary (sporadic or hereditary) or secondary to a variety of inherited disorders[5,6] (Box 10-2). Many of these disorders are the result of mutations of enzymes of metabolism or of mitochondrial DNA. These disorders may perturb metabolism of the renal cell or be related to the deposition of toxic materials (galactose-1-phosphate

> **Box 10-2. Classification of Proximal Renal Tubular Acidosis (Type II)**
> Proximal (type II)
>   Isolated
>   Sporadic
>   Hereditary
> Fanconi syndrome
>   Primary
>   Sporadic
>   Hereditary
>   Cystinosis
>   Lowe syndrome
>   Galactosemia
>   Tyrosinemia
>   Fructosemia
>   Fanconi-Bickel syndrome
>   Wilson disease
>   Mitochondrial diseases
>   Dent disease (X-linked nephrolithiasis)
>   Secondary
>   Heavy metals, outdated tetracycline, gentamicin, ifosfamide, cyclosporine/tacrolimus

or fructose-1-phosphate) or heavy metals (ie, copper in Wilson disease, lead from environmental exposure).

The diagnosis of Fanconi syndrome is usually made by a cluster of signs and symptoms such as muscle weakness and pain (from hypokalemia), bone pain and bowing (from hypophosphatemic rickets and acidosis), poor weight and height gain (from bone disease and acidosis), polyuria as a result of hypokalemia, damage to sites of ADH action on urine concentration, and lactic acidosis, especially in disorders of mitochondrial DNA. Two disorders, cystinosis and Lowe syndrome, can also result in renal failure. Hence, patients with these disorders may have mild to moderate renal insufficiency.

Infantile nephropathic cystinosis is the most common form of the renal Fanconi syndrome in children, which usually develops at 18 months of age.[1,4,6] In this disorder, the molecular defect is found in the lysosomal membrane transporter, called *cystinosin*, which leads to the efflux of intralysosomal cystine from nearly all organs in the body, including kidneys, liver, spleen, skeletal muscle, and thyroid. With a defective transporter, cystine accumulates. Because cystine is a highly insoluble amino acid, it precipitates within the lysosome, leading to release of lysosomal hydrolases. Over time, tissue damage intensifies, resulting in organ failure, especially of the kidney and the thyroid gland. In addition to general therapy of Fanconi syndrome, listed later, patients with cystinosis are treated with cysteamine, which permits cystine egress through the lysosome membrane by forming a mixed disulfide with cystine.

Lowe syndrome is an X-linked disorder that results in a cluster of symptoms including severe mental retardation, a peculiar sloping forehead, glaucoma, and other ocular defects caused by mutations in the OCRLI gene that codes for the phosphatidylinositol 5-phosphatase protein. This results in abnormalities of vesicular transport in the Golgi apparatus. These alterations are presumably responsible for the relatively nonspecific tubulointerstitial alterations and thickened glomerular basement membrane and proximal tubular mitochondria evident in renal biopsy samples.[1,4-6] Therapy of Lowe syndrome is symptomatic and does not change the renal findings. Among clinical features that require attention are behavioral changes including tantrums, obsessions, swaying, and stereotypy; unfortunately, therapy is not especially effective.

Therapy of all forms of Fanconi syndrome includes sufficient sodium bicarbonate to reverse acidosis, neutral phosphate solutions, and insulin in those patients with acquired diabetes mellitus. No attempts are made to replace amino acids or glucose. The doses of sodium bicarbonate and neutral phosphate are comparable to those needed to reverse acidosis in proximal (type II) RTA and the phosphate needed in X-linked hypophosphatemia, respectively.[4-6]

Several other forms of Fanconi syndrome deserve mention. Three hereditary forms—galactosemia, hereditary fructose intolerance, and tyrosinemia—affect both the liver and the kidney. In tyrosinemia, patients are treated with both a liver and kidney transplant. Dent disease, or X-linked hypercalciuric nephrolithiasis, is a proximal renal tubular disorder with low-molecular-weight proteinuria, hypercalciuria, nephrocalcinosis, metabolic bone disease, and progressive renal failure. It is caused by a mutation in the CLCN5 chloride transporter gene, which is coded on the X chromosome.

❧ Pearl

Fanconi syndrome is characterized by glucosuria, generalized aminoaciduria, phosphaturia, proximal RTA, and low-molecular-weight proteinuria.

Two toxins can cause sporadic Fanconi syndrome: outdated tetracy-cline and ifosfamide. Ifosfamide, used in patients with solid tumors, causes Fanconi syndrome with some or all its symptoms in approximately 15% of patients. Removal of these toxins usually reduces or fully reverses the clinical aspects of the syndrome.[1-6]

Distal Tubular Disorders

Type I or Distal Renal Tubular Acidosis

Impaired hydrogen ion (or proton) secretion by distal nephron sites occurs in certain proton-secreting processes, especially those that influence the H^+/adenosinetriphosphatase or the H^+/Cl^- anion exchangers.[1,7] As a result of impaired hydrogen ion excretion, urine pH remains higher than 6, despite metabolic acidosis. Patients with distal RTA have reduced serum bicarbonate, chronic non–anion gap metabolic acidosis, and hypokalemia. Patients also can demonstrate hypocitraturia with hypercalciuria and often nephrocalcinosis. Bone disease is relatively common because bone bicarbonate and other anions serve as a buffer against H^+ excess.

Several clinical forms are found: sporadic, autosomal dominant, autosomal recessive, or acquired. A typical patient has growth failure in addition to hyperchloremic non–anion gap metabolic acidosis. The various forms of distal RTA are listed in Box 10-3. One form of type I RTA involves sensorineural deafness.

One other variant of distal RTA can occur in subjects with Beckwith-Weidemann syndrome who develop medullary sponge kidney. These patients develop a caliectasis of the distal portions of the collecting duct near the renal pyramids. Medullary nephrocalcinosis may be marked. In general, this does not occur in infancy; it occurs in adolescence and is associated with frequent urinary tract infections. The dilation of the collecting ducts is developmental in origin but can impair proton secretion by distal tubule sites.[2-6]

A number of conditions that result in renal interstitial damage can be associated with distal RTA, and these are listed in Box 10-3. All of these chronic conditions damage or destroy cells that are important in hydrogen ion secretion and acidification of the urine.

Box 10-3. Distal Renal Tubular Acidosis (Type I)
Primary
   Sporadic
   Hereditary
Secondary
   Interstitial nephritis
   Obstructive uropathy
   Vesicoureteral reflux
   Pyelonephritis
   Transplant rejection
   Sickle cell nephropathy
   Ehlers-Danlos syndrome
   Lupus nephritis
   Nephrocalcinosis
   Medullary sponge kidney
   Hepatic cirrhosis
Toxins/medications
   Amphotericin B, lithium, toluene (glue sniffing), cisplatin

---

ತ Pearl

Patients with type I distal RTA have hyperchloremic non–anion gap metabolic acidosis and growth failure.

The therapeutic approach to type I RTA is the provision of sodium bicarbonate at 1 to 4 mEq/kg/d given in divided doses. If a patient adheres to the prescribed dosage, the biochemical features are reversed and bone disease improves. Provision of adequate sodium bicarbonate will reverse hypokalemia and hypercalciuria as well.

Type IV or Hyperkalemic Renal Tubular Acidosis

Because of sodium bicarbonate wasting, the kidneys work to conserve sodium by increasing apparent sodium-potassium exchange, resulting in increased urinary potassium excretion and hypokalemia. However, a number of patients with RTA have associated hyperkalemia. This is referred to as *type IV RTA*[1-6] (Box 10-4).

The fundamental pathogenic mechanism is that the action of aldosterone on the renal tubule to secrete hydrogen ions and to enhance potassium secretion is impaired, either as a result of an absence of aldosterone or of its hormonal action. Hence, the tubule does not secrete hydrogen ions and potassium. This can result from Addison disease or congenital adrenal

Box 10-4. Hyperkalemic Renal Tubular Acidosis (Type IV)
Primary
   Sporadic
   Hereditary
Secondary
   Hypoaldosteronism
      Addison disease
      Congenital adrenal hyperplasia
   Pseudohypoaldosteronism (type I or II)
   Obstructive uropathy
   Pyelonephritis
   Interstitial nephritis
   Diabetes mellitus
   Sickle cell nephropathy
   Trimethoprim-sulfamethoxazole
   Angiotensin-converting enzyme inhibitors
   Cyclosporine

hyperplasia (which reduces aldosterone levels) or, alternately, to unresponsiveness of the renal cell to aldosterone. The tubule is often unresponsive after an acute episode of pyelonephritis, with acute urinary obstruction or with chronic obstructive uropathy. Systemic lupus erythematosus and diabetes mellitus may also be associated with mild to moderate renal insufficiency. In patients with tubular unresponsiveness to aldosterone, potassium levels and aldosterone levels are elevated in plasma, which by definition is type IV RTA.

A hereditary condition known as *pseudohypoaldosteronism (type I)* occurs when mutations of the sodium channel (ENaC) permit sodium wasting with dehydration and volume depletion; electrolyte levels indicate impressive hyponatremia, hyperkalemia, and acidosis. Growth failure is prevalent because it begins during infancy. Less severe pseudohypoaldosteronism occurs with mutations on the mineralocorticoid receptor. Another variant, termed *pseudohypoaldosteronism (type II)* or Gordon disease, develops in older children and is autosomal dominant in inheritance.[1,4-6]

As mentioned in Chapter 12 and Appendix I, the anion gap is measured by adding the serum sodium and serum potassium and subtracting from the total the serum chloride and serum bicarbonate:

$$(Na^+ + K^+) - (Cl^- + HCO_3^-)$$

If the anion gap is 12 or less, this is a non–anion gap acidosis. If the number exceeds 18, then a lactic or other metabolic acidosis (usually from diabetes or an inborn error of metabolism) is pertinent. In patients with a non–anion gap acidosis, the bicarbonate wasting from anion losses within the gut as a result of acute or chronic diarrhea may be the culprit. These children may need reevaluation after diarrhea has abated. If the non–anion gap acidosis persists, then the 3 major distinctions in typing RTA are (1) a urine pH greater than 5.5 despite acidosis (serum bicarbonate <18 mEq/L) in proximal RTA (type II); (2) hypokalemia and a urine pH greater than 5.5 in distal RTA (type I); (3) hyperkalemia and a urine pH greater than 5.5 in type IV RTA.[6,7]

Appendix III contains many formulas used in defining the various types of RTA. The therapy for type IV RTA is similar to that for type I, using bicarbonate doses between 1 and 4 mEq/kg/24 hours. Patients with hereditary pseudohypoaldosteronism may require sodium chloride supplementation. Some patients with this rare condition will have marked reduction in their hyponatremia in the second or third year of life. Such patients are those with mineralocorticoid receptor mutations.

Bartter Syndrome

Bartter syndrome is rare, and it consists of a group of disorders characterized by hypokalemic metabolic alkalosis, often with hypercalciuria. In very young children, an antenatal form of Bartter syndrome may be found, called *hyperprostaglandin E syndrome*. Patients often show marked salt wasting and have a history of polyhydramnios.[4–6]

A milder variant is found in older children, who may demonstrate recurrent episodes of dehydration and failure to thrive, and have distinct facial features. At times antenatal Bartter syndrome may also show sensioneural deafness and chronic renal failure. The inheritance pattern is usually autosomal recessive.[2–4]

From a biochemical standpoint, findings in children with Bartter syndrome resemble the clinical findings following furosemide administration (or other loop of Henle active diuretics) with urinary losses of chloride, sodium, and potassium. Volume depletion following these urinary ion losses leads to stimulation of the renin-angiotensin-aldosterone axis. Further urinary potassium excretion follows aldosterone action with enhanced proton secretion as well, which accentuates metabolic alkalosis. At least 3 separate ion channels are mutated in various forms of Bartter syndrome: Variant forms of either the NaK_2Cl transporter ($NKCC_2$) or the luminal potassium channel (ROMK) are evident in antenatal Bartter syndrome, and an effect on the basolateral membrane chloride channel protein a (CLCKA) or b (CLCKB) is found in classic Bartter syndrome.

The antenatal variant is often found in the offspring of consanguineous unions. With the classic form, infants have a history of polyhydramnios and exhibit large batlike ears, a triangular face, and a drooping mouth. Hypercalciuria accompanies increased urinary losses of sodium, potassium, and chloride. Because of volume depletion, serum renin, aldosterone, and prostaglandin E are also elevated. Nevertheless, because of volume depletion, hypertension is rare.[1,4,6]

Among the other features of Bartter syndrome are profound hypokalemia, often below 2 mEq/L; massive chloride losses in the urine; and, whenever renal tissue is available to examine, juxtaglomerular hyperplasia.

A nonhereditary condition, or pseudo-Bartter syndrome, can be found in individuals who abuse laxatives or diuretics or those who have bulimia. This form is not usually found in children; it is common in young adult women.[3–6] In distinction to elevated urinary chloride values in hereditary Bartter syndrome, the urine chloride concentration is low in pseudo-Bartter syndrome.

Treatment of Bartter syndrome is focused on correction of volume defects, hypokalemia, and improved nutrition. Some patients may also require indomethacin treatment, especially those with the antenatal variant. Potassium doses are often high, and children often will have cravings for potassium-rich foods, such as potatoes or pickles.

❧ Pearl

Bartter syndrome consists of a group of disorders characterized by hypokalemic metabolic alkalosis, massive urinary chloride losses, and often hypercalciuria.

Gitelman Syndrome

Another Bartter-like condition occurring more commonly in adolescents or young adults is Gitelman syndrome. Its unique features are a hypokalemic metabolic alkalosis with hypocalciuria and hypomagnesemia. Biochemically, the Gitelman syndrome situation can be accomplished in normal subjects with chronic use of thiazide diuretics, which act on the NCCT, located in the distal convoluted tubule. Mutations in the gene for NCCT are found in patients with this autosomal recessive disorder.[3-6]

Muscle cramps are often a presenting sign and are the result of reduced serum magnesium values. Dehydration is not usual. Laboratory values reveal a hypokalemic metabolic alkalosis with marked hypermagnesuria and notable hypocalciuria, the latter being in distinct contrast to Bartter syndrome.

Therapy is directed at replacement of potassium and magnesium. In contrast to Bartter syndrome, sodium supplements and indomethacin therapy are almost never required.[3-6]

Liddle Disease

Liddle disease is an autosomal dominant disorder characterized by hypertension and hypokalemic metabolic alkalosis. It is associated with a gain-of-function mutation of the epithelial sodium channel in the collecting duct. Because of enhanced distal overaccumulation of sodium, these patients manifest hypokalemia, suppressed aldosterone secretion, and vascular volume overload.

Ironically, a loss-of-function mutation in this same collecting duct sodium channel causes a disorder discussed previously—pseudohypoaldosteronism—with features of hyperkalemia and marked urinary sodium wasting. A further ironic result of these mutations in the collecting duct sodium channel is that with gain of function, the "clinical" features of excess aldosterone prevail, whereas, in reality, aldosterone values are diminished. Conversely, with a loss-of-function mutation, the features of reduced aldosterone secretion are apparent, but aldosterone values are high. These differences demonstrate that mutations at a site of aldosterone action can mimic the findings of aldosterone excess or deficiency. Effective therapy of Liddle syndrome includes thiazide diuretics.[3-6]

Disorders of Water Transport

An uncommon inherited disorder of water transport is nephrogenic DI. Nephrogenic DI is most commonly X-linked and occurs in males, but an autosomal recessive form has also been described. Nephrogenic DI is a condition in which patients have massive polyuria, dilute urine, resistance to the action of ADH action, and hypernatremia, especially before thirst habits are formed. Nonhereditary variants occur with damage to the collecting duct such as occur with cystic disorders, obstructive uropathy, nephrocalcinosis, or interstitial nephritis. In nonoliguric renal failure, the collecting duct may be unresponsive to ADH. Several toxins, including lithium and amphotericin B, can result in nephrogenic DI, as does profound hypokalemia.

Urine concentration is dependent on an intact concentration gradient in the renal medulla and the ability to open or close water channels in the collecting tubule. Antidiuretic hormone acts by binding to the vasopressin receptor, termed *V2* (AVPR2), on the basolateral membrane of the collecting tubule. With ADH vasopressin receptor binding, a cyclic adenosine monophosphate signaling pathway is activated, and water channels (aquaporin 2) are inserted in the apical membrane of the collecting tubule, which allows water movement. The X-linked form of nephrogenic DI relates to mutation of the V2 receptor and the autosomal recessive form to mutations in aquaporin 2.[4-6]

Hereditary nephrogenic DI usually develops in infants who have bouts of severe dehydration, hypernatremia, ongoing polyuria, and fever. These infants also have constipation and failure to thrive. The need for drinking volumes of water tends to suppress the appetite of the child. Because the V2 receptor defect is far more common (the X-linked form), most patients are males. Because of bouts of hypernatremic dehydration, patients frequently have behavioral issues and hyperactivity.[4-6] Failure of the kidney to respond to ADH is the pathogenic mechanism. The classic test used in diagnosing DI is the water deprivation test. This test should be performed in a hospital setting where the patient's vital signs can be closely monitored and should be performed with caution in small infants because water deprivation in these individuals may lead to circulatory collapse. The procedure may be performed as follows:

1. In the morning, empty bladder and weigh patient. Patient should take nothing by mouth.
2. Obtain hourly weight measurements, urine volume, sg and osmolality, and plasma sodium and osmolality. Stop this part of the test if body weight decreases by more than 3%, plasma Na^+ >150 mEq/L, or Posm greater than 300 mOsm/kg water. At the completion of the aforementioned steps
   a. Collect blood for ADH level.
   b. Give 1 g/m² aqueous vasopressin intramuscularly or 10 g desmopressin (DDAVP, Sanofi-Aventis, Bridgewater, NJ) intranasally.
   c. Obtain 2 consecutive 30-minute specimens for urine sg and osmolality and Posm.

In normal individuals, water deprivation leads to progressive decrease in urine flow and increased Uosm up to 500 to 1,400 (700–800 in newborns) mOsm/kg water, whereas Posm remains normal. Following dehydration, Uosm remains less than Posm in complete central and nephrogenic DI (Uosm <200 mOsm/kg water), whereas Uosm increases in partial central DI (Uosm greater than Posm). Patients with psychogenic polydipsia will always have Uosm greater than Posm.

Antidiuretic hormone administration in normal individuals produces no further increase in urine sg and osmolality (≤5% change) or decrease in urine volume. In a child with complete central DI, Uosm increases 50% or less and serum osmolality gradually increases. Patients with nephrogenic DI do not respond to ADH, and there is no change in Uosm or volume or Posm. In patients with nephrogenic DI, a 10-fold dose of ADH should be given to differentiate between the partial and complete forms. When the water deprivation test is inconclusive, a hypertonic saline infusion test may distinguish between central DI, nephrogenic DI, and primary polydipsia. Five percent saline is given intravenously for 2 hours at the rate of 0.04 to 0.05 mL/kg/min. Plasma samples for osmolality and ADH assays are collected at 30-minute intervals, and results are plotted on a nomogram. In patients with central DI, plasma ADH is subnormal relative to Posm and volume, whereas it is normal in patients with primary polydipsia and nephrogenic DI.

The mainstays of therapy are the use of adequate fluid (permitting a child free access to water), the use of a low-sodium and low-solute diet, and the use of medications to reduce urine output. Thiazide diuretics, in combination with amiloride, reduce urinary water losses. This is valuable because water reabsorption in the proximal tubule and intermedullary collecting duct is not dependent on ADH. Nonsteroidal anti-inflammatory drugs can be employed if the aforementioned measures do not work.

ᕒ Pearl

Nephrogenic DI is characterized by massive polyuria, very dilute urine, resistance to ADH action, and hypernatremia.

References

1. Guay-Woodford LM, Sedor JR. Syllabus: genetic diseases of the kidney. *NephSAP.* 2007;6(1):1–53

2. Chesney RW. Noncystic hereditary diseases of the kidney. In: Brady HR, Wilcox CS, eds. *Therapy in Nephrology and Hypertension.* London, UK: Saunders; 2003:503–511

3. McKusick-Nathans Institute for Genetic Medicine, Johns Hopkins University (Baltimore, MD) and National Center for Biotechnology Information, National Library of Medicine (Bethesda, MD). Online Mendelian Inheritance in Man (OMIM). http://www.ncbi.nlm.nih.gov/omim/. Accessed February 9, 2007

4. Kaplan BS. Disorders of renal tubular function. In: Kaplan BS, Meyers KEC, eds. *Pediatric Nephrology and Urology: The Requisites in Pediatrics.* Philadelphia, PA: Elsevier Mosby; 2004:231–238

5. Chesney RW. Specific renal tubular disorders. In: Goldman L, Ausiello D, eds. *Cecil Textbook of Medicine.* 22nd ed. Philadelphia, PA: Saunders; 2004:745–750

6. Jones DP, Chesney RW. Tubular function. In: Avner ED, Harmon WE, Niaudet P, eds. *Pediatric Nephrology.* 5th ed. Baltimore, MD: Lippincott, Williams & Wilkins; 2004:45

7. Section VI: Tubular disease. In: Avner ED, Harmon WE, Niaudet P, eds. *Pediatric Nephrology.* 5th ed. Baltimore, MD: Lippincott, Williams & Wilkins; 2004:665–817

Chapter 11

■ Water and Electrolyte Disorders

Aaron Friedman

Introduction

Body fluids (water and the electrolytes or solutes suspended within it) are tightly regulated in human and all mammalian tissue. A newborn is nearly 75% water by weight, but within the first year of life, this percentage reaches adult levels of approximately 60%. Intracellular fluid makes up two-thirds of the total body fluid, and one-third is in the extracellular space (interstitial and plasma fluid). The constituent electrolyte composition of each space is quite different and plays an important homeostatic and functional role in each fluid space. The predominant cation in intracellular fluid is potassium, whereas the predominant cation in extracellular fluid is sodium. There is little or no protein in interstitial fluid but considerable amounts in intracellular fluid and plasma. Chloride and bicarbonate are the predominant extracellular anions, but this is not so in the intracellular space, where protein, phosphate, sulfates, and smaller concentrations of bicarbonate predominate[1] (Figure 11-1).

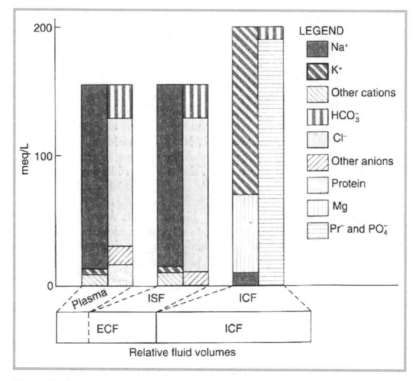

Figure 11-1.

Composition of body fluids. ECF indicates extracellular fluid; ICF, intracellular fluid; ISF, interstitial fluid. (Reprinted with permission from Ford DM. Fluid, electrolyte, and acid-base disorders and therapy. In: Hay WW, Levin MJ, Sondheimer JM, Deterding RR, eds. *Current Diagnosis and Treatment in Pediatrics.* 18th ed. New York, NY: Lange and McGraw–Hill; 2004:1274–1282.)

Because cell function and metabolism require the careful regulation of water and solute movement through all fluid spaces, understanding body fluid physiology and disorders of body fluid physiology are important to successfully managing patients.

Fluid and Electrolyte Therapy

Water movement across most cell membranes is not restricted. Exceptions to this include cells in the loop of Henle and the collecting duct of the kidneys, where restricted and more tightly regulated water movement is needed. Water moves across permeable cell membranes influenced by the osmolality of fluid inside and outside the cell. Osmolality is determined by the solute concentrations within the intracellular and extracellular compartments. Thus molecules—such as sodium and chloride or glucose (in hyperglycemia settings)—are restricted to the extracellular space and exert an osmotic force on water. Counterbalancing these, and restricted largely to the intracellular space, are cations and anions such as potassium, magnesium, and various proteins. The effective osmolality (or tonicity) of extracellular fluid can be estimated using the following formula:

$$\text{mOsm (kg H}_2\text{O)} = [2\,(\text{Na}^+\,\text{mEq/L})] + [\text{glucose (mg/dL)}/18] + [\text{urea (mg/dL)}/2.8]$$

Because urea is permeable across cell membranes, it does not influence water movement unless it is infused quickly. Also glucose in the normal serum concentrations adds little more than 5 mOsm to extracellular osmolality, making sodium and anions, such as chloride and bicarbonate, effectors of extracellular osmolality in most clinical situations. Although these small ions influence osmolality and water movement between the intracellular and extracellular fluid spaces, the movement of fluid within the extracellular space, between plasma and interstitial fluid, is influenced by oncotic forces generated by macromolecules, such as albumin, and hydrostatic forces generated by arteriolar, venous, and interstitial pressures.

Other important factors that influence ion and water balance include the following:

1. Thirst and the control of water intake. Patients who cannot perceive thirst as a result of injury in centers in the brain can develop serious problems with fluid balance.

2. Antidiuretic hormone. This is the hormone that increases water reabsorption in the distal tubule and collecting duct of the kidney. Without ADH, the urine produced is dilute. The stimuli for ADH release from the hypothalamus are an increased serum osmolality (osmotic release of ADH) and decreased effective plasma volume or other stimuli, such as pain, medications, anesthetic agents, or nausea (nonosmotic release of ADH). Antidiuretic hormone is responsible for helping create the internal environment in the kidneys for producing concentrated urine and for signaling the kidneys to open water channels in the distal tubule, allowing water to be reabsorbed. Water losses also occur through skin, such as losses because of sweating or breakdown of the normal, intact

skin barrier (such as in a burn) and water losses through breathing. These 2 factors highlight a fundamental point in the understanding of water metabolism. The regulation of water metabolism is a balance between intake and output.

3. Aldosterone. This increases renal reabsorption of sodium and increases excretion of potassium. Aldosterone is stimulated in states of extracellular volume depletion.

4. Natriuretic peptides (ANP, BNP). Atrial natriuretic peptide may play a role in the excretion of sodium and some water in situations of extracellular and plasma volume excess.

What do we do when children cannot ingest water? How do we maintain water balance? This question was addressed in the 1950s, and an approach was published in 1957 to help physicians maintain water in patients and, to some extent, electrolyte balance. A method called *maintenance fluid therapy* was developed to provide fluid, calories, and some electrolytes to hospitalized patients for anticipated 24-hour needs.[2] The maintenance fluid therapy equation ties water requirements to caloric needs and suggests electrolyte replacement based on average daily losses (Table 11-1). Maintenance fluid therapy is designed to provide anticipated physiologic losses over the next 24 hours. It is not a fluid prescription for replacement of abnormal losses, such as vomiting or diarrhea. It is not a fluid prescription for the restoration of body fluids in the dehydrated patient. Finally, maintenance fluid therapy presumes euvolemia and no other signals for the nonosmotic release of ADH. Therefore, a patient with concentrated urine should have the volume of maintenance fluid reduced to half the suggested volume and

Table 11-1. Maintenance Fluid Calculation		
Body Weight (kg)	**mL of water/kg/24 hours**	**mL of water/kg/h**
3–10	100	4
11–20	1,000 + 50 mL/kg for each kg >10 and ≤20	40 + 2 mL/kg for each kg >10 and ≤20
>20	1,500 + 20 mL/kg for each kg >20	60 + 1 mL/kg for each kg >20
or		
H$_2$O requirement = 1,500 mL/m² body surface area/24 hours Electrolytes: Na$^+$ = 2–3 mEq/100 mL of water; K$^+$ = 2 mEq/100 mL of water		

Abbreviations: Na$^+$, sodium; K$^+$, potassium.

should undergo treatment to restore extracellular fluid volume if appropriate. Another approach to maintenance fluid therapy has recently been suggested.[3] This approach recommends volumes identical to the Holliday-Segar approach, but it uses isotonic saline as the solution. It is posited that this approach will prevent severe hyponatremia and brain injury in those patients for whom nonosmotic ADH release would result in potentially rapid falls in serum sodium when a hypotonic solution is administered intravenously. This approach has not been tested in many patients for whom intravenous maintenance fluid therapy might be used.

೫ Pearl

Factors that influence ion and water balance include thirst, ADH, aldosterone, and natriuretic peptides. Maintenance fluid therapy is designed to provide anticipated physiologic losses over the next 24 hours.

Dehydration

Dehydration is a broad term meaning depletion of body fluids. Although its literal meaning is "loss of water," it has come to mean "loss of body fluids" and is generally applied to conditions in which extracellular volume is the predominant site of loss (eg, diarrheal dehydration). Dehydration is common in children and is the result of infectious diseases leading to gastroenteritis with resultant abnormal fluid losses because of vomiting, diarrhea, fever, and upper respiratory infections with fever and increased respiratory rate. In both examples, a contributor to dehydration is the inability to keep up with losses resulting from anorexia and decreased intake. Other causes of dehydration include diabetes mellitus, DI, or renal disease with loss of concentrating ability. In diabetes mellitus, an intercurrent illness such as gastroenteritis or urinary tract infection can result in hyperglycemia with resultant osmotic diuresis and loss of water and electrolytes in the urine. Diabetes insipidus, whether central (little or no ADH release from the hypothalamus) or nephrogenic (inability of the kidney to respond to ADH) results in large or even massive losses of water in urine. In DI, a patient's ability to keep up with the losses by primarily ingesting water determines whether the patient develops dehydration. Another at-risk group for dehydration is breastfed newborns. Early on a mother's volume of breast milk may not be sufficient to keep up with a newborn's needs, especially during hot weather.

The approach to dehydration depends on determining the degree of dehydration and then developing a plan for restoration of body fluids. When body weight is accurately known just prior to the recent illness, the amount of weight loss is a good indicator of the amount of dehydration. A 20-kg child who currently weighs 18 kg (2 kg loss) is 10% dehydrated. Unfortunately, precise weight measurements often are not available, and as a result, other, less precise indicators of dehydration are used (Table 11-2). These indicators include moistness of mucous membranes, skin color and turgor, production of tears, the presence of a depressed fontanelle (in infants), hemodynamic signs (pulse rate, blood pressure, capillary refill), and urine output and urine concentration. Hemodynamic changes, especially a very rapid pulse, significant slowing of the capillary refill time, and a drop in blood pressure or orthostatic hypotension, occur later in children but are signs of severe extracellular volume depletion. This requires immediate aggressive treatment.

The treatment for severe extracellular volume depletion with evidence of hemodynamic insufficiency is intravenous fluids. Isotonic saline or LR solutions are the best choices. In rare instances, a colloid solution (5% albumin in isotonic saline) may be useful. Dehydration resulting in hemodynamic

Table 11-2. Clinical Signs of Dehydration			
Clinical Signs	**Degree of Dehydration**		
	Mild	**Moderate**	**Severe**
Decrease in body weight	3%–5%	6%–10%	11%–15%
Skin turgor	N	Decreased	Very decreased
Skin color	N	Pale	Very pale, mottled
Mucous membrane	Dry	Dry	Mottled, parched
Tears	Decreased	Decreased	Absent
Pulse	N	Increased	Very increased
Capillary refill	2–3 sec	3–4 sec	>4 sec
Blood pressure	N	N or slight decrease	Decreased
Urine output	Slightly decreased	Decreased	Very decreased or anuria
Urine specific gravity	>1.020	<1.020	Anuria
Urine Na+	<20 mEq/L	<20 mEq/L	Anuria

Abbreviations: N, normal; Na+, sodium.

changes usually does not develop until a patient is 7% dehydrated or more. Seven percent means body fluids losses of 70 mL/kg or more in body weight. With hemodynamic changes, most physicians recommend intravenous fluid as described previously, with a starting amount of 20 mL/kg infused over 30 minutes to 1 hour. Given that 20 mL/kg is less than half of the estimated loss, it is likely that a second bolus of 20 mL/kg of isotonic saline or LR will be needed before measurable improvement in hemodynamic indicators is appreciated. It is important to recognize that rapid restoration of extracellular fluids has salutary effects above and beyond a decrease in heart rate and improved peripheral capillary filing. Restoration of extracellular fluid volume will also improve organ perfusion of the gastrointestinal tract and the kidney.[4] Improved gastrointestinal tract perfusion will permit a more rapid switch to the oral route for continuing to restore body fluids and keeping up with losses or the provision of maintenance fluids. Once at least half the estimated loss is replenished, further restoration therapy can be provided more slowly. The traditional approach to restoration therapy was to provide half the loss in the first 8 hours and the other half over the next 16 hours. Recently, more rapid restoration with completion of the restoration in 8 to 12 hours has been advocated.[4]

Planning fluid therapy for dehydrated patients requires attention to ongoing losses and maintenance fluid needs along with restoration therapy from previous losses. The composition of fluids that commonly makes up losses is listed in Table 11-3. When using intravenous replacement, a solution that delivers fluids at a rate and with an electrolyte composition similar to that which is lost is desirable. Finally, one should provide maintenance fluid at the recommended amounts if urine volume is above 1 to 2 mL/kg/h and urine concentration is 300 mOsm/kg H_2O or less (sg <1.012). If Uosm and/or urine sg is high or urine volume is low, then give only half the calculated maintenance fluid volume and replace urine volume and urine electro-

Table 11-3. Electrolyte Composition of Body Fluids			
	Na⁺ (mEq/L)	K⁺ (mEq/L)	HCO₃⁻ (mEq/L)
Diarrhea	50–90	10–50	40
Gastric	10–40	5–20	0
Small intestine	50–140	5–15	40

Abbreviations: K⁺, potassium; Na⁺, sodium; HCO₃⁻, bicarbonate.

lytes milliliter for milliliter until euvolemia is restored. Other conditions that increase the volume of maintenance fluids needed include fever (increase by 10%–12% per degrees Centigrade over 38), hyperventilation (10%–50% increase depending on respiratory rate), and percent humidity of inspired air. A patient on a ventilator is inspiring 100% humidified air and needs no maintenance fluid to replace losses of water as a result of breathing.

For mild and even moderate dehydration, oral restoration may be used and is used extensively in parts of the world. Clear liquids or those with high sugar content are not as effective as commercially available solutions that adhere more closely to World Health Organization recommendations for electrolytes and glucose. Glucose or similar sugars should not exceed 2% to 2.5%. Sodium concentrations vary from 40 to 90 mEq/L, with the most readily available commercial products in the United States providing 40 to 45 mEq/L of sodium. The potassium concentration is approximately 30 mEq/L of the citrate or bicarbonate salt. Frequent, small aliquots (5–15 mL) should be given so as to provide 40 to 50 mL/kg over 4 to 6 hours for mild dehydration and 70 to 100 mL/kg over 6 to 8 hours for moderate dehydration. For severe dehydration—in the comatose patient, in the patient with an acute surgical abdomen, or in the patient with profound hyponatremia (Na^+ <120 mEq/L) or hypernatremia (Na^+ >160 mEq/L)—intravenous restoration should be given first with consideration of switching to oral restoration, if appropriate, to complete the restoration regimen.

> ## ᴥ Pearl
>
> Fluid therapy for dehydrated patients should include ongoing losses, maintenance fluids, and previous losses, delivering intravenous fluids with the rate and composition of the fluids lost.

Hyponatremia

Serum sodium below 135 mEq/L is generally considered hyponatremia. Although often associated with volume depletion, hyponatremia can, in fact, occur without volume depletion or with volume excess (Table 11-4). The most common presentation of hyponatremia is associated with gastroenteritis and is hyponatremia with volume depletion. The approach is to estimate fluid loss and begin (as noted previously) with extracellular volume restoration (isotonic saline or LR). The reason that hyponatremia occurs in the

Table 11-4. Etiology of Hyponatremia		
Volume Depletion	**Euvolemia**	**Volume Expansion**
• Dehydration • Cystic fibrosis • Renal insufficiency (obstructive uropathy) • Cerebral salt wasting • Hyperglycemia • Decreased sodium intake (rare)	• Vasopressin excess (SIADH) • Fictitious hyponatremia (hyperlipidemia)	• Vasopressin excess (SIADH) • Cirrhosis • Nephrotic syndrome • Heart failure

Abbreviation: SIADH, syndrome of inappropriate antidiuretic hormone release.

face of volume losses, such as gastroenteritis, is 2-fold. Volume losses include sodium, chloride, and bicarbonate (diarrhea). However, the fluid ingested during an episode of gastroenteritis often is hypotonic (clear liquids). Nausea, vomiting, and plasma volume depletion all contribute to the nonosmotic release of ADH. This results in the avid reabsorption of water at the same time that both sodium and water are lost because of gastroenteritis. In combination, extracellular sodium concentrations fall in situations of volume depletion. When the serum sodium is below 130 mEq/L and especially below 125 mEq/L, one might need to add additional sodium to correct the deficit. The generally accepted equation to determine the amount of sodium is as follows:

$$Na^+ \text{ deficit} = [Na^+ \text{ decreased} - Na^+ \text{ observed}] \times \text{body weight (kg)} \times 0.6$$

When treating a patient with hyponatremia, correct the serum sodium to 135 mEq/L, which is the lower limit of the normal range. This approach will reduce the risk of raising the serum sodium too rapidly. Further, because the first course of therapy is to replace extracellular volume and the therapy is isotonic saline or LR, recheck the serum sodium after providing at least half of the extracellular restoration fluid to see how much sodium should be replaced. If the serum sodium is rising, continuing extracellular fluid restoration, holding any maintenance therapy until restoration is nearly complete and waiting to see if additional sodium added to maintenance therapy is needed is prudent.

A far more complicated situation is the rare instance of cerebral salt wasting. It is thought that this situation results from natriuretic peptides (ANP or BNP) elaborated with brain injury, which result in high urine sodium outputs. In this condition, salt and perhaps water replacement are needed because extracellular volume depletion is associated with the condition.

Hyponatremia associated with euvolemia or hypervolemia can occur in edema states—nephrotic syndrome, cirrhosis, and congestive heart failure. These are conditions with lower urine volumes, low urine sodium, and high Uosm. The treatment is sodium and some water restriction. Syndrome of inappropriate release of ADH, therefore vasopressin excess, may be truly inappropriate as in situations of brain injury, malignancy, elaboration of an ADH-like substance or anesthesia, and so on. Syndrome of inappropriate release of ADH is often used to describe the nonosmotic release of ADH such as that which can occur with extracellular volume depletion, nausea and vomiting, or lung disease with decreased filling of the left atrium. Urine findings include lower urine volumes, high urinary sodium (50–100 mEq/L or higher), and concentrated urine. The treatment is water restriction. Finally, patients with water intoxication—high fluid intake—may have hyponatremia, but they are not volume depleted and they produce large volumes of dilute urine. The treatment is water intake reduction.

Severe hyponatremia (generally serum Na^+ <120 mEq/L or rapid falls in serum Na^+) can be associated with central nervous system symptoms, such as lethargy, confusion, obtundation, coma, and brain herniation. When symptoms are noted, the approach is to (1) increase the serum to above 120 to 125 mEq/L and (2) increase serum sodium until alleviation of symptoms and improved mental status or the serum sodium has been raised by 15 mEq in 24 hours. The commonly used solution is 3% NaCl (513 mEq/L). Approximately 1 mL/kg of 3% NaCl will increase the serum sodium by 1 mEq/L. As noted previously, safe correction of severe hyponatremia (serum Na^+ increase of 15 mEq/L/24 hours) is desired.

᠊᠊᠊ Pearl

When treating a patient with hyponatremia, serum sodium should be corrected to 135 mEq/L.

Hypernatremia

Hypernatremia is less common than hyponatremia and results from fluid loss without adequate replacement of water. This can occur with diarrhea and vomiting but may also be the result of poor fluid intake or excessive water loss as may be seen with DI. Only rarely is hypernatremia the result of too much sodium chloride or sodium bicarbonate. The approach to hypernatremia is crucial because too rapid a correction can result in cerebral edema with central nervous system morbidities or death. Hypernatremic dehydration generally occurs over a number of days. During that time, water shifts from the intracellular to extracellular space. In addition, osmolytes are produced intracellularly, including amino acids such as taurine. When water is provided, these osmolytes must be metabolized or transported out of the intracellular space, which is a slow process. Too rapid a replacement of water (serum Na^+ fall of >15–20 mEq/L/24 hours; approximately 1 mEq/L/h) or fall in serum osmolality of >40 mOsm/24 hours (>2 mOsm/h) can lead to cerebral edema. The approach should be as follows:

1. Any patient with dehydration and a serum sodium greater than 150 mEq/L should be considered as having hypernatremic dehydration. The patient should also be considered at least 10% dehydrated. Patients with hypernatremia have the appearance of being clinically less dehydrated than they are.

2. Provide isotonic saline or LR to restore at least 50 mL/kg over the first 4 hours.

3. Check serum sodium (and/or serum osmolality) every 2 hours to be sure to not decrease the serum sodium/osmolality too rapidly.

4. After the replacement of at least 50 mL/kg, recheck the serum sodium/ osmolality and consider this the starting point for any additional hypotonic solution, which might be used to further decrease the serum sodium/osmolality.

5. To gradually decrease the serum sodium/osmolality, calculate the water deficit: 4 mL/kg of water for every milliequivalent of sodium above 145 mEq.

6. Metabolic acidosis and hyperglycemia may accompany hypernatremic dehydration. Hyperglycemia improves with fluid restoration, especially with isotonic saline or LR. If giving hypotonic solution with hyperglycemia, consider 2.5% glucose with electrolytes. Metabolic acidosis may improve with volume restoration. If sodium bicarbonate is being considered, provide it slowly.

7. If DI is the cause of the hypernatremic dehydration, a more rapid restoration of extracellular fluid volume is needed and the institution of hypotonic fluids should begin sooner.

?♥ Pearl

Too rapid correction of hypernatremic dehydration can lead to cerebral edema.

Patients with hypernatremia dehydration generally are thirsty. Careful observation and counting of oral fluids must be performed and even oral fluid restriction maintained to avoid too rapid a fall in serum sodium/osmolality.

Disorders of Potassium

Potassium is the major intracellular cation. Intracellular potassium concentrations are maintained by Na^+-K^+-ATPase (sodium potassium adenosine triphosphatase), but the concentration can be altered by decreased extracellular pH leading to a shift of potassium out of cells into the extracellular fluid and an increase in extracellular pH, which causes a shift of potassium from the extracellular fluid into cells. A commonly used estimate is that for every 0.1 change in pH there is a concomitant 0.7 mEq change in extracellular potassium. Because the cell membrane potential is dependent on the ratio of intracellular to extracellular potassium shifts, depletion or rapid extracellular changes can affect muscle (especially cardiac) or renal function. Potassium is filtered by the glomerulus, reabsorbed by the proximal tubule, and excreted by the distal tubule. Distal tubule secretion and total urinary potassium are influenced by aldosterone. Except for situations of abnormal loss, such as prolonged diarrhea, potassium balance is the result of dietary intake and renal excretion.

Hypokalemia

Table 11-5 describes the cause of low extracellular potassium (hypokalemia). Once hypokalemia develops, it can be assumed that the intracellular pool of potassium is quite low and the total body potassium (overwhelmingly in the intracellular space) is depleted. In most instances of gastrointestinal disease associated with hypokalemia, the potassium loss from the gut is less than the loss in the urine as a result of chronic volume depletion. Clinically, hypokalemia will eventually result in weakness or paresis; decreased peristal-

Table 11-5. Hypokalemia (Serum Potassium <3.5 meq/L)	
Elevated Urinary Potassium	**Low Urinary Potassium**
Elevated blood pressure	Anorexia nervosa or bulimia
Renovascular disease	Gastrointestinal losses
Primary hyperaldosteronism	Laxative abuse
Renin excess	
Cushing syndrome	
Normal blood pressure	
Renal tubular acidosis	
Bartter syndrome	
Fanconi syndrome	
Diabetes	
Increased insulin	
Antibiotics	
Metabolic alkalosis	

sis; or even ileus, hyporeflexia, rhabdomyolysis, and arrhythmia. The electro-cardiographic changes associated with hypokalemia are rarely seen in other conditions and include a flattened T-wave, a U-wave, and shortened PR interval. Arrhythmias include premature ventricular contraction, tachycardias, and even ventricular fibrillation. The treatment depends on the severity of the symptoms. If cardiac arrhythmias, obvious U-waves, and profound muscle weakness or respiratory compromise are present, intravenous potassium may be indicated. In some patients (eg, those with anorexia nervosa), phosphate may be low as well and potassium phosphate may be a good choice for admin-istration. Intravenous potassium should be given with cardiac monitoring, and the phosphate salt may cause a decline in serum calcium. Intravenous potassium should be given at a dose no greater than 0.5 mEq/kg/h. If the dosage exceeds a concentration of 40 mEq/L, it can cause peripheral vein irritation and injury. Oral potassium is generally safe, although bitter tasting. Doses of 2 to 3 mEq/kg/d will eventually replete body stores. Weeks of oral therapy may be needed to fully replenish potassium stores.

๑ Pearl

Intravenous potassium should be given at a dose no greater than 0.5 mEq/kg/h.

Hyperkalemia

Hyperkalemia is the result of renal insufficiency or decreased renal potassium excretion, mineralocorticoid insufficiency or unresponsiveness, and the release of intracellular stores as may be seen in crush injury or hypoperfusion. Hyperkalemia can cause muscle weakness or paresis, paresthesia, and cardiac arrhythmias. The classic description of changes in the electrocardiogram include peaked T-wave, widening of the QRS complex (with findings such as bradycardia, atrioventricular or idioventricular rhythms), and ventricular tachycardia or ventricular fibrillation. The severity of cardiac abnormalities is associated with the degree of hyperkalemia, but the status of other electrolytes and the pH of the extracellular fluid will profoundly affect the severity of the cardiac picture. Associated acidosis, hyponatremia, hypocalcemia, or the presence of digoxin will worsen the picture. If the aforementioned electrocardiogram features are present, immediate action is needed. This includes the following:

1. Providing calcium to stabilize cell membranes—intravenous 10% calcium gluconate 0.2 to 0.5 mL/kg over 2 to 10 minutes in a monitored patient.

2. Increasing extracellular pH with intravenous sodium bicarbonate 1 to 2 mEq/kg over 5 minutes to help shift potassium into the intracellular space.

3. In patients who are not diabetic, 0.5 g/kg of intravenous glucose over 1 hour will help shift potassium into cells. Concomitant insulin as a drip may be needed with careful monitoring of glucose.

4. Beta-agonists, such as albuterol, may work to shift potassium into the intracellular space.

Steps 1 through 4 move potassium into the intracellular space or stabilize membranes. These measures are short acting (Table 13-1).

◈ Pearl

Hyperkalemia results from renal or mineralocorticoid insufficiency and release of intracellular potassium (crush injury or hypoperfusion).

To remove potassium from the body, one needs to reestablish renal function. If renal function is reasonable, a loop diuretic such as furosemide at 1 to 2 mg/kg intravenously will increase potassium excretions. Exchange resins (sodium for potassium) such as sodium polystyrene sulfonate orally (0.5 g/kg) or as an enema (1 g/kg) will result in the excretion of potassium through the stool. Finally, dialysis may need to be considered to remove potassium.

References

1. Ford DM. Fluid, electrolyte, and acid-base disorders and therapy. In: Hay WW, Levin MJ, Sondheimer JM, Deterding RR, eds. *Current Diagnosis and Treatment in Pediatrics*. 18th ed. New York, NY: Lange and McGraw-Hill; 2004:1274–1282

2. Holliday MA, Segar WE. The maintenance need for water is parenteral fluid therapy. *Pediatrics*. 1957;19:823–832

3. Moritz ML, Ayers JC. Prevention of hospital acquired hyponatremia: a case for using isotonic saline. *Pediatrics*. 2003;111:227–230

4. Holliday MA. Extracellular fluid and its proteins: dehydration, shock and recovery. *Pediatr Nephrol*. 1999;13:989–995

Chapter 12

Acid-Base Disturbances

Fumio Niimura and Iekuni Ichikawa

Abbreviations

A-aDO$_2$	Alveolar-arterial oxygen gradient
AG	Anion gap
BUN	Blood urea nitrogen
CKD	Chronic kidney disease
HCO$_3^-$	Bicarbonate
FiO$_2$	Fractional inspired oxygen
P$_A$O$_2$	Alveolar oxygen partial pressure
PaCO$_2$	Arterial carbon dioxide partial pressure
PaO$_2$	Arterial oxygen partial pressure
PCO$_2$	Carbon dioxide partial pressure
PiO$_2$	Partial oxygen in inspired air
RTA	Renal tubular acidosis
tCO$_2$	Total carbon dioxide

Introduction

Acidemia is a status with arterial pH less than 7.35, and alkalemia is a status with pH greater than 7.45. Acidosis is defined as a pathophysiologic process that, if unopposed, will lead to acidemia. Likewise, alkalosis is a pathophysiologic process that, if unopposed, will lead to alkalemia. Of note, -*osis* is commonly used to mean -*emia*. The metabolic process includes addition of exogenous acid or alkali, loss of endogenous acid or alkali, overproduction of endogenous acid, and inability of the kidneys to excrete acid properly (ie, primary process affecting the bicarbonate concentration). The respiratory process includes altered excretion of carbon dioxide through the lungs, leading to an excess or deficit of carbonic acid in the body fluid. Compensation is a secondary process to minimize the alteration in blood pH caused by primary acid-base disturbances. Compensation takes place through metabolic or respiratory processes. Compensation brings pH toward, but not to, normal level, which will help determine what is the primary event and what kind of compensation is operating.

Approach to the Diagnosis of Acid-Base Disturbances

The diagnosis consists of recognizing the necessity for the analysis of acid-base status of the patient, taking a clinical history, performing a physical examination, and analyzing the laboratory data.

When to Consider Acid-Base Disturbances

There are many clinical settings that warrant diagnosis of acid-base disorders in pediatric practice. Critically ill patients often have metabolic acidosis. If a patient is intoxicated with some chemicals, such as salicylates or methanol, prompt diagnosis and treatment will lead to a good prognosis. The most common cause of acid-base disorder seen in children is dehydration secondary to diarrhea, which might be associated with metabolic acidosis. Diabetic ketoacidosis is not rare in pediatric practice and is suspected by the history of polydipsia, polyuria, and loss of weight. History of kidney disease and stunted

> **♒ Pearl**
>
> The most common cause of acid-base disorder in children is metabolic acidosis secondary to dehydration.

growth suggests CKD with reduced renal function or RTA. Respiratory distress may be associated with retention of carbon dioxide, hence respiratory acidosis. Hyperventilation may be a primary event causing respiratory alkalosis or a secondary process to represent a respiratory compensation in metabolic acidosis. Vomiting or diuretic use may cause metabolic alkalosis through loss of chloride and hydrogen ion due in part to secondary hyperaldosteronism that develops as a result of dehydration. Analysis for acid-base disturbances should also be performed in children with urolithiasis or electrolyte disturbances, especially hypokalemia or hyperkalemia. Thus when acid-base disorder is found, clinical history-taking and physical examination should include child intoxication, bowel habit, vomiting, polydipsia, polyuria, growth chart, weight gain or loss, blood pressure, peripheral circulation, respiratory distress, hyperventilation, and child abuse.

Blood Gas Data (pH, HCO_3^-, and $PaCO_2$)

The arterial or venous pH and PCO_2 are measured directly by a blood gas analyzer. The plasma HCO_3^- concentration cannot be measured directly. The value of plasma HCO_3^- concentration is calculated from the measured pH and $PaCO_2$ values, being automatically performed by a blood gas analyzer. The tCO_2 is a measure of blood HCO_3^-, dissolved carbon dioxide gas, and carbonic acid combined. Within the clinically relevant range of $PaCO_2$ values, the difference between tCO_2 and HCO_3^- is negligible, so that they are considered interchangeable. The pH and HCO_3^- from venous blood closely correlate with those from arterial blood when extremities are adequately perfused. The pH and PCO_2 of venous samples are approximately 0.05 U lower and 6 mm Hg higher, respectively.[1] Note that the parameters, especially $PaCO_2$ and HCO_3^-, in healthy children somewhat differ according to their age, as shown in Table 12-1.[2,3]

The acid-base map[4] (Figure 12-1), which is applicable to school-aged children, is helpful in promptly analyzing the acid-base status using available blood gas data. The equations listed in Box 12-1 are also useful in determining the adequacy of respiratory and renal (or metabolic) compensatory responses versus concurrent existence of other acid-base disorders.

Table 12-1. Acid-Base Parameters as a Function of Age[a]

Age	pH	PaCO₂ (mm Hg)	HCO₃⁻ (mEq/L)
1 month (term infant)	7.39 ± 0.02	31 ± 1.5	20 ± 0.7
3–24 mos	7.39 ± 0.03	34 ± 4.0	21 ± 2.0
1.5–3.4 mos	7.35 ± 0.05	37 ± 4.0	20 ± 2.5
3.5–5.4 mos	7.39 ± 0.04	38 ± 3.0	22 ± 1.5
5.5–12.4 mos	7.40 ± 0.03	38 ± 3.0	23 ± 1.0
12.5–17.4 mos	7.38 ± 0.03	41 ± 3.0	24 ± 1.0
Adults	7.40 ± 0.02	41 ± 3.5	25 ± 1.0

Abbreviations: PaCO₂, arterial partial pressure of carbon dioxide; HCO₃⁻, bicarbonate.

[a]All values are arterial blood measurements. (Data from Albert MS, Winters RW. Acid-base equilibrium of blood in normal infants. *Pediatrics.* 1966;37:728–732 and Cassels DE, Morse M. Arterial blood gases and acid-base balance in normal children. *J Clin Invest.* 1953;32:824–836.)

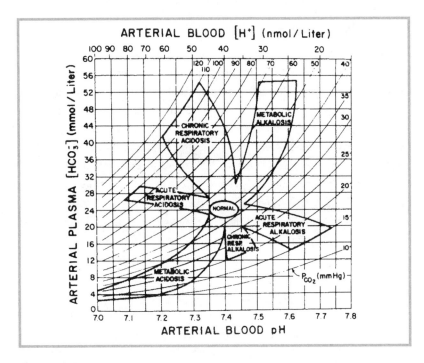

Figure 12-1.

Acid-base map. The shaded areas represent normalcy of compensatory metabolic or respiratory response in the presence of respiratory or metabolic acid-base disorders, respectively. If a patient has acid-base parameters falling outside of the shaded area, the presence of a mixed acid-base disturbance is indicated. (Reprinted with permission from Cogan MG, Rector FC Jr. Acid-base disorders. In: Brenner BM, Rector FC Jr, eds. *The Kidney.* Philadelphia, PA: WB Saunders; 1991:753–804.)

Box 12-1. A Few Rules for Memory to Assess the Adequacy of Compensatory Responses[a]

If respiratory compensation is intact in metabolic acidosis:
$$PaCO_2 = 1.5 \times [HCO_3^-] + 8 \pm 2$$
If respiratory compensation is intact in metabolic alkalosis:
$$\Delta PaCO_2 = 0.4 \text{ to } 0.7 \times \Delta[HCO_3^-]$$
If metabolic compensation is intact in respiratory disturbances:

In acute respiratory acidosis:
$$\Delta[HCO_3^-] = 0.1 \times \Delta PaCO_2$$
In chronic respiratory acidosis:
$$\Delta[HCO_3^-] = 0.35 \times \Delta PaCO_2$$
In acute respiratory alkalosis:
$$\Delta[HCO_3^-] = 0.2 \times \Delta PaCO_2$$
In chronic respiratory alkalosis:
$$\Delta[HCO_3^-] = 0.5 \times \Delta PaCO_2$$

Abbreviations: $PaCO_2$, arterial partial pressure of carbon dioxide; HCO_3^-, bicarbonate.

[a]Compensatory mechanisms bring pH toward, but not to, normal level. Δ indicates the degree of deviation from normal value.

Data That Need to Be Collected Other Than Blood Gas Parameters

In addition to defining the type of acid-base disturbance from the blood gas data, as mentioned previously, it often becomes important to clarify the pathophysiologic mechanism underlying acid-base disturbances. There are many conditions that cause metabolic acidosis, respiratory acidosis, metabolic alkalosis, and respiratory alkalosis, as summarized in Tables 12-2 and 12-3, and Boxes 12-2 and 12-3, respectively. To identify the specific condition or conditions, there are a few tools, such as AG, urinary AG, osmolar gap, A-aDO$_2$, blood chemistry (including BUN, creatinine, glucose, sodium, potassium, calcium, and phosphate), and urinary electrolytes.

ᕫ Pearl

Tools used to identify acid-base problems include AG, osmolar gap, A-aDO$_2$, and blood and urine chemistries.

Anion Gap[5-7]

The AG is calculated as follows:

$$AG = [Na^+ + K^+] - [Cl^- + HCO_3^-]$$

In normal individuals, the AG is approximately 11 mEq/L and is attributed primarily to negatively charged proteins, particularly albumin, because the charges of other ions (potassium, sodium, magnesium, etc, versus phosphate, etc) are mutually offsetting. Anion gap of 14 or more is considered abnormal, and one should seek such unmeasured anions as lactate and ketone. (See also Chapter 4.) Thus elevation in AG in a patient with metabolic acidosis suggests an existence of some of the conditions listed in Table 12-2.[8] However, the AG can increase or decrease without changes in such nonvolatile acids in the plasma. For example, the AG decreases when cations, such as potassium, calcium, mag-

Pearl

Anion gap in normal individuals is approximately 11 mEq/L.

Table 12-2. Causes of Metabolic Acidosis		
Cause of the Disorder	**Anion Gap**	
	Normal	**High**
Loss of Bicarbonate		
Diarrhea	♦	
Pancreatic drainage	♦	
Biliary drainage	♦	
Neonatal ileostomy		♦
Urinary diversion	♦	
Carbonic anhydrase inhibition	♦	
Dilutional acidosis	♦	
Addition of Acid		
Hydrochloric acid, ammonium chloride	♦	
Cationic amino acid	♦	
Lactic acidosis		♦
Diabetic ketoacidosis		♦
Starvation ketoacidosis	♦	♦
Alcoholic ketosis		♦
Organic alcohol ingestion		♦
Paraldehyde ingestion		♦
Salicylate intoxication		♦
Organic acid		♦
Failure of Acid Excretion		
Renal tubular acidosis, type 1, 2, 4	♦	
Renal insufficiency		♦

Table 12-3. Causes of Respiratory Acidosis	
Acute	**Chronic**
Airway obstruction	**Airway obstruction**
Aspiration of foreign body or vomitus	Chronic obstructive lung disease
Laryngospasm	Cystic fibrosis
Generalized bronchospasm	**Bronchopulmonary dysplasia**
Epiglottitis and croup	
Respiratory center depression	**Respiratory center depression**
General anesthesia	Primary alveolar hypoventilation
Drug overdose	Pickwickian syndrome, sleep apnea
Cerebral trauma, tentorial herniation	Brain tumor
Circulatory catastrophes	**Neuromuscular defects**
Cardiac arrest	Poliomyelitis
Severe pulmonary edema, pneumonitis	Multiple sclerosis
Neuromuscular defects	Amyotrophic lateral sclerosis
High cervical cordotomy	Diaphragmatic paralysis
Botulism, tetanus	Myopathic diseases
Hypokalemic myopathy	**Restrictive defects**
Guillain-Barré syndrome	Kyphoscoliosis
Myasthenia gravis crisis	Interstitial fibrosis
Drugs or toxic agents	Decreased diaphragmatic movement—ascites, obesity
Restrictive defects	**Congenital defects**
Pneumothorax	Cyanotic congenital heart disease
Hemothorax	Congenital diaphragmatic hernia
Flail chest	
Mechanical ventilation	

nesium, and lithium (iatrogenic), increase in concentration because sodium decreases to maintain electroneutrality. A decrease in serum albumin, which is negatively charged, is associated with elevation of chloride and causes "innocent" decrease in the AG. Innocent decrease in AG occurs not only as a result of increased cations and hypoalbuminemia, but also as a result of hypergammaglobulinemia (globulins being cations), which obligates an increase in chloride. Hyperalbuminemia, by decreasing both chloride and bicarbonate (again, to maintain electroneutrality), will in turn cause an

Box 12-2. Causes of Metabolic Alkalosis

Exogenous alkali administration (normal BP)
1. Ingestion of large quantities of bicarbonate
2. Excessive acetate in hyperalimentation
3. Exchange transfusions
4. Recovery from organic acidosis
5. Soybean formula diet
6. Milk alkali syndrome; combined therapy with nonresorbable alkali and exchange resins

Chloride-responsive alkalosis (normal or low BP)
1. Gastric losses
2. Diuretic therapy
3. Posthypercapnic state
4. Congenital chloridorrhea
5. Cystic fibrosis

Chloride-resistant alkalosis

High BP
1. Primary aldosteronism
2. Congenital adrenal hyperplasia
3. Cushing syndrome

Normal BP
1. Bartter and Gitelman syndromes

Miscellaneous causes of metabolic alkalosis
1. Penicillin administration and refeeding during fasting

Abbreviation: BP, blood pressure.

innocent rise in AG. Alkalemia alone can increase AG up to 5 mEq/L. This is partly a result of increased lactate concentration resulting from alkali-induced activation of phosphofructokinase in the glycolytic pathway and from increased negative charge of serum proteins.[9]

Serum Potassium

High serum potassium strongly suggests the presence of metabolic acidosis. However, we should be aware of the following limitations in interpreting serum potassium:
1. Patients with severe tissue breakdown may have hyperkalemia regardless of their acid-base status.
2. When metabolic acidosis develops in patients with potassium depletion, serum potassium may be normal or low.

Box 12-3. Causes of Respiratory Alkalosis

Anxiety, hysteria
Fever
Drugs
  Salicylate intoxication
  Nicotine
Central nervous system diseases
  Cerebrovascular accident
  Trauma
  Infection
  Tumor
Intrathoracic processes
  Congestive heart failure
  Pneumonitis
  Asthma
  Pulmonary fibrosis
  Pulmonary emboli
  Foreign body

Hypoxia
  Lowered barometric pressure
  Increased venous admixture
  Marked ventilation-perfusion
    abnormalities
Hepatic insufficiency
Gram-negative sepsis
Pregnancy
Mechanical ventilation

---

3. In high AG metabolic acidosis, the level of serum potassium tends to be only modestly high because of organic acid accumulation.

4. In some forms of normal AG metabolic acidosis, typically RTA and diarrhea (except for type 4 RTA), potassium may be normal or low.

> **☙ Pearl**
>
> High serum potassium strongly suggests the presence of metabolic acidosis.

Blood Urea Nitrogen, Creatinine, and Phosphate

Renal excretion of ammonium ion varies directly with the level of the glomerular filtration rate. Thus patients with CKD (ie, high BUN and serum creatinine) are invariably acidotic. Unless tubular damage is advanced, the ability to acidify the urine (ie, to achieve high urinary concentration of free hydrogen) is relatively well preserved. However, net acid excretion is markedly depressed as a result of reduced synthesis of ammonia (hydrogen binder), hence excretion of ammonium ion. Abnormal plasma phosphate level, when accompanied by metabolic acidosis, is often suggestive of a presence of certain pathologic conditions. Hyperphosphatemia occurs when renal function is reduced, and hypophosphatemia develops in proximal renal tubular dysfunction.

Alveolar-Arterial O_2 Gradient

Alveolar-arterial O_2 gradient is calculated as:

$$P_AO_2 - PaO_2 = PiO_2 - 1.25 \times (PaCO_2 - PaO_2)$$

PiO_2 is calculated as $713 \times FiO_2$, so PiO_2 of room air ($FiO_2 = 0.21$) is 150 mm Hg. Normal young individuals have A-aDO_2 of about 5 mm Hg, which represents a portion of the pulmonary blood flow that escapes the interface with the inspired air, owing to pulmonary arteriovenous shunts and underventilated areas of the lung. Values over 15 mm Hg in pediatric patients reflect an increased ventilation-perfusion mismatch, which may be accompanied by respiratory acidosis. Note that in central hypoventilation or disorders involving ventilatory muscles, respiratory failure may develop; however, because ventilation-perfusion mismatching does not occur, respiratory acidosis may develop in the absence of an increased A-aDO_2. Thus A-aDO_2 may provide us with the etiologic background of respiratory failure in some patients.

Urinary Electrolytes and Urinary Anion Gap

Hypovolemia stimulates renal sodium chloride reabsorption. Thus metabolic alkalosis caused by vomiting, nasogastric suction, prior use of diuretics, and iatrogenic rapid correction of chronic hypercapnia characteristically manifest urinary chloride concentration below 15 mEq/L.[10] The syndromes of primary aldosteronism, ongoing diuretic use, alkali administration, or severe deficits of total body potassium may be associated with urinary chloride concentration above 20 mEq/L.

Urinary AG,[11] a simple indicator of urinary excretion of ammonium, is calculated as follows:

$$(U_{Na^+} + U_{K^+}) - U_{Cl^-}$$

The kidneys excrete acid as free hydrogen ions and ammonium ions. The capacity of the kidneys to excrete free hydrogen ions is estimated by urine pH during acidemia. However, the capacity to excrete ammonium is much greater than the capacity to excrete free hydrogen ions. Thus urinary AG is an indicator of renal acid excretion, and in this regard is more sensitive than urine pH. Ammonium ion is an unmeasured cation that reflects the difference between measured cations (sodium and potassium) and measured anion (chloride). Negative urinary AG

❧ Pearl

Urinary AG ([$U_{Na^+} + U_{K^+}$] − U_{Cl^-}) is more sensitive than urine pH as an indicator of renal acid excretion.

(ie, [Na$^+$] + [K$^+$] < [CL$^-$]) in acidemia indicates that the kidney is normally responding to internal or external acid load by increasing urinary ammonium excretion. Acidosis with normal serum AG and positive urinary AG (ie, [Na$^+$] + [K$^+$] ≥ [CL$^-$]) suggests the presence of several specific disorders, including RTA.

Metabolic Acidosis

Epidemiology

The causes of metabolic acidosis are classified into 3 pathophysiologic categories (as presented in Table 12-2): (1) loss of bicarbonate, (2) addition of acid, and (3) failure of renal acid excretion.[8] The most common cause is diarrhea-related dehydration in which bicarbonate is excessively excreted through the bowel. However, the acidosis may recover spontaneously along with rehydration and improvement of the underlying enterocolitis. Diabetic ketoacidosis, on the other hand, should be appropriately diagnosed and treated, or it may result in critically ill status, including death. Renal tubular acidosis requires life-long treatment (Chapter 10).

> **Pearl**
>
> Metabolic acidosis may result from the loss of bicarbonate, addition of acid, or failure of renal acid excretion.

Presenting Symptoms

The clinical manifestations of metabolic acidosis vary depending on the cause, severity, and duration of metabolic acidosis. Increased ventilation and hypocapnia are noted as an intrinsic physiologic response to hypobicarbonatemia, resulting in amelioration of acidemia. Metabolic acidosis from any cause may lead to tissue hypoperfusion with cellular hypoxia; outpouring of lactic acid further exacerbates the acidosis and culminates in shock. Gastrointestinal disturbances, including nausea and vomiting, are common consequences of certain metabolic acidosis, particularly diabetic ketoacidosis and uremia. Polydipsia and polyuria with progressive loss of body

> **Pearl**
>
> Metabolic acidosis from any cause may lead to tissue hypoperfusion with cellular hypoxia; outpouring of lactic acid further exacerbates the acidosis and culminates in shock.

weight may precede the onset of diabetic ketoacidosis. Young infants with inborn errors of metabolism[12,13] come to medical attention in early childhood because of their lethargy, poor feeding, apnea or tachypnea, vomiting, hypotonia, seizures, and coma, although these symptoms are nonspecific. Children with RTA may often present with stunted growth.

Physical Examination

Increased respiratory rate may reflect compensatory response to metabolic acidosis. The presence of symptoms of dehydration, such as dry lips and oral cavity, decreased skin turgor, and prolonged capillary refilling time, is suggestive of diarrhea-related metabolic acidosis, diabetic ketoacidosis, and other conditions with decreased circulating volume.

Differential Diagnosis

High AG metabolic acidosis includes lactic acidosis, diabetic ketoacidosis, various organic alcohol ingestion, salicylate intoxication, and overproduction of organic acid resulting from inborn errors of metabolism. The most frequent cause of clinical lactic acidosis is tissue hypoxia exemplified by shock, severe exercise, generalized seizures, asphyxia, carbon monoxide poisoning, and chronic low circulatory flow states. Various drugs and toxins are associated with increased blood lactate levels. Ethanol may interfere with hepatic metabolism of lactate. Methanol, salicylates, and cyanide may affect intermediary metabolism of lactate. Diabetic ketoacidosis is usually associated with hyperglycemia (blood glucose >300 mg/dL), ketonemia, and arterial pH less than 7.30 or bicarbonate less than 15 mEq/L. Maple syrup urine disease and other organic acid metabolic diseases, including propionic acidemia and methylmalonic acidemia, may cause high AG metabolic acidosis. Renal insufficiency can be the cause of high AG metabolic acidosis resulting from accumulation of organic acid that would be otherwise excreted through the kidney.

Normal AG acidosis, or hyperchloremic acidosis, is divided into 2 types, extrarenal and renal hyperchloremic acidosis. Extrarenal hyperchloremic acidosis is defined by negative urinary AG (ie, intact renal acid and ammonium ion excretion). This condition includes diarrheal diseases, drainage of pancreatic and biliary secretions, and urinary diversion (eg, bowel augmentation cystoplasty). Although hyperchloremic acidosis is the most common disturbance in children with acute diarrheal diseases, coexisting high AG metabolic acidosis can be revealed in some clinical settings in which the decrease in serum bicarbonate exceeds the increase in the AG. This may be caused by additional organic acid production by starvation and lactic acid production by hypovolemia-induced tissue hypoxia. Renal hyperchloremic acidosis includes proximal, distal, and type 4 RTA (Chapter 10).

Treatment

The treatment of the underlying conditions must be initiated promptly. Immediate correction of acidotic state with alkali administration is usually limited to an acute acidotic state with blood pH <7.10, in which acidosis itself could be life threatening. There are several reasons for not correcting the less severe acidotic state. These include paradoxical lowering of intracellular pH after administration of bicarbonate[14] and reduction of cardiac output resulting from lowered ionized calcium associated with elevation of pH after bicarbonate administration. In diabetic ketoacidosis, sodium bicarbonate administration provides no beneficial effects on morbidity and mortality, rather increasing the risk for cerebral edema, which is an important cause of death in children with diabetic ketoacidosis. Children with diabetic ketoacidosis should receive appropriate rehydration and insulin administration under close monitoring of glucose and acid-base state by physicians familiar with this complicated clinical condition.

> **ᏆᎼ Pearl**
>
> Immediate correction of acidotic state with alkali administration is usually limited to an acute acidotic state with blood pH less than 7.10.

Respiratory Acidosis

Epidemiology

Respiratory acidosis refers to the acid-base disturbance caused by carbon dioxide retention and hypercapnia associated with alveolar hypoventilation. The causes for respiratory acidosis are listed in Table 12-3[15] according to

> **ᏆᎼ Pearl**
>
> Respiratory acidosis refers to the acid-base disturbance caused by carbon dioxide retention and hypercapnia associated with alveolar hypoventilation.

the mode of onset and mechanism of hypoventilation. Acute respiratory failure that accompanies cardiac arrest is a common cause of acute hypercapnia in children.

Presenting Symptoms

The clinical manifestations of respiratory acidosis vary widely depending on the rapidity with which the hypercapnia develops. Acute hypercapnia is associated with marked anxiety, disorientation, confusion, and severe breathlessness, with coma or stupor in severe cases. Chronic hypercapnia is better tolerated, but it is often responsible for confusion, memory loss, and somnolence. Concomitant hypoxemia may also be an important factor in causing these symptoms.

Physical Examination

Physical examination reveals dyspnea in various severities. Concomitant hypoxemia can be recognized by visible cyanosis on the lips and fingertips or by pulse oximetry. The patient might be critically ill with circulatory failure.

Differential Diagnosis

Clinical history-taking can differentiate acute from chronic respiratory distress. One can determine whether a patient with respiratory acidosis is in acute phase or chronic phase by blood gas analysis. The onset of acute hypercapnia is followed by an immediate increase in plasma bicarbonate concentration that is completed within 5 to 10 minutes (acute steady state). As hypercapnia becomes chronic, body bicarbonate stores are augmented by renal synthesis or retention (chronic steady state). The extent of the increase in bicarbonate in acute or chronic steady state can be calculated using the equations listed in Box 12-1. As mentioned previously, A-aDO$_2$ is helpful in distinguishing between poor respiratory effort and intrinsic lung disease.

Treatment

Treatment of respiratory acidosis includes mechanical ventilation, bronchodilators, and stimulation of respiration by drugs. In patients with chronic respiratory acidosis, respiratory stimulation is driven by hypoxia rather than hypercapnia. So excessive use of oxygen often blunts the respiratory drive in patients with chronic respiratory acidosis, causing further elevation of $PaCO_2$. This is why oxygen should be used cautiously in these patients. Administration of sodium bicarbonate to normalize the acidic pH in patients with respiratory acidosis is not recommended.

Metabolic Alkalosis

Epidemiology

Metabolic alkalosis is an acid-base disturbance initiated by an increase in the plasma bicarbonate concentration. The various causes of metabolic alkalosis are classified into 4 groups as listed in Box 12-2.[8] Loss of gastric juice from nasogastric suction or vomiting (eg, pyloric stenosis) is a common cause of metabolic alkalosis in children.

Presenting Symptoms

In chloride-responsive alkalosis, in which volume depletion and low urinary chloride concentration (<15 mEq/L) are present, thirst and lethargy may be the presenting symptoms. In contrast, chloride-resistant alkalosis, in which expanded extracellular fluid volume and urinary chloride greater than 20 mEq/L are present, is often associated with hypertension. Hypokalemia, which is an important concomitant electrolyte abnormality in metabolic alkalosis, is associated with muscle weakness. In some tubular disorders presenting with metabolic alkalosis, short stature may be a presenting symptom. In infants with congenital adrenal hyperplasia with excessive mineralocorticoids, hypertension or hypertension-related convulsion with or without pigmented ambiguous genitalia might be a presenting symptom.

Physical Examination

The presence or absence of hypertension is important in the differential diagnosis of metabolic alkalosis, as described later in this chapter.

Differential Diagnosis

Measurement of urinary chloride concentration is indispensable in the differential diagnosis of metabolic alkalosis. Low urinary chloride concentration (<15 mEq/L) in patients with metabolic alkalosis and without hypertension is suggestive of volume depletion resulting from diuretic use or gastric losses. High urinary chloride concentration (>20 mEq/L) in patients with metabolic alkalosis suggests the presence of expanded extracellular fluid volume. Patients with Bartter and Gitelman syndromes are normotensive despite the high urinary chloride concentration (ie, volume expansion). The causes of high blood pressure with high urinary chloride concentration in patients with metabolic alkalosis include primary aldosteronism, some forms of congenital adrenal hyperplasia, Cushing syndrome, renovascular disease, and renin-secreting tumor, which are all associated with the excess of mineralocorticoid function. Measurement of plasma renin activity, aldosterone, cortisol, and adenocorticotropic hormone is also important in those patients.

Treatment

Most children with mild metabolic alkalosis (HCO_3^- <32 mEq/L) do not require any intervention. In children with moderate to severe metabolic alkalosis, some intervention may be required depending on the etiology in each patient. The nasogastric tube could be removed in some patients, or administration of proton pump inhibitor should be considered. Dosage of diuretics could be reduced in some patients, or addition of spironolactone, a blocker of mineralocorticoid receptor, is helpful in ameliorating both hypokalemia and alkalosis without altering the volume status. For children with Bartter and Gitelman syndromes, potassium supplementation along with angiotensin-converting enzyme inhibitor or mineralocorticoid receptor blocker is indicated (Chapter 10).

Respiratory Alkalosis

Epidemiology

Primary hyperventilation with alkalemia is synonymous with respiratory alkalosis because increased alveolar ventilation is the only process that results in reduction of $PaCO_2$. The causes of respiratory alkalosis are listed in Box 12-3.[15] A common benign cause of acute respiratory alkalosis is the anxiety-hyperventilation syndrome.

Presenting Symptoms

Acute hypocapnia includes light-headedness, confusion, paresthesia of extremities, chest tightness, and circumoral numbness. Additional manifestations are related to the underlying disease.

Physical Examination

Increased ventilation is present, although it is often hard to be clinically detected when metabolic compensation is completed. Hypoxia, which is a well-known cause of hyperventilation, may be detected by visible cyanosis or by pulse oximetry, although mild hypoxia is difficult to recognize. Other findings related to lung and central nervous system disease and others are listed in Box 12-3.

Differential Diagnosis

Clinical history-taking usually reveals the etiology of respiratory alkalosis. Within 5 to 10 minutes after the acute reduction of $PaCO_2$, secondary adaptive reduction of bicarbonate immediately takes place. If hypocapnia persists, a further reduction in plasma bicarbonate occurs through reduced reabsorption of bicarbonate and excretion of net acid, being completed in 2 to 4 days. The extent of physiologic reduction of bicarbonate in acute and chronic respiratory alkalosis can be calculated using the equations listed in Box 12-1. Deviation of bicarbonate beyond the aforementioned physiologic reduction suggests the presence of primary metabolic process (ie, metabolic acidosis or metabolic alkalosis). Diagnostic imaging of the lung and central nervous system may be helpful. Hepatic failure, especially in the presence of elevated ammonia concentration, causes respiratory alkalosis. Tissue hypoxia resulting from carbon monoxide poisoning or Gram-negative sepsis is also considered one of the causes of respiratory alkalosis.

Treatment

No specific treatment for respiratory alkalosis is necessary. One should focus on the treatment of underlying disorders. During an acute episode of anxiety-hyperventilation, rebreathing into a paper bag is often effective in increasing the patient's $PaCO_2$, and hence decreasing the clinical symptoms. Pulse oximetry during the paper bag rebreathing is required to avoid hypoxia. In this regard, paper bag instead of plastic bag is preferred.

Rebreathing needs to be performed only when other causes of hyperventilation are eliminated.

References

1. Weisberg HF. pH and blood gases. In: Hicks JM, Boeckx RL, eds. *Pediatric Clinical Chemistry.* Philadelphia, PA: WB Saunders Co; 1984:87–106
2. Albert MS, Winters RW. Acid-base equilibrium of blood in normal infants. *Pediatrics.* 1966;37:728–732
3. Cassels DE, Morse M. Arterial blood gases and acid-base balance in normal children. *J Clin Invest.* 1953;32:824–836
4. Cogan M, Rector FC Jr. Acid-base disorders. In: Brenner BM, Rector FC Jr, eds. *The Kidney.* Philadelphia, PA: WB Saunders; 1991:753–804
5. Emmett M, Narins RG. Clinical use of the anion gap. *Medicine.* 1977;56:38–54
6. Oh MS, Carroll HJ. The anion gap. *N Engl J Med.* 1977;297:814–817
7. Lorenz JM, Kleinman LI, Markarian K, Oliver M, Fernandez J. Serum anion gap in the differential diagnosis in critically ill newborns. *J Pediatr.* 1999;135:751–755
8. Ichikawa I, Narins RG, Harris HW. Acid-base disorders. In: Ichikawa I, ed. *Pediatric Textbook of Fluids and Electrolytes.* Baltimore, MD: Williams & Wilkins; 1990:187–217
9. Madias NE, Ayus JC, Adrogue HJ. Increased anion gap in metabolic alkalosis: the role of plasma-protein equivalency. *N Engl J Med.* 1979;300:1421–1423
10. Kassirer JP, Schwartz WB. The response of normal man to selective depletion of hydrochloric acid. Factors in the genesis of persistent gastric alkalosis. *Am J Med.* 1966;40:10–18
11. Batlle DC, Hizon M, Cohen E, Gutterman C, Gupta R. The use of the urinary anion gap in the diagnosis of hyperchloremic metabolic acidosis. *N Engl J Med.* 1988;318:594–599
12. Burton BK. Inborn errors of metabolism in infancy. *Pediatrics.* 1998;102:e69
13. Wraith JE. Diagnosis and management of inborn errors of metabolism. *Arch Dis Child.* 1989;64:1410–1415
14. Ritter JM, Doktor HS, Benjamin N. Paradoxical effect of bicarbonate on cytoplasmic pH. *Lancet.* 1990;335:1243–1246
15. Cohen JJ, Madias NE. Acid-base disorders of respiratory origin. In: Brenner BM, Stein JH, eds. *Acid-Base and Potassium Homeostasis.* New York, NY: Churchill Livingstone; 1978:150

Acute Kidney Injury

Sharon P. Andreoli

Abbreviations

ACE	Angiotensin-converting enzyme
AIN	Acute interstitial nephritis
AKI	Acute kidney injury
ATN	Acute tubular necrosis
BUN	Blood urea nitrogen
CKD	Chronic kidney disease
CVVHD	Continuous venovenous hemodiafiltration
HD	Hemodialysis
HUS	Hemolytic uremic syndrome
MAG3	Mercaptoacetyl triglycine
NS	Nephrotic syndrome
NSAID	Nonsteroidal anti-inflammatory drug
PD	Peritoneal dialysis
RPGN	Rapidly progressive glomerulonephritis
Tc-99m	Technetium 99
Uosm	Urine osmolality
WBC	White blood cell

Introduction

Acute kidney injury, previously called acute renal failure, is characterized by a reversible increase in the blood concentration of creatinine and nitrogenous waste products and by the inability of the kidney to appropriately regulate fluid and electrolyte homeostasis. There are many causes of AKI, and the more common ones are listed in Box 13-1. With some diseases (such as the tumor lysis syndrome, drug-induced interstitial nephritis, aminoglycoside nephrotoxicity, and other toxic nephropathies), recovery from AKI is usually complete, whereas other diseases such as RPGN may have similar

Box 13-1. Common Causes of Acute Kidney Injury

Prerenal Failure
  Decreased true intravascular volume
  Decreased effective intravascular volume

Intrinsic Renal Disease
  Acute tubular necrosis (vasomotor nephropathy)
    Hypoxic-ischemic insults
    Drug-induced
    Toxin-mediated
      Endogenous toxins—hemoglobin, myoglobin
      Exogenous toxins—ethylene glycol, methanol

  Uric acid nephropathy and tumor lysis syndrome

  Interstitial nephritis
    Drug-induced
    Idiopathic

  Glomerulonephritis

  Vascular lesions
    Renal artery thrombosis
    Renal vein thrombosis
    Cortical necrosis
    Hemolytic uremic syndrome

  Hypoplasia/dysplasia with or without obstructive uropathy
    Idiopathic
    Exposure to nephrotoxic drugs in utero

  Hereditary renal disease
    Autosomal dominant polycystic kidney disease
    Autosomal recessive polycystic kidney disease
    Alport syndrome
    Sickle cell nephropathy
    Juvenile nephronophthisis

Obstructive Uropathy
  Obstruction in a solitary kidney
  Bilateral ureteral obstruction
  Urethral obstruction

symptoms as AKI but rapidly evolve into CKD. Several renal diseases, such as HUS, Henoch-Schönlein purpura, and obstructive uropathy with associated renal dysplasia, may present as AKI with improvement of renal function to normal or near-normal levels, but a child's renal function may slowly deteriorate, leading to CKD several months to years later.

Epidemiology

Although the precise incidence and prevalence of AKI in pediatric patients is unknown, the incidence of AKI in hospitalized children appears to be increasing.[1-8] In a pediatric tertiary care center, 227 children received dialysis therapy during an 8-year interval, for an overall incidence of 0.8 per 100,000 total population.[2] Very low birth weight (<1,500 g), a low Apgar score, a patent ductus arteriosus, and maternal administration of antibiotics and NSAIDS have been associated with the development of AKI.[4,6,9] In addition to environmental factors, some children may have genetic risk factors for AKI.

Presenting Symptoms

The presenting symptoms of AKI in children are quite variable. Because of the rapid development of the metabolic derangement characteristic of AKI, children with AKI typically present with symptoms of uremia, acidosis, anemia, and fluid overload (Chapter 14). Children with AKI owing to hypoxic-ischemic insults, HUS, acute nephritis, or other causes are more likely to demonstrate oliguria or anuria (urine output <400–500 mL/24 hours in older children or urine output <0.5–1.0 mL/kg/h in younger children and infants).[10] Children with AIN, nephrotoxic renal insults including amino-glycoside nephrotoxicity, and contrast nephropathy are more likely to have AKI with normal urine output.[10] If uremia is advanced, a child may have significant nausea and vomiting. None of the presenting symptoms of AKI are specific for kidney disease, and the establishment of AKI rests on the typical laboratory findings of elevated BUN and creatinine levels.

Physical Examination Findings

The physical examination findings in children with AKI are also quite variable, and most findings on physical examination are nonspecific. Children may present with signs and symptoms of fluid overload if they have had a history of oliguria. Children with HUS may be quite pale as a result of the associated hemolytic uremia. Children with hypocalcemia associated with AKI of any cause may have physical examination findings of tetany and seizures. In the presence of severe acidosis, a child may have Kusmall respiration as a respiratory compensation for severe metabolic acidosis. If uremia is advanced, a child may have a pericardial friction rub associated with uremia-induced pericarditis. If the etiology of AKI is obstructive uropathy, a child may present with flank masses and/or a palpable bladder.

Differential Diagnosis

Establishing the diagnosis of AKI is relatively easy once the BUN and creatinine have been determined to be elevated by standard blood tests. The challenge is to determine the etiology of the AKI. Box 13-1 provides a partial listing of the many different and diverse causes of AKI in children. A renal ultrasound, Tc-99m-MAG3 renal scan, and other specialized radiographic studies are important in determining the etiology of AKI in children. A renal ultrasound should be performed promptly in a child with AKI to evaluate for obstructive uropathy, which can be treated by relieving the obstruction.

Renal failure can be divided into prerenal failure; intrinsic renal disease, including vascular insults; and obstructive uropathies (see Box 13-1). Some causes of AKI, such as cortical necrosis and renal vein thrombosis, occur more commonly in neonates, whereas HUS is more common in young children and RPGN generally occurs in older children and adolescents. An important cause of AKI in neonates is exposure in utero to maternal drugs that interfere with nephrogenesis, such as ACE inhibitors, angiotensin receptor blockers, and NSAIDS.[11,12]

ॐ Pearl

A renal ultrasound should be performed promptly in a child with AKI to evaluate for obstructive uropathy, which can be treated by relieving the obstruction.

The history, physical examination, and laboratory studies, including a urinalysis and appropriate radiographic studies, can establish the likely cause or causes of AKI. In some instances, such as AKI occurring in hospitalized children, multiple factors are likely to be implicated in the etiology of AKI.

Prerenal Failure

Prerenal failure occurs when blood flow to the kidney is reduced as a result of true intravascular volume contraction or to a decreased effective blood volume. The kidneys are intrinsically normal, and prerenal failure is reversible once the blood volume and hemodynamic conditions are restored to normal. Prolonged prerenal failure can result in intrinsic AKI resulting from hypoxic-ischemic ATN. The evolution of prerenal failure to intrinsic renal failure is not sudden, and several compensatory mechanisms maintain renal perfusion when renal hemodynamics are not optimal. When renal perfusion is compromised, the afferent arteriole relaxes its vascular tone to decrease renal vascular resistance and maintain renal blood flow. During renal hypoperfusion, the intrarenal generation of vasodilatory prostaglandins, including prostacyclin, mediates vasodilatation of the renal microvasculature to maintain renal perfusion.[13] Administration of cyclooxygenase inhibitors such as aspirin or NSAIDS can inhibit this compensatory mechanism and precipitate acute renal insufficiency. Similarly, when renal perfusion pressure is low, as in renal artery stenosis, the intraglomerular pressure necessary to drive filtration is in part mediated by increased intrarenal generation of angiotensin II to increase efferent arteriolar resistance. Administration of ACE inhibitors in these conditions can eliminate the pressure gradient needed to drive filtration and precipitate AKI. Thus administration of medications that can interfere with compensatory mechanisms to maintain renal perfusion can precipitate AKI in certain clinical circumstances.

Prerenal failure results from renal hypoperfusion resulting from true volume contraction from hemorrhage, dehydration as a result of gastrointestinal losses, salt-wasting renal or adrenal diseases, central or nephrogenic diabetes insipidus, increased insensible losses as occurs with burns, and in disease states associated with third space losses such as sepsis, NS, traumatized tissue, and capillary leak syndrome. Decreased effective blood volume occurs when the true blood volume is normal or increased but renal perfusion is decreased as a result of diseases such as congestive heart failure, cardiac tamponade, and hepatorenal syndrome. Whether prerenal failure is caused by true volume depletion or decreased effective blood volume, correction of the underlying disturbance will return renal function to normal.

Several urinary parameters, including Uosm, urine sodium concentration, the fractional excretion of sodium, and the renal failure index, have all been proposed to help differentiate prerenal failure from vasomotor nephropathy. Renal tubules work properly in prerenal failure and are able to conserve salt and water appropriately, whereas in vasomotor nephropathy the tubules have progressed to a state of irreversible injury and are unable to conserve salt appropriately. During prerenal failure, the tubules are able to respond to decreased renal perfusion by appropriately conserving sodium and water such that the Uosm is greater than 400 to 500 mOsm/L, the urine sodium is less than 10 to 20 mEq/L, and the fractional excretion of sodium (see the following equation) is less than 1%:

$$\text{FENa}^+ (\%) = [\text{UNa}^+/\text{SNa}^+] \times [\text{SCr/UCr}] \times 100$$

Because the renal tubules in newborns and premature infants are relatively immature compared with those in older infants and children, the corresponding values suggestive of renal hypoperfusion are Uosm greater than 350 mOsm/L, urine sodium less than 20 to 30 mEq/L, and a fractional excretion of sodium of less than 2.5%.[14] When the renal tubules have sustained injury, as occurs in ATN, they cannot conserve sodium and water appropriately, so the Uosm is less than 350 mOsm/L, the urine sodium is greater than 30 to 40 mEq/L, and the fractional excretion of sodium is greater than 2.0%. However, the use of these numbers to differentiate prerenal failure from ATN requires that the patient have normal tubular function initially.

❧ Pearl

Administration of medications that can interfere with compensatory mechanisms to maintain renal perfusion can precipitate AKI.

Although this may be the case in some children, newborns with immature tubules and children with preexisting renal disease or salt-wasting renal adrenal disease, as well as other diseases, may have prerenal failure with urinary indices suggestive of ATN. Therefore, it is essential to consider the state of the function of the tubules before the potential onset that might precipitate vasomotor nephropathy or ATN.

Intrinsic Renal Disease

Hypoxic-Ischemic Acute Tubular Necrosis

Hypoxic-ischemic ATN is also called vasomotor nephropathy because the renal failure is characterized by early vasoconstriction followed by patchy cortical necrosis. In hypoxic-ischemic ATN, the urinalysis is usually unremarkable or may demonstrate low-grade proteinuria and granular casts, whereas urine indices of tubular function demonstrate an inability to conserve sodium and water, as described previously. The creatinine typically increases by about 0.5 to 1.0 mg/dL/d. Radiographic studies demonstrate kidneys of normal size with loss of corticomedullary differentiation, whereas a radionucleotide renal scan with Tc-99m-MAG3 will demonstrate normal or slightly decreased renal blood flow with poor function and delayed accumulation of the radioisotope in the renal parenchyma without excretion of the isotope in the collecting system (Figure 13-1A).

Some children with ATN will begin to recover renal function within days of the onset of renal failure, whereas recovery may not occur for several weeks in other children. Recovery of renal function may be accompanied by a diuretic phase with voluminous urine output at a time when the tubules are beginning to recover but have not recovered sufficiently to reabsorb solute and water appropriately. When the diuretic phase does occur, close attention to fluid and electrolyte balance is essential.

❧ Pearl

In the diuretic phase of ATN, close attention to fluid and electrolyte balance is essential.

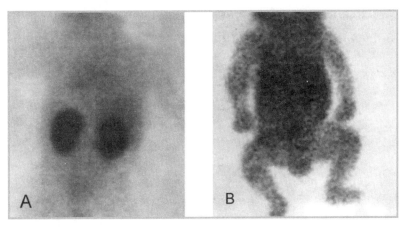

Figure 13-1.
Technetium 99 mercaptoacetyl triglycine renal scan in a newborn with acute tubular necrosis (ATN) and in a newborn with cortical necrosis. Each scan is at 4 hours after injection of isotope. **A.** This scan shows delayed uptake of isotope with parenchymal accumulation of isotope with little to no excretion of isotope into the collecting system in a neonate with ATN. **B.** In contrast, this image demonstrates no renal parenchymal uptake of isotope in a neonate with cortical necrosis. (Reprinted with permission from Andreoli SP. Clinical aspects and management of acute renal failure in children. In: Barratt TM, Avner ED, Harmon WE, eds. *Pediatric Nephrology*. Baltimore, MD: Williams & Wilkins, Inc.; 1998:1119–1124.)

Nephrotoxic Renal Failure

Medications associated with AKI include aminoglycoside antibiotics, intravascular contrast media, amphotericin B, chemotherapeutic agents (such as ifosfamide and cisplatin), acyclovir, and acetaminophen, whereas other medications have been implicated less commonly. Children with acute lymphocytic leukemia and B-cell lymphoma are at high risk of AKI resulting from uric acid nephropathy and/or the tumor lysis syndrome.[15-17] A common cause of AKI in patients with leukemia is the development of tumor lysis syndrome during chemotherapy.[16,17] Tumor lysis syndrome results in rapid increases in the serum potassium, BUN, purine metabolite products, and phosphorus, with a reciprocal decrease in the serum calcium as tumor cells are lysed.

Acute Interstitial Nephritis

Acute interstitial nephritis may cause renal failure as a result of a reaction to a drug or because of an idiopathic AIN. Children with AIN may have rash, fever, arthralgias, eosinophilia, and pyuria with or without eosinophiluria. Radiographic studies demonstrate large echogenic kidneys, and a kidney biopsy demonstrates interstitial infiltrate with many eosinophils. Medications commonly associated with AIN include methicillin and other penicillin analogues, cimetidine, sulfonamides, rifampin, and NSAIDS, whereas other drugs have been associated with AIN less commonly.[18] Acute interstitial nephritis associated with NSAIDS may also present with high-grade proteinuria and NS. Specific therapy for AIN includes withdrawal of the drug implicated in causing AIN. In addition, corticosteroids may aid in the resolution of the renal failure.

Rapidly Progressive Glomerulonephritis

Any form of glomerulonephritis in its most severe degree can present with AKI and RPGN. The clinical features include hypertension, edema, hematuria that is frequently gross, and a rapidly rising BUN and creatinine. The characteristic pathologic finding in RPGN is extensive crescent formation. Serologic tests, including antinuclear antibody, antineutrophil cytoplasmic antibody, anti–glomerular basement membrane titers, and complement studies, are required to evaluate the etiology of the RPGN. Because specific therapy will depend on the pathologic findings, a biopsy should be performed relatively promptly when a child presents with clinical characteristics suggestive of RPGN.

Vascular Insults

Large blood vessel insults, such as renal artery thrombosis and renal vein thrombosis, will present with AKI only if bilateral or if they occur in a solitary kidney. Microvascular insults occur in cortical necrosis, in typical (diarrhea-positive) and atypical (diarrhea-negative) HUS, and in HUS after bone marrow transplantation.

Cortical necrosis as a cause of AKI is much more common in young children, particularly in the neonate. Cortical necrosis is associated with hypoxic-ischemic insults resulting from perinatal anoxia, placenta abruption, and twin-twin or twin-maternal transfusions with resultant activation of the coagulation cascade. Children and newborns with cortical necrosis usually have gross or microscopic hematuria and oliguria and may have hypertension. In addition to laboratory features of an elevated BUN and creatinine, thrombocytopenia may also be present as a result of the microvascular injury. Radiographic features include a normal renal ultrasound in the early phase, and ultrasound in the later phases may show that the kidney has undergone atrophy and substantially decreased in size. A radionuclide renal scan will show decreased to no perfusion with delayed or no function (Figure 13-1B) in contrast to the delayed function that is observed in ATN (Figure 13-1A). The prognosis for cortical necrosis is much worse than that for ATN. Children with cortical necrosis may have partial recovery or no recovery at all. Typically, children with cortical necrosis will need short-term or long-term dialysis therapy, but children who do recover sufficient renal function are at risk for the late development of CKD.

Hemolytic uremic syndrome is a common cause of AKI in children and leads to substantial morbidity and mortality and long-term complications that may not become apparent until adulthood.[19] Typical HUS usually follows a gastrointestinal illness characterized by hemorrhagic colitis associated with shiga-like, toxin-producing *Escherichia coli* infection, of which O157:H7 is the most common serotype. At the time the diarrhea is subsiding, a child appears pale and lethargic as a result of the hemolytic anemia. Oliguria and anuria occur in about 30% to 50% of children, and about 40% to 75% of children will need dialysis therapy.

Hemolytic uremic syndrome is a systemic disease in which the kidney and gastrointestinal tract are the organs most commonly affected; however, evidence of central nervous system, pancreatic, skeletal, and myocardial involvement may also be present.[20,21] Gastrointestinal involvement may lead to rectal prolapse, ischemic colitis, and transmural colonic necrosis. Pancreatic involvement manifested as elevated pancreatic enzymes occurs in 10% to 20% of children, and glucose intolerance resulting from pancreatic islet cell involvement occurs in less than 10% of children. Central nervous system disease may present as seizures, coma, lethargy, and irritability. Laboratory studies demonstrate that the characteristic triad of HUS includes microangiopathic hemolytic anemia, thrombocytopenia, and renal disease. Renal disease is manifested as hematuria and/or proteinuria with elevated BUN and creatinine in most children. A high polymorphonuclear neutrophil with a prominent left shift is typical of the disease, and a high WBC count is associated with more severe disease and a worse outcome.[22]

Some studies have shown that administration of antibiotics to children with hemorrhagic colitis associated with shiga-like toxin-producing *E coli* significantly increased the odds of a child developing HUS.[23] However, a meta-analysis did not demonstrate that antibiotic therapy was harmful.[24] It has been thought that antibiotic therapy has the theoretical potential to alter the bacterial production of toxin, resulting in increased release of toxin.

ᕉ Pearl

The prognosis for cortical necrosis is much worse than that for ATN.

Similarly, antimotility agents are also not indicated because they may increase the systemic absorption of toxin as a result of the slower gastrointestinal transit time. Unfortunately, therapy for HUS is only supportive.

Obstructive Uropathy

Obstruction of the urinary tract can cause AKI if the obstruction occurs in a solitary kidney, if it involves the ureters bilaterally, or if there is urethral obstruction. Obstruction can result from congenital malformations, such as posterior urethral valves, bilateral ureteropelvic junction obstruction, or bilateral obstruction ureteroceles. Acquired urinary tract obstruction can result from passage of kidney stones or, rarely, tumors. It is important to evaluate for obstruction because the management of secondary AKI is to promptly relieve the obstruction. Obstructive uropathy is discussed in more detail in Chapters 5 and 18.

Management

Preventive Measures

Two recent studies from different geographic regions of Nigeria demonstrated that the most common cause of AKI in children was volume depletion and that the AKI was the result of preventable cause.[25,26] Because dialytic resources were scarce, the mortality rate in these studies was quite high.[25,26] Thus, on a global scale, the prevention of AKI is likely to have a larger impact on mortality than other measures.

Once intrinsic renal failure has become established, management of the metabolic complications of AKI requires meticulous attention to fluid balance, electrolyte status, acid-base balance, and nutrition. Additional renal injury from hypoperfusion and hypoxic-ischemic and nephrotoxic insults that could delay and complicate recovery should be prevented as much as possible.

Diuretics and Dopamine

Diuretics and renal-dose dopamine are commonly used to prevent or limit AKI. Several clinical studies using mannitol, diuretics, and renal-dose dopamine for AKI have been reported, but none are conclusive.[27,28] Stimulating urine output eases management of AKI, but conversion of oliguric to nonoliguric AKI has not been shown to alter the course of renal failure.[28] Lasix can be given as a bolus (1–5 mg/kg/dose) or as a continuous intravenous drip (0.1–1.0 mg/kg/h). Although the use of renal-dose dopamine (0.5 to 3.5 μg/kg/min) to improve renal perfusion is common in AKI, there are no definitive studies to demonstrate that low-dose dopamine is effective in decreasing the need for dialysis or improving survival in patients with AKI.[27,28]

Fluid, Electrolyte, and Acid-Base Balance

Depending on the etiology of AKI and the presence or absence of associated symptoms, such as vomiting or diarrhea, children with AKI may present with hypovolemia, euvolemia, or fluid overload and pulmonary edema.

When assessing fluid status, blood pressure, heart rate, skin turgor, and capillary refill are each used to assess the intravascular volume. In children who are intravascularly volume depleted, 10 to 20 mL/kg normal saline solution can be infused to reestablish intravascular volume. If urine output does not increase and azotemia does not improve after fluid resuscitation, then central venous pressure monitoring may be necessary to further guide fluid therapy. If a child has fluid overload, fluid restriction and/or fluid removal with dialysis or hemofiltration may be instituted if the child does not respond to diuretics.

Once normal intravascular volume has been reached, euvolemia can be maintained by providing the child with fluid to replace normal water losses from the skin and respiratory and gastrointestinal tracts (insensible losses, 400 mL/m^2/24 hours). Excess stool losses (as may occur with diarrhea) or excess skin and respiratory tract loss (as may occur with hyperthermia) should be accounted for as well and replaced with the appropriate fluid. Urinary losses may also be replaced milliliter for milliliter with the appropriate fluid, usually determined by measuring urine electrolytes. Ongoing fluid therapy is guided by daily weights, blood pressure, accurate fluid input and output records, physical examination, and nutritional needs of the child.

Mild hyponatremia is common in AKI and may be the result of dehydration, but fluid overload with dilutional hyponatremia is more common. If the serum sodium is greater than 120 mEq/L, fluid restriction or water removal by dialysis or hemofiltration will correct the serum sodium. If the serum sodium is less than 120 mEq/L, a child is at higher risk for seizures resulting from hyponatremia, and correction to a sodium level of approximately 125 mEq/L with hypertonic saline solution should be considered. Hypertonic saline is usually infused over several hours to avoid rapid correction of the serum sodium, which in adults with chronic hyponatremia has been associated with neurologic injury, particularly central pontine myelinolysis. Restriction of free water will further correct hyponatremia.

Because the kidneys regulate potassium balance and excrete approximately 90% of dietary potassium intake, hyperkalemia is a common and potentially life-threatening electrolyte abnormality in AKI. Hyperkalemia results from decreased filtration, impaired tubular secretion, altered distribution of potassium by acidosis that shifts potassium from the intracellular to the extracellular compartment, and release of intracellular potassium resulting from the associated catabolic state. The serum potassium level may be falsely elevated if the technique of the blood drawing is traumatic, if hemolysis occurs during the blood draw, or if a child has a high WBC or platelet count that can falsely elevate the potassium.[29] True hyperkalemia results in disturbances of cardiac rhythm by its depolarizing effect on the cardiac conduction pathways. The concentration of serum potassium that results in arrhythmia is dependent on the acid-base balance and the other serum electrolytes. For example, hypocalcemia that is common in renal failure exacerbates the adverse effects of the serum potassium on cardiac conduction pathways. Electrophysiologic findings of hyperkalemia include tall, peaked T-waves and prolongation of the PR interval on electrocardiogram, whereas flattening of P-waves and widening of QRS complexes are later abnormalities. Severe hyperkalemia will eventually lead to ventricular tachycardia and fibrillation.

Therapy for hyperkalemia is indicated if cardiac conduction abnormalities are noted or if levels are greater than 6 to 7 mEq/L; therapy for hyperkalemia is summarized in Table 13-1. Sodium bicarbonate (0.5–1.0 mEq/kg/dose) will transfer potassium into cells, but this therapy may precipitate seizures and tetany if the serum calcium level is low, resulting in a decreased ionized calcium level. Intravenous glucose and insulin also transfer potas-

Table 13-1. Treatment of Hyperkalemia

Agent	Mechanism	Dose	Onset	Complications
Sodium bicarbonate	Shifts K+ into cells	1 mEq/kg IV over 10–30 min	15–30 min	Hypernatremia, change in ionized calcium
Albuterol	Shifts K+ into cells	400 µg by nebulizer	30 min	Tachycardia, hypertension
Glucose and insulin	Shifts K+ into cells	Glucose 0.5 gm/kg	30–120 min	Hypoglycemia
Calcium gluconate, 10%	Stabilizes membrane potential	0.5–1 mL/kg IV over 5–15 min	Immediate	Bradycardia, arrhythmias, and hypercalcemia
Kayexalate		1 g/kg PO or PR in sorbitol	30–60 min	Hypernatremia, constipation, colonic membrane irritation (PR)

Abbreviations: IV, intravenously; PO, orally; K+, potassium; PR, rectally.

sium from the extracellular to the intracellular compartment. Intravenous calcium gluconate will increase the threshold potential of the excitable myocardial cells and counteract the depolarizing effect of the hyperkalemia. Administration of albuterol given as a nebulizer will acutely lower the serum potassium level by stimulating intracellular uptake of potassium. Each of these is a temporizing measure and does not remove potassium from the body. Sodium polystyrene sulfonate (Kayexalate) given orally (by nasogastric tube) or rectally will exchange sodium for potassium in the gastrointestinal tract and result in potassium removal. Complications of this therapy include possible hypernatremia, sodium retention, and constipation. Depending on the degree of hyperkalemia and the need for correction of other metabolic derangements in AKI, hyperkalemia frequently requires the initiation of dialysis or hemofiltration.

Because the kidneys excrete net acids generated by diet and intermediary metabolism, acidosis is common in AKI. Severe acidosis can be treated with intravenous or oral sodium bicarbonate, oral sodium citrate solutions, and/ or dialysis therapy. It is important to consider the serum ionized calcium level when considering therapy for acidosis. Approximately half the total calcium is protein bound and half is free and in the ionized form, which is what determines the transmembrane potential and electrochemical gradient. Hypocalcemia is common in AKI, and acidosis will increase the fraction of total calcium to the ionized form. Treatment of acidosis can then shift the ionized calcium to a more normal ratio, decreasing the amount of ionized calcium and precipitating tetany and/or seizures. Thus base therapy for acidosis should not be considered without knowledge of the total and ionized calcium levels. When giving base therapy, 0.5 to 1 mEq/kg over approximately 1 hour is reasonable. Administering sodium bicarbonate generates carbon dioxide, and an intact respiratory system to excrete the excess generated carbon dioxide is required for bicarbonate therapy to be effective.

ॐ Pearl

Hyperkalemia is common and potentially life threatening in AKI.

Calcium and Phosphate Balance

Because the kidneys excrete a large amount of ingested phosphorus, hyperphosphatemia is a common electrolyte abnormality noted during AKI. Hyperphosphatemia should be treated with dietary phosphorus restriction and with oral calcium carbonate or other calcium compounds to bind phosphorus and prevent gastrointestinal absorption of phosphorus. Aluminum-containing compounds should be avoided because several studies have demonstrated that orally administered aluminum-containing phosphorus binders result in substantial aluminum absorption, leading to severe aluminum intoxication. As described previously, acid-base balance has a profound effect on the ionized calcium level, and interpretation of the calcium level and consideration of therapy should take into consideration the degree of acidosis. If hypocalcemia is severe and/or if bicarbonate therapy is necessary for hyperkalemia, therapy with 10% calcium gluconate (100 mg/kg up to a maximum of 1 g or 1 mL/kg up to a maximum of 10 mL) should be given over 30 to 60 minutes with continuous electrocardiographic monitoring.

Nutritional Therapy

Acute kidney injury can be associated with severe anorexia, and malnutrition can develop rapidly. Proper nutrition is essential in the management of the child with AKI. If the gastrointestinal tract is intact and functional, enteral feedings with formula (Similac PM 60/40 for newborns and infants) should be instituted as soon as possible. In older children, a diet of high biologic value protein, low phosphorus, and low potassium foods can be used. Infants should receive maintenance calories (120 kcal/kg/d), and older children should receive appropriate maintenance calories or higher if needed due to catabolic state and malnutrition. If a child is oliguric or anuric and sufficient calories cannot be achieved while maintaining appropriate fluid balance and growth, earlier initiation of dialysis should be considered.

Renal Replacement Therapy

The purpose of renal replacement therapy is to remove endogenous and exogenous toxins and to maintain fluid, electrolyte, and acid-base balance until renal function improves. Renal replacement therapy may be provided by PD, intermittent HD, or hemofiltration with or without a dialysis circuit. Many factors, including the age and size of the child, the cause of renal failure, the degree of metabolic derangements, blood pressure, and nutritional needs, are considered in deciding when to initiate renal replacement therapy and the modality of therapy. During AKI it is important to initiate renal replacement therapy in a timely manner; initiation when a child has severe fluid overload has been associated with increased mortality.

The indications to initiate renal replacement therapy are not absolute and take into consideration a number of factors, including the cause of renal failure, the rapidity of the onset of renal failure, the severity of fluid and electrolyte abnormalities, and the age of the child. Because infants and younger children have less muscle mass than older children, they require initiation of renal replacement therapy at lower serum levels of serum creatinine and BUN. The presence of fluid overload unresponsive to diuretic therapy and the need for enteral feedings or hyperalimentation to support nutritional needs are important factors in considering the initiation of renal replacement therapy. The highlights of the different forms of renal replacement therapy for AKI follow.

Peritoneal dialysis has been a major modality of therapy for AKI, particularly in neonates and small children when vascular access may be difficult to maintain. Advantages of PD are that it is relatively easy to perform, it does not require heparinization, and children do not need to be hemodynamically stable. The disadvantages include a slower correction of metabolic parameters and the potential for peritonitis. To increase the efficiency of PD, frequent exchanges as often as every hour and use of dialysate with higher glucose concentrations will remove more solute and water, respectively. Relative contraindications include recent abdominal surgery and massive organomegaly or intra-abdominal masses, as well as ostomies, which may increase the risk of peritonitis. Complications include peritonitis and fluid and electrolyte abnormalities.

Hemodialysis has also been used for several years in the treatment of AKI in children. Hemodialysis has the advantage that metabolic abnormalities can be corrected rather quickly, and hypervolemia can be corrected by rapid ultrafiltration as well. The disadvantages of HD include the requirement for heparinization, the need for maximally purified water by a reverse osmosis system, and the need for skilled nursing personnel. Relative contraindications include hemodynamic instability or severe hemorrhage.

Renal replacement therapy for AKI with hemofiltration—including continuous venovenous hemofiltration or, with the addition of a dialysis circuit to the hemofilter, CVVHD—have become increasingly used for the treatment of AKI in children. Hemofiltration without dialysis follows the principle of removal of large quantities of ultrafiltrate from plasma with replacement of an isosmotic electrolyte solution, whereas CVVHD also results in solute removal via the added dialysis circuit.

Hemofiltration (with or without a dialysis circuit) can result in rapid fluid removal; it does not require the patient to be hemodynamically stable when a pump is inserted into the circuit; and it is continuous, avoiding rapid solute and fluid shifts, as occur in HD. Disadvantages of hemofiltration include that it may require constant heparinization, and there is a potential for severe fluid and electrolyte abnormalities owing to the large volume of fluid removed and subsequently replaced.

Prognosis

The prognosis of AKI is highly dependent on the underlying etiology of the disease.[1-8] Children who have AKI as a component of multisystem failure have a much higher mortality rate than children with intrinsic renal disease, such as HUS, RPGN, and AIN. Children who have suffered substantial loss of nephrons, as in HUS or RPGN, are at risk for late development of renal failure long after the initial insult. Thus children who have had cortical necrosis during the neonatal period and recovered renal function or children with an episode of severe Henoch-Schönlein purpura or HUS are clearly at risk for the late development of renal complications. Acute kidney injury from any cause can be a concern for later kidney disease.

≥❧ *Pearl*

Patients with AKI need lifelong monitoring of their renal function, blood pressure, and urinalysis.

Importantly, AKI is likely to be especially deleterious when the kidneys are not yet grown to adult size and/or before the full complement of nephrons have developed. Because nephrogenesis is not complete until approximately 34 weeks' gestation, AKI during this interval might lead to a decreased nephron number, and indeed studies have suggested that AKI during nephrogenesis results in decreased nephron number and subsequent glomerulomegaly.[30,31] Studies in older children have also shown that AKI leads to CKD in a higher percentage of children than previously appreciated.[32] Thus children with a history of AKI need lifelong monitoring of their renal function, blood pressure, and urinalysis.

References

1. Andreoli SP. Acute renal failure. *Curr Opin Pediatr.* 2002;14:183–188
2. Moghal NE, Brocklebank JT, Meadow SR. A review of acute renal failure in children: incidence, etiology and outcome. *Clin Nephrol.* 1998;49:91–95
3. Andreoli SP. Acute renal failure in the newborn. *Sem Perinatol.* 2004;28:112–123
4. Karlowivz MG, Adelman RD. Nonoliguric and oliguric acute renal failure. *Pediatr Nephrol.* 1995;9:718–722
5. Martin-Ancel A, Garcia-Alix A, Gaya F, Cabañas F, Burgueros M, Quero J. Multiple organ involvement in perinatal asphyxia. *J Pediatr.* 1995;127:786–793
6. Cataldi L, Leone R, Moretti U, De Mitri B, Fanos V. Potential risk factors for the development of acute renal failure in preterm newborn infants: a case controlled study. *Arch Dis Child Fetal Neonatal Ed.* 2005;90:F14–F19
7. Hui-Stickle S, Brewer ED, Goldstein SL. Pediatric ARF epidemiology at a tertiary care center from 1999 to 2001. *Am J Kidney Dis.* 2005;45:96–101
8. Aggarwal A, Kumar P, Chowkhary G, Majumdar S, Narang A. Evaluation of renal function in asphyxiated newborns. *J Trop Pediatr.* 2005;51:295–299
9. Cuzzolin L, Fanos V, Pinna B, et al. Postnatal renal function in preterm newborns: a role of diseases, drugs and therapeutic interventions. *Pediatr Nephrol.* 2006;21:931–938
10. Andreoli SP. Acute renal failure: clinical evaluation and management. In: Avner ED, Harmon WE, Niaudet P, eds. *Pediatric Nephrology.* Baltimore, MD: Williams & Wilkins, Inc.; 2004:1233–1254
11. Cooper WO, Hernandez-Diaz S, Arbogast PG, Dudley JA, Dyer S. Major congenital malformations after first trimester exposure to ACE inhibitors. *N Engl J Med.* 2006; 354:2443–2451
12. Benini D, Fanos V, Cuzzolin L, Tatò L. In utero exposure to nonsteroidal anti-inflammatory drugs: neonatal acute renal failure. *Pediatr Nephrol.* 2004;19:232–234
13. Badr KF, Ichikawa I. Prerenal failure: a deleterious shift from renal compensation to decompensation. *N Engl J Med.* 1988;319:623–628
14. Ellis EN, Arnold WC. Use of urinary indexes in renal failure in the newborn. *Am J Dis Child.* 1982;136:615–617
15. Andreoli SP. Clinical aspects and management of acute renal failure in children. In: Avner ED, Harmon WE, Niaudet P, eds. *Pediatric Nephrology.* Baltimore, MD: Williams & Wilkins, Inc.; 1998:1119–1124
16. Stapleton FB, Strother DR, Roy S, Wyatt RJ, McKay CP, Murphy SB. Acute renal failure at onset of therapy for advanced stage Burkitt lymphoma and B cell acute lymphoblastic lymphoma. *Pediatrics.* 1988;82:863–869

17. Jones DP, Mahmoud H, Chesney RW. Tumor lysis syndrome: pathogenesis and management. *Pediatr Nephrol.* 1995;9:206–212

18. Vohra S, Eddy A, Levin AV, Taylor G, Laxer RM. Tubulointerstitial nephritis and uveitis in children and adolescents. *Pediatr Nephrol.* 1999;13:426–432

19. Garg AX, Suri RS, Barrowman N, et al. Long-term renal prognosis of diarrhea associated hemolytic uremic syndrome: a systematic review, meta-analysis and meta-regression. *JAMA.* 2003;290:1360–1370

20. Andreoli SP, Bergstein JM. Development of insulin-dependent diabetes mellitus during the hemolytic-uremic syndrome. *J Pediatr.* 1983;100:541–545

21. Siegler RJ. The spectrum of extrarenal involvement in post-diarrheal hemolytic-uremic syndrome. *J Pediatr.* 1994;125:511–518

22. Walters MDS, Matthei IU, Kay R, Dillon MJ, Barratt TM. The polymorphonuclear leucocyte count in childhood hemolytic uraemic syndrome. *Pediatr Nephrol.* 1989;3:130–134

23. Wong CS, Jelacic S, Habeeb RL, Watkins SL, Tarr PI. Risk of hemolytic uremic syndrome after antibiotic treatment of *Escherichia coli* O157:H7 infections. *N Engl J Med.* 2000; 342:1930–1936

24. Safdar N, Said A, Gangnon RE, Maki DG. Risk of hemolytic uremic syndrome after antibiotic treatment of *Escherichia coli* O157:H7 enteritis: a meta-analysis. *JAMA.* 2002; 288:996–1001

25. Anochie I, Eke F. Acute renal failure in Nigerian children: Port Harcourt experience. *Pediatr Nephrol.* 2005;20:1610–1614

26. Olowu WA, Adelusola KA. Pediatric acute renal failure in southwestern Nigeria. *Kidney Int.* 2004;66:1541–1548

27. Cantarovich F, Rangoonwwala, B, Loremz H, Verho M, Esnault LM. High dose furosemide for established ARF: a prospective, randomized, double blind, placebo-controlled trial. *Am J Kidney Dis.* 2004;44:402–409

28. Friedrich JO, Adhikari N, Herridge MS, Beyene J. Meta-analysis: low dose dopamine increases urine output but does not prevent renal dysfunction or death. *Ann Int Med.* 2005;142:510–524

29. Rodriguez-Soriano J. Potassium homeostasis and its disturbances in children. *Pediatr Nephrol.* 1995;9:364–374

30. Abitbol CL, Bauer CR, Montane B, Chandar J, Duara S, Zilleruelo G. Long-term follow-up of extremely low birth weight infants with neonatal renal failure. *Pediatr Nephrol.* 2003;18:887–893

31. Polito C, Papale MR, LaManna AL. Long-term prognosis of acute renal failure in the full term newborn. *Clin Pediatr.* 1998;37:381–386

32. Askenazi DJ, Feig DI, Graham NM, Hui-Stickle S, Goldstein S. 3-5 year longitudinal follow-up of pediatric patients after acute renal failure. *Kidney Int.* 2006;69:184–189

Chapter 14

▉ *Chronic Kidney Disease*

Mouin G. Seikaly and Nina Salhab

Abbreviations

ACE	Angiotensin-converting enzyme
ARB	Angiotensin receptor blocker
BUN	Blood urea nitrogen
CKD	Chronic kidney disease
DRI	Dietary reference intake
DTPA	Diethylene triamine penta-acetic acid
ESRD	End-stage renal disease
GFR	Glomerular filtration rate
GN	Glomerulonephritis
HD	Hemodialysis
K/DOQI	Kidney Disease Outcomes Quality Initiative
NAPRTCS	North American Pediatric Renal Trials and Collaborative Studies
NS	Nephrotic syndrome
PD	Peritoneal dialysis
PTH	Parathyroid hormone
rhGH	Recombinant human growth hormone
SD	Standard deviation
Tc-99m	Technetium 99

Introduction and Definition

Healthy People 2010, a public health mandate issued by the Surgeon General of the United States, outlines critical health initiatives for US citizens.[1] In this document a section is devoted to CKD, which is the precursor of ESRD. It underscores the significant societal burden of CKD as a result of its complications, disability, death, and economic cost. Early recognition and treatment of CKD can reduce its morbidity. The availability of a single quantifiable measure that can predict renal health and monitor its progression remains elusive. Several biomarkers of renal well-being are used to assess kidney function and its morphology. Today GFR and interstitial fibrosis are considered the best available markers of renal health.[2,3]

Recently the National Kidney Foundation published the K/DOQI. These guiding principles introduced a new nomenclature for CKD and developed clinical practice guidelines for its management.[4] The K/DOQI definition of CKD hinges on persistent structural or functional evidence of renal damage (Table 14-1 and Figure 14-1). The whole CKD paradigm revolves around the hypothesis that certain complications of CKD develop at certain levels of reduced GFR.

> **☙ Pearl**
>
> The definition of CKD hinges on persistent structural or functional evidence of renal damage.

Epidemiology and Etiology

The true prevalence of CKD in children is uncertain. The third National Health and Nutrition Examination Survey estimates that 4.3% of the US population has a GFR less than 60 mL/min/1.73 m[2].[2-5] The study mainly included adults with a subset of individuals between 12 and 19 years of age. Serum creatinine greater than 1.5 mg/dL is prevalent in 2% of the US population between 12 and 19 years of age. Among black males in this age

Table 14-1. Symptoms and Action Plan by Chronic Kidney Disease Stage			
Stages of CKD	Estimated GFR (mL/min/ 1.73 m²)	Symptoms	Action Plan
Stage 1	>90	Symptoms of primary disease	Treat primary disease
Stage 2	89–60	Symptoms of primary disease	Treat primary disease
Stage 3	59–30	Symptoms of primary disease, ± fluid retention, ± hypertension	Treat primary disease + manage comorbid conditions
Stage 4	29–15	Same as above + hyperparathyroidism, renal osteodystrophy, anemia, acidosis, growth delay	Treat primary disease + manage comorbid conditions; consider preemptive renal transplant when GFR <20 mL/min/1.73 m²
Stage 5	<15	Same as above + uremic syndrome	Initiate dialysis, workup for renal transplant

Abbreviations: CKD, chronic kidney disease; GFR, glomeruler filtration rate.

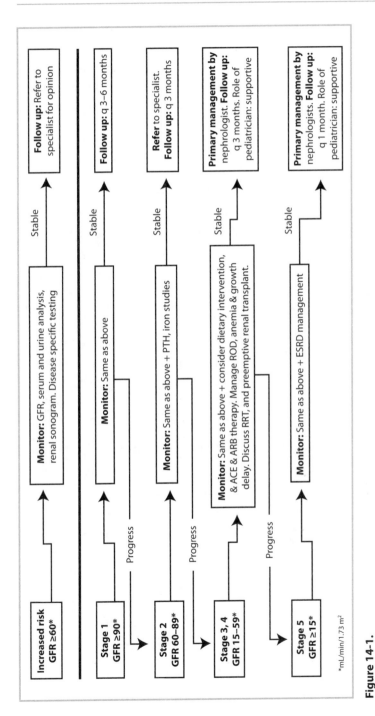

Figure 14-1.

Practice guidelines for referral and follow-up of children with chronic kidney disease. GFR, indicates glomerular filtration rate; q, every; PTH, parathyroid hormone; ACE, angiotensin-converting enzyme; ARB, angiotensin receptor blocker; ROD, renal osteodystrophy; RRT, renal replacement therapy; ESRD, end-stage renal disease.

Contents of figure:

Increased risk GFR ≥60*
Monitor: GFR, serum and urine analysis, renal sonogram. Disease specific testing
Stable → **Follow up:** Refer to specialist for opinion

Stage 1 GFR ≥90*
Monitor: Same as above
Stable → **Follow up:** q 3–6 months
Progress →

Stage 2 GFR 60–89*
Monitor: Same as above + PTH, iron studies
Stable → **Refer** to specialist. **Follow up:** q 3 months
Progress →

Stage 3, 4 GFR 15–59*
Monitor: Same as above + consider dietary intervention, & ACE & ARB therapy. Manage ROD, anemia & growth delay. Discuss RRT, and preemptive renal transplant.
Stable → **Primary management by** nephrologist. **Follow up:** q 3 months. Role of pediatrician: supportive
Progress →

Stage 5 GFR ≥15*
Monitor: Same as above + ESRD management
Stable → **Primary management by** nephrologists. **Follow up:** q 1 month. Role of pediatrician: supportive

*mL/min/1.73 m²

ઈ✥ *Pearl*

Congenital renal abnormalities of the urinary tract are the most prevalent cause of CKD in young children, whereas GN is more prevalent in adolescents.

group, the prevalence is as high as 5.2%. The etiology of CKD in children is listed in Table 14-2. Causes of CKD vary with age of onset. Congenital renal abnormalities of the urinary tract are the most prevalent cause of CKD in young children, whereas GN is more prevalent in adolescents.[6]

Presenting Symptoms and Physical Signs

Early in the course of CKD, clinical signs vary depending on the primary diagnosis (see Table 14-2). As CKD progresses, the presenting symptoms vary depending on the degree of renal insufficiency at the time of diagnosis.

ઈ✥ *Pearl*

Uremic syndrome results from hormonal and physiologic derangements that develop with progressive deterioration of renal function.

Cystic kidney disease presents with abdominal mass; obstructive uropathy with urinary tract infection; and GN with hematuria, proteinuria, edema, and hypertension. Uremic syndrome results from hormonal and physiologic derangements that develop with progressive deterioration of renal function, and it presents with fatigue, anorexia, failure to thrive, itchiness,

Table 14-2. Primary Diagnosis in Stages 2 to 4 Chronic Kidney Disease	
Diagnosis	**Percentage**
Obstructive uropathy	23
Aplastic/hypoplastic/dysplastic kidneys	18
Reflux nephropathy	9
Focal segmental glomerulosclerosis	8
Polycystic kidney disease	4
Systemic immunologic disease	4
Syndrome of agenesis of abdominal musculature	3
Renal infarct	3
Hemolytic uremic syndrome	2
Cystinosis	2
Others, such as chronic GN, familial and interstitial nephritis	24

Abbreviation: GN, glomerulonephritis.

pallor, easy bruising, bone pain, and fractures. If undiagnosed, advanced CKD can present with encephalopathy, coma, congestive heart failure, and pericarditis. With improved health care, uremic syndrome is a rare presentation of CKD.

Workup

Diagnostic testing in children with CKD should be initially directed at the primary disease. The discussion in this chapter will focus on evaluating renal function and structure related to monitoring progression of CKD.

Urine Tests

Urinary findings vary depending on the type of primary renal disease and the stage of CKD. The degree of proteinuria and hematuria increases as CKD progresses. When dipstick for protein is abnormal, further testing is warranted. A biochemical analysis is performed to quantitate urine protein and creatinine. The ratio of protein/creatinine in the urine provides a good estimate of quantitative urinary protein excretion per day; the normal is less than 0.20 for children 6 years and older and as high as 0.86 for infants.[7]

Collection of urine for 24 hours can be analyzed for protein, urea nitrogen, and creatinine. The presence of excessive protein in the urine (>4 mg/h/m^2) indicates hyperfiltration or kidney damage. The amount of creatinine and urea excretion in the urine can also be used to estimate GFR.

Blood Tests

Serum creatinine and BUN are the most commonly used blood biomarkers to screen and monitor renal disease. Creatinine is a breakdown product of normal muscle. Serum creatinine could be disproportionately elevated compared with the degree of renal dysfunction in certain conditions, including rhabdomyolysis and increased meat intake.

Urea is a by-product of protein metabolism. Blood urea nitrogen level is not only dependent on kidney function but also can be elevated during dehydration, increased catabolism (such as high fever, gastrointestinal bleeding, steroid therapy), and high protein intake. As renal function deteriorates, the level of these markers in the blood rises.

Kidney dysfunction causes serum electrolyte imbalance, especially potassium, bicarbonate, phosphorus, and calcium (Chapter 11). Rise in serum potassium is a late development in CKD. Acid-base balance is usually disrupted as CKD progresses, resulting in metabolic acidosis. The proximal tubule has the 1α-hydroxylase enzyme necessary for the final hydroxylation of 1,25-dihydroxyvitamin D, the active form of vitamin D. Decreased production of 1,25-dihydroxyvitamin D can decrease serum calcium, which results in osteomalacia and increased levels of PTH. Increased PTH level results in bone resorption and increased serum calcium and phosphorous. Inability to excrete phosphorus by failing kidneys, combined with hyperparathyroidism, causes its levels in the blood to rise, resulting in extra skeletal deposition. Osteomalacia and hyperparathyroidism will result in bone disease manifesting with pain and fractures. Treatment of hyperphosphatemia and hyperparathyroidism will be discussed later in this chapter.

❧ Pearl

Serum creatinine and BUN are the most commonly used blood biomarkers to screen and monitor renal disease.

Imaging Studies

Ultrasound is commonly used to diagnose kidney disease. Ultrasound is a noninvasive technique that provides information about the size, shape, texture, and presence of solid or cystic masses of the kidneys. At birth, a kidney normally measures around 5 cm in its maximum longitudinal dimension, and it reaches around 12 cm in length in adults. Normative values for kidney size with SD scores are available to the radiologist for size comparison (Appendix II). Although the kidneys are enlarged in acute conditions, they are often small in most patients with CKD. Patients with CKD secondary to autosomal dominant polycystic kidney disease, diabetic nephropathy, and amyloidosis may have enlarged kidneys. Neonatal kidneys are lobular and become smooth later in infancy. Abnormality in kidney contour can occur in patients with reflux nephropathy. The kidney texture could be echogenic in CKD. Ultrasound may also be used to diagnose urinary obstruction and kidney stones and to assess the renal blood flow.

Renal scans are often used to diagnose specific kidney conditions. Static renal scans (Tc-99m-dimercaptosuccinic acid) are indicated in the diagnosis of renal scarring (reflux nephropathy) and differential renal function between the right and left kidney. Normally renal function is equally distributed between each kidney. A discrepancy in renal function more than 55% in one and 45% in the other is seen in renal dysplasia, hypoplasia, multicystic dysplastic kidneys, and reflux nephropathy. Dynamic imaging (Tc-99m-DTPA), or Tc-99m-mercaptoacetyl triglycine is often used to diagnose obstructive uropathy, especially when used in conjunction with furosemide. Other specialized dynamic renal scans include the use of captopril to diagnose renal artery thrombosis or stenosis, and Tc-99m DTPA to measure GFR (Chapter 5).

Renal Biopsy

Early in the course of CKD, a percutaneous renal biopsy is indicated to delineate the etiology of renal disease. Some of the indications for renal biopsy include persistent gross hematuria or persistent isolated microscopic hematuria (>12 months), hematuria combined with proteinuria, excessive proteinuria (>40 mg/hr/m^2) not responsive to immunosuppression, unexplained stage 2 CKD or greater, renal involvement in systemic disease such as staging nephropathy in systemic lupus erythematosus, and evaluation of kidney dysfunction in a renal transplant. In the presence of solitary kidney or when excessive bleeding is anticipated, open rather than percutaneous renal biopsy is recommended.

Percutaneous renal biopsy is a safe procedure. Rare complications include hematuria, perirenal hematoma, arteriovenous fistula, and renal infection. The biopsy should be avoided when the kidneys are small because the risks of bleeding from the procedure increases and the potential information obtained may not contribute further to the management of CKD. At our institution, we often perform renal biopsies under intravenous sedation and ultrasonographic guidance. Overnight observation in the hospital is required following this procedure.

Measurement of Glomerular Filtration Rate

Renal clearance of solutes and toxins is the best overall index of renal function in health and disease. Glomerular filtration rate is the most commonly used marker of renal function. Glomerular filtration rate is defined as the volume of blood that a 1-minute excretion of urine suffices to completely clear inulin (a substance that is freely filtered, not secreted, reabsorbed, or metabolized by the nephron). Glomerular filtration rate is an excellent biomarker of renal function because it can be accurately and reproducibly measured.[8] At birth, GFR is 30 mL/min/1.73 m^2 and by 2 weeks it increases to 75 mL/min/1.73 m^2. The normal GFR in adults (100–140 mL/min /1.73 m^2 in men and 85–115 mL/min/1.73 m^2 in women) is not reached until the first or second year of life. Glomerular filtration rate is also sensitive in detecting small decrements in renal function. Glomerular filtration rate is a good indicator of the ability of the kidney to clear plasma from toxins of uremia and potentially harmful solutes.[9] Moreover, GFR often predicts the onset of clinical signs and symptoms of CKD; as GFR drops below 30 mL/min/1.73 m^2, anemia and hyperparathyroidism develop. Signs of uremic syndrome develop when GFR is below 10 mL/min/1.73 m^2, even when acidosis and electrolyte imbalance are corrected.[10,11] Glomerular filtration rate changes in response to therapeutic interventions and pathologic processes, making it a good gauge for CKD progression.

Clinically, several biomarkers have been used to estimate GFR; most commonly used is serum creatinine. Unfortunately, serum creatinine is relatively insensitive in detecting changes in renal function. Serum creatinine does not rise until GFR decreases by at least 30%. Formulae are available to estimate GFR using calculations that include height,[12] but they have been shown to be inaccurate in predicting renal function, especially at lower levels of GFR[13] (see Appendix II). The GFR may be calculated from the 24-hour urine clearance of endogenously produced substances, such as creatinine and urea.

> ### ❧ Pearl
>
> Glomerular filtration rate is the best and most commonly used biomarker of renal function.

Creatinine is secreted by the nephron, hence it overestimates GFR, whereas urea is reabsorbed and thus underestimates GFR. The average of creatinine and urea clearances is closer to true GFR than each one alone. The exact measurement of GFR is at times necessary for management of CKD. Inulin clearance is the gold standard, but it is difficult to perform and hence impractical in clinical medicine. Radiolabeled iothalamate is among the more popular exogenous biomarkers used to measure GFR in children.[14]

Treatment

Treatment Aimed at the Primary Disease

As renal disease is diagnosed, management strategies should be aimed at treating the primary disease. It is imperative that reversible causes of renal failure (eg, obstructive uropathy, prerenal causes, medications, and others) be identified and reversed as early as feasible. Glomerulonephritis often requires immunosuppressive therapy. Obstructive uropathy and vesicoureteral reflux require surgery to correct urologic anomalies.

Treatment Aimed at Slowing Down Clinical Progression

Chronic kidney disease is at times destined to progress to ESRD. The mechanisms for progression of kidney disease are not well delineated but seem multifactorial. A seemingly common path to CKD progression is glomerular hyperfiltration. This is an adaptive process that develops to compensate for lost function as nephron mass decreases. However, hyperfiltration in itself causes glomerular injury and further deterioration of renal function. Glomerular permeability and proteinuria are invariable consequences of hyperfiltration.[15] Proteinuria, a marker of progression of CKD, has the potential to encourage tubulointerstitial damage.[16]

Increased PTH also seems to play a role in the progression of CKD by causing hypercalcemia and hyperphosphatemia. These in turn are associated with arterial calcification.[17] Parathyroid hormone is also one of several presumed toxins of uremia.[18] These toxins are known to activate inflammatory cytokines and oxygen free radicals leading to the development of atherosclerosis, glomerulosclerosis, and degeneration of tubular epithelial cells.[19] Hence, one could speculate that PTH and other uremic toxins accumulating in CKD could stimulate inflammatory processes that accelerate progression into ESRD. Dyslipidemias can also play a role in the initiation and progression of CKD.[20]

Control of progression of CKD often requires the use of certain medications, such as ACE inhibitors, ARBs, statins, phosphate binders, and vitamin D analogues. Recent studies suggest that ACE inhibitors and ARBs, especially when used in combination, are beneficial in CKD even in the absence of hypertension. This is mainly because of evidence suggesting that both classes of medications (1) delay the progression of renal damage in glomerular hypertension; (2) decrease proteinuria in patients with NS[21]; and (3) improve blood flow to the heart, brain, and kidneys despite lowering the blood pressure. Cardiovascular disease, a major comorbid condition in adults with CKD, often starts in children. Children with CKD often have hypercholesterolemia and hyperlipidemia. Collective recent review and meta-analysis indicate that statins slow down progression of renal disease (1.22 mL/min/y) and decrease proteinuria in adult subjects with nondiabetic CKD.[22,23] As mentioned elsewhere in this chapter, both elevated serum phosphorous and PTH can accelerate progression of CKD. Phosphate binders and vitamin D analogues used to manage these comorbid conditions will be discussed later in this chapter.

Nutrition is an essential part of the management plan of a child with CKD. Studies have repeatedly suggested that children with CKD have several nutrient imbalances and protein-energy malnutrition.[24] Early nutrition intervention has a positive impact on progression of renal disease to ESRD.[25] As renal function deteriorates, several dietary restrictions have to be implemented. Renal diets include high biologic value protein at amounts guided by DRI for height, age, low phosphate, low potassium, and no added salt. These renal diets could be used individually or in combination. These diets are aimed at managing electrolyte disturbances, controlling hypertension and edema, and delaying the progression of renal failure while promoting optimal growth and development.[26] Studies in adults have suggested that high-protein diet can hasten the progression of renal failure, whereas a moderately low protein diet (0.6 g protein/kg/d) might slow the progression of CKD to ESRD.[27] Results of such studies were not replicated in children. Occasionally some departure from these diets is warranted (eg, a child who has sodium-losing nephropathy or obstructive uropathy requires sodium supplemententation). Fluid restriction is often not necessary in the early stages of CKD. However, in certain kidney diseases, such as NS, fluid retention is excessive and can be treated with any of a number of diuretics.

Children with CKD stage 3 or greater have special vitamin requirements. Current K/DOQI guidelines recommend limiting vitamin and mineral supplements to whenever clinically indicated. Most water-soluble vitamins need to meet 100% of the DRI for thiamin, riboflavin, pyridoxine, and vitamin

B_{12}. Vitamins A, C, E, and K should also meet 100% of the recommended daily allowance. Folic acid, on the other hand, should be supplemented at a higher level than that required in children without CKD, especially while on dialysis.[28] Vitamin A tends to accumulate in CKD stage 3 or greater.

ᶓᴥ *Pearl*

Early detection and intervention may delay progression of CKD. Renal diets include high biologic value protein, low phosphate, low potassium, and no added salt.

Hypervitaminosis A will manifest as vomiting, diplopia, cranial nerve palsies, and pseudotumor cerebri. Although the current recommendation is not to restrict dietary vitamin A, further supplementation should be avoided. All vitamin preparations given to children with CKD stage 3 or greater should contain no additional vitamin A. Vitamin C supplementation should not exceed 100 mg because it can lead to oxalate stone formation.

The kidney is responsible for the 1α-hydroxylation of the final step in the production of calcitriol, the active form of vitamin D. Calcitriol is commercially available and needs to be supplemented to patients with CKD stage 3 and greater. Commercially available vitamin preparations for use in CKD patients contain vitamin C, thiamin, riboflavin, folic acid, B_{12}, biotin, and pantothenic acid with or without iron. Recently a liquid renal vitamin preparation became available for use in younger children (Nephronex®, Llorens Pharmaceuticals, Miami, FL).

Treatment Aimed at Comorbid Conditions

Studies in adults with CKD indicate that patients are not routinely identified early in their clinical courses and are not treated with adequate attention to dietary protein, anemia, hypertension, and other comorbid events.[29] Children with CKD have added comorbid conditions that are not encountered in adults. Chronic kidney disease may influence physiologic and cognitive maturation of children. The metabolic alterations associated with CKD in children result in stunted growth, delayed pubertal development, and impaired neurocognitive functions. In adults, CKD is independently associated with increased risks of death and cardiovascular events.[30] Some of the complications of CKD are listed in Table 14-3.

Hypertension is a common comorbid condition in children with CKD (Chapter 15). Uncontrolled hypertension often accelerates progression of

Table 14-3. Comorbid Conditions Associated With Chronic Kidney Disease	
Cardiovascular	Hypertension, myocardial dysfunction, pulmonary edema, uremic pericarditis
Gastrointestinal	Anorexia, dysgeusia, nausea, gastroesophageal reflux, gastritis
Endocrine	Growth retardation, gynecomastia, increased prolactin levels, irregular menses, anovulatory cycles, decreased libidinal drives, impotence, decreased testosterone levels
Neuromuscular	Myopathy, peripheral neuropathy, encephalopathy
Psychological	Learning disability, attention disorder, depression, issues with body image
Dermatologic	Sallow skin color, pruritus, dry skin
Hematologic	Bleeding, platelet aggregation dysfunction, anemia
Immunologic	Predisposition to infection

CKD.[4] High blood pressure can be treated with any of a large number of medications. The choice of antihypertensives should be based on understanding of its pathogenesis in a particular clinical setting. Converting enzyme inhibitors or ARBs are used as first-line therapy in the presence of high plasma renin activity, unilateral renovascular hypertension, renal parenchymal disease, proteinuria, congestive heart failure, and diabetes mellitus. These drugs should be avoided in pregnancy. Tight control of hypertension combined with the use of converting enzyme inhibitors reduces the rate of decline of renal function by 3 to 4 mL/min/y.[31]

Calcium channel blockers (nifedipine) may be used as the first-line therapy in patients with emergency hypertension, diabetes mellitus, chronic obstructive lung disease, bronchopulmonary dysplasia, gout, hyperlipidemia, and peripheral vascular disease, and in black patients. Beta-blockers (propranolol, nadolol) are used for patients with contracted intravascular volume, high plasma renin activity, hyperdynamic circulation, anxiety, migraine, hyperthyroidism, and neuroadrenergic tumors. Beta-blockers should be avoided in athletes and diabetics. Diuretics as an adjunct second-line drug should be used for patients with volume overload, NS, acute glomerulonephritis, low plasma renin activity, oral contraceptive therapy, and congestive heart failure. Diuretics should be avoided in athletes.

The cause of anemia in CKD is multifactorial. When GFR declines below 30 mL/min/1.73 m^2, the life span of the red blood cells decreases, and as tubulointerstitial nephritis progresses, the synthesis of erythropoietin decreases. Other causes of anemia include aluminum, medications, folate and B_{12} deficiency, occult blood loss, and iron deficiency. Treatment with erythropoietin reverses anemia of renal failure, improves quality of life, retards progression of CKD, and decreases cardiovascular risk factors associated with CKD.[32,33] Anemia of CKD is often normochromic and normocytic; however, as CKD progresses, anorexia and subsequently iron deficiency develop. Oral iron is often poorly absorbed in children with CKD, but its absorption can be enhanced by the use of ascorbic acid. As GFR declines, parenteral iron use is needed to maintain the transferrin saturation index at or above 30%. With advanced renal disease, uremic toxins build up and antifolates accumulate, thus increasing daily folic acid requirement to 1 mg from the regular 200 µg in healthy children.

Chronic metabolic acidosis is a frequent comorbid clinical condition associated with advanced stages of CKD. Metabolic acidosis can affect growth by inducing resistance to the anabolic action of growth hormone, calcium efflux from bone, suppression of albumin synthesis, and degradation of muscle protein.[33] Control of acidosis helps maintain bone mineralization and subsequently growth because excess hydrogen resorbs bone.[34,35] Eighty-eight percent of children with CKD and growth retardation are acidemic.[36] In CKD, the relationship between growth delay and acidosis is not clear because there is a lack of consistent improvement in growth with correction of acidosis.[37]

1,25-dihydroxyvitamin D_3 (calcitriol) levels begin to decline at an early stage of CKD. As GFR declines to lower than 45 mL/min/1.73 m², synthesis of 1,25-dihydroxyvitamin D_3 declines below the lower limits of normal. As GFR declines further (<30 mL/min/1.73 m²), hyperparathyroidism develops. Decline in the synthesis of 1,25-dihydroxyvitamin D_3 leads to hypocalcemia and osteomalacia; both conditions are treated with calcitriol or another vitamin D analog that does not require 1α-hydroxylation by the kidneys. Hyperparathyroidism leads to a characteristic bony disease called *osteitis fibrosa cystica.* Treatment of hyperparathyroidism consists of controlling serum phosphorous and pharmacologically suppressing PTH. Vitamin D and its analogues, such as calcitriol or paricalcitol, are used to suppress PTH. Another class of drugs called *calcimimetic agents* (cinacalcet) that mimics calcium at its receptors recently has been used to control PTH.

Controlling serum phosphorous requires dietary intervention (as discussed previously) and the use of phosphate binders. Phosphate binders are either calcium-containing (calcium carbonate, calcium acetate, calcium citrate), calcium-free (sevelamer, lanthanum carbonate), or contain aluminum (aluminum hydroxide). Aggressive suppression of PTH is not recommended because it can result in a dynamic bone disease. Osteomalacia, osteitis fibrosa cystica, and adynamic bone disease, alone or in combination, cause renal osteodystrophy.

It was recently reported that 36.9% of children with CKD had statural growth impairment at the time of enrollment into the NAPRTCS registry.[38] The etiology of growth delay in children with CKD is multifactorial. Several non–growth hormone-related factors have been proposed by previous studies as single risk factors; these include age at onset of CKD, primary renal disease, residual renal function, protein-calorie malnutrition, increased protein catabolism, metabolic acidemia, renal osteodystrophy, anemia, urinary sodium losses and other electrolyte abnormalities, and prior use of corticosteroids.[39] In children with CKD, the pituitary hypothalamic axis is intact. Insulin-like growth factor-binding protein −1, −2, −4, −6 levels are elevated[40] as a result of decreased clearance or increased hepatic synthesis.[41] The rela-

> **Pearl**
>
> Hypertension, anemia, acidosis, and growth delay occur with CKD and need early treatment.

tion between various factors and height at entry into the registry in children with CKD was further evaluated, and it was found that older patients, those with GFR higher than 50 mL/min/1.73 m², black patients, and patients with focal segmental glomerulosclerosis were at lower risk of being short at entry.[34] Anemia with a hematocrit below 33% is an independent risk factor for short stature. Acidosis, serum phosphorous, calcium, albumin, and PTH at registration are poor predictors of short stature. Short stature should be treated by managing nutritional deficiencies, acidosis, anemia, and renal osteodystrophy. Despite adequate metabolic control, growth retardation persists and will require the daily use of rhGH. Controlled clinical trials evaluating the effect of rhGH on height SD score in children with CKD have shown definite beneficial effect on catch-up growth.[42]

Treatment to Replace Renal Function

End-stage renal disease is a term used to designate the time reached to initiate renal replacement therapy (ie, dialysis or transplant). It does not refer to a specific level of GFR but rather the time of occurrence of signs and symptoms of uremic syndrome. End-stage renal disease is an administrative term used as a stipulated condition for health care reimbursement by the Centers for Medicare & Medicaid Services ESRD program in the United States. When GFR drops to 20 mL/min/1.73 m², preemptive renal transplant should be considered. According to the NAPRTCS 2006 annual report, up to 25% of children who have a transplant have a preemptive transplant.[43] It has become axiomatic that renal transplant is the treatment of choice for all children with ESRD. In children from birth to 14 years of age, there is an improvement of up to 30 years in life expectancy in those who have transplants compared with those undergoing dialysis.[44] In 2005, 6.4% of renal transplants (890 of 14,794 transplants procured from either deceased or living donors) were in children 17 years of age or younger.[45] With the introduction of newer and more potent immunosuppressive therapy, 1-year graft survival for deceased and living donor kidneys is 93% and 95%, respectively, and 5-year graft survival is 77% and 85%, respectively.[39] Complications of transplant include cardiovascular disease, opportunistic infection, and malignancy.

Dialysis should be initiated when GFR drops to below 15 mL/min/1.73 m² or when symptoms of uremia set in. According to the US Renal Data Registry, the point incident rate of ESRD in children in 2004 was 14.4 per million children (0–19 years) corresponding to incident count of 1,212 children.[40] The point prevalent rate is 81.7 per million children corresponding to point prevalent count of 6,730 children on dialysis per calendar year in the United States. Two types of dialysis are available

⊅ Pearl

Renal transplantation is the treatment of choice in children with ESRD.

in children: peritoneal dialysis and HD. Peritoneal dialysis is the preferred modality for young children. The development of automated PD made home dialysis possible. The main complication of PD is peritonitis. Hemodialysis is usually performed in a dialysis unit. Vascular access for HD remains a challenge, especially in young children. Although arteriovenous fistulae are the access of choice for older HD patients, this goal is difficult to achieve in small patients. The use of hemodialysis catheters placed in the internal jugular is often inevitable in children weighing less than 20 kg. Complications of hemodialysis include disequilibrium syndrome, seen with aggressive first dialysis session, accesses failure, and infection. Disequilibrium syndrome occurs during or shortly after dialysis and often results from intracellular fluid shifts following rapid osmotic solute removal. Clinically it presents with lethargy, obtundation, headache, or seizure.

When to Refer to a Specialist

Studies in adult CKD have observed that patients are not routinely identified early in their clinical courses and are not treated with adequate attention to dietary protein, anemia, hypertension, and other comorbid events. Recently, Nissenson and colleagues[46] reviewed a large health maintenance organization database to identify an adult patient population with CKD. Care in most of these patients (88%) was primary physician based, with only 22% of the patients seen by a nephrologist during the first year after entry into the study cohort. Referral to the adult nephrologist usually occurred when the serum creatinine values reached 3 mg/dL. Although similar data are not available in children, the prevalent opinion is that all children with CKD should be seen by a nephrologist. It is highly recommended that affected children 14 years of age and younger are seen by a pediatric nephrologist who can better address their comorbid conditions and especially their growth and development needs. Figure 14-1 presents a practice guideline as to the time of referral and frequency of follow-up.

> **Pearl**
>
> Patients with stage 1 CKD with persistent hematuria and proteinuria or radiologic evidence of renal disease and those with stage 2 CKD or higher should be referred to a pediatric nephrologist.

Natural History and Prognosis

Recently, the chronic renal insufficiency arm of the NAPRTCS database was reviewed.[6] The rate of progression of this cohort to ESRD (ie, required dialysis or preemptive renal transplant) was analyzed. (Mechanisms of progression of CKD to ESRD were discussed previously.) In this analysis, 62% of patients with CKD progressed to ESRD; the median time to dialysis or transplantation was 353 days. The rate of progression to ESRD in this sub-

group at 1, 2, and 3 years was 51%, 69%, and 78%, respectively. The risk factors for progression to ESRD were recently shown to include low hematocrit, hypoalbuminemia, hyperphosphatemia, and hyperparathyroidism. Primary clinical diagnosis, degree of GFR, and the age at entry into the registry were additional risk factors.[6]

References

1. National Institute of Diabetes and Digestive and Kidney Disease. *Healthy People 2010: Chronic Renal Disease.* Bethesda, MD: National Institutes of Health, National Institute of Diabetes and Digestive and Kidney Disease; 2000

2. Filler G, Browne R, Seikaly MG. Glomerular filtration rate as a putative surrogate endpoint for renal transplant clinical trials in children. *Pediatr Transplant.* 2003;7:18–24

3. Nicholson ML, McCulloch TA, Harper SJ. Early measurement of interstitial fibrosis predicts renal function and graft survival in renal transplantation. *Br J Surg.* 1996;83: 1082–1085

4. National Kidney Foundation. K/DOQI clinical practice guidelines for chronic kidney disease evaluation, classification and stratification. *Am J Kidney Dis.* 2002;39(suppl 1): S1–S266

5. Jones CA, McQuillan GM, Kusek JW, et al. Serum creatinine levels in the US population: Third National Health and Nutrition Examination Survey. *Am J Kidney Dis.* 1998;32: 992–999

6. Seikaly MG, Ho PL, Emmett L, Fine R, Tejani A. Chronic renal insufficiency in children. The 2001 annual report of the NAPRTCS. *Pediatr Nephrol.* 2003;18:796–804

7. Suzuki MM. Nephrology. In: Siberry GK, Iannone R, eds. *The Harriet Lane Handbook.* 5th ed. St Louis, MO: Mosby; 2000:439–459

8. Filler G, Browne R, Seikaly MG. GFR as a candidate "surrogate end-point" in renal transplant. *Pediatr Transplant.* 2003;7:18–24

9. Schainuck LI, Striker GE, Cutler RE, Benditt EP. Structure-functional correlations in renal disease: II. *Hum Pathol.* 1970;1:631–641

10. Levey AS. Use of glomerular filtration rate to assess the progression of renal disease. *Semin Nephrol.* 1989;9:370–379

11. Shemesh O, Golbetz H, Kriss JP, Myers BD. Limitations of creatinine as filtration marker in glomerulopathic patients. *Kidney Int.* 1985;28:830–838

12. Schwartz GJ, Brion LP, Spitzer A. The use of plasma creatinine concentration for estimating glomerular filtration rate in infants, children and adolescents. *Pediatr Clin North Am.* 1987;34: 571–590

13. Seikaly MG, Browne R, Bajaj G, Arant BS Jr. Limitations of body length/serum creatinine ratio as an estimate of glomerular filtration in children. *Pediatr Nephrol.* 1996;10:709–711

14. Bajaj G, Alexander S, Sakarcan A, Browne R, Seikaly MG. ^{125}Iodine-iothalamate clearance in children. A simple method to measure GFR. *Pediatr Nephrol.* 1996;10:25–28

15. Remuzzi G, Bertani T. Pathophysiology of progressive nephropathies. *N Engl J Med.* 1998;339:1448–1456

16. Nath K. The tubulointerstitium in progressive renal disease. *Kidney Int.* 1998;54:992–994

17. Goodman WG, Goldin J, Kuizon BD, et al. Coronary-artery calcification in young adults with end-stage renal disease who are undergoing dialysis. *N Engl J Med.* 2000;342:1478–1483

18. Massry SG, Smogorzewski M. Mechanisms through which parathyroid hormone mediates its deleterious effects on organ function in uremia. *Semin Nephrol.* 1994;14:219–231

19. Scwelder S, Schnizel R, Vaith P, Wanner C. Inflammation and advanced glycation end products in uremia: simple coexistence, potentiation or causal relationship? *Kidney Int.* 2001;59:S32–S36

20. Campese VM, Nadim MK, Epstein M. Are 2-hydroxy-3 methylglutaryl-CoA reductase inhibitors renoprotective? *J Am Soc Nephrol.* 2005;16(supp):S11–S17

21. Tanaka H, Suzuki K, Nakahata T, et al. Combined therapy of enalapril and losartan attenuates histologic progression in immunoglobulin A nephropathy. *Pediatr Int.* 2004;46(5):576–579

22. Agarwal R. Effect of statins on renal function. *Am J Cardio.* 2006;97:748–755

23. Sandhu S. Do statins have a beneficial effect on the kidney? *J Am Soc Nephrol.* 2006;17:206–216

24. Wong CS, Gipson DS, Gillen DL, et al. Anthropometric measures and risk of death in children with end stage renal disease. *Am J Kidney Dis.* 2000;36:811–819

25. Ledermann SE, Shaw V, Trompeter RS. Long-term enteral nutrition in infants and young children with chronic renal failure. *Pediatr Nephrol.* 1999;13:870–875

26. Rodriguez-Soriano J, Arant BS, Rodehl J, Norman ME. Fluid and electrolyte imbalances in children with chronic renal failure. *Am J Kidney Dis.* 1986;7:268–274

27. Wingen AM, Fabian-Bach C, Mehls O. Multicentre randomized study on the effect of a low protein diet on the progression of renal failure in childhood: one-year results. *Miner Electrolyte Metab.* 1992;18:303–308

28. National Kidney Foundation Kidney Disease Outcomes Quality Initiative. Clinical practice guidelines for nutrition in chronic renal failure. *Am J Kidney Dis.* 2000;35 (6 suppl 2):S1–S140

29. Obrador GT, Pereira BJG. Early referral to the nephrologist and timely initiation of renal replacement therapy: a paradigm shift in the management of patients with chronic renal failure. *Am J Kidney Dis.* 1982;31:398–417

30. Go AS, Chertow GM, Fan D, McCulloch CE, Hsu C-Y. Chronic kidney disease and the risks of death, cardiovascular events, and hospitalization. *N Engl J Med*. 2004; 352:1296–1305

31. Levi M. Do statins have a beneficial effect on the kidney? *Nat Clin Pract Nephrol*. 2006; 2:666–667

32. Kuryama S, Tomonari H, Yoshida H, Hashimoto T, Kawaguchi Y, Sakai O. Reversal of anemia by erythropoietin therapy retards the progression of chronic renal failure especially in non-diabetic patients. *Nephron*. 1997;77:176–185

33. Maniar S, Kleinknecht C, Zhou X, Motel V, Yvert JP, Dechaux M. Growth hormone action is blunted by acidosis in experimental uremia or acid load. *Clin Nephrol*. 1996;46:72–76

34. Bushinsky DA, Frick KK. The effect of acid on bone current opinion. *Nephrol Hyperten*. 2000;9:369–379

35. Nash MA, Torrado AD, Greifer I, Spitzer A, Edelmann CM Jr. Renal tubular acidosis in infants and children. Clinical course, response to treatment and prognosis. *J Pediatr*. 1972;80:738–748

36. Betts PR, Magrath G. Growth pattern and dietary intake of children with chronic renal insufficiency. *Br Med J*. 1974;2:189–193

37. Potter DE, Greifer I. Statural growth of children with renal disease. *Kidney Int*. 1978; 14:334–339

38. Seikaly MG, Salhab N, Gipson D, Liu V. Stature in children with chronic kidney disease: analysis of NAPRTCS Database. *Pediatr Nephrol*. 2006;21:793–799

39. Stickler GB, Bergen BJ. A review: short stature in renal disease. *Pediatr Res*. 1973;7:978–982

40. Tonshoff B, Kiepe D, Ciarmatori S. Growth hormone/insulin like growth factor system in children with chronic renal failure. *Pediatr Nephrol*. 2005;20:279–289

41. Tonshoff B, Mehls O. Growth retardation in children with chronic renal insufficiency: current aspects of pathophysiology and treatment. *J Nephrol*. 1995;8:133–142

42. Fine RN, Khaut EC, Brown D, Perlman AJ. Growth after recombinant human growth hormone therapy in children with chronic renal failure: report of a multi-center and double-blind placebo-control study. *J Pediatr*. 1994;124:374–382

43. North American Pediatric Renal Trials and Collaborative Studies. *2006 Annual Report*. http://www.NAPRTCS.org. Accessed January 2007

44. United States Renal Data System. *2006 Annual Data Report: Atlas of the End-stage Renal Disease in the United States*. Bethesda, MD: National Institute of Diabetes and Digestive and Kidney Disease; 2006

45. US Organ Procurement and Transplantation Network and the Scientific Registry of Transplant Recipients. *2006 Annual Report of the US Organ Procurement and Transplantation Network and the Scientific Registry of Transplant Recipients: Transplant Data 1996–2005*. Rockville, MD: Health Resources and Services Administration, Healthcare Systems Bureau, Division of Transplantation; 2006

46. Nissenson AR, Collins AJ, Hurley J, Petersen H, Pereira BJ, Steinberg EP. Opportunities for improving the care of patients with chronic renal insufficiency: current practice patterns. *J Am Soc Nephrol*. 2001;12:1713–1720

■ *Hypertension*

Deborah P. Jones

Definition

Hypertension in children and adolescents is defined by BP levels persistently greater than the 95th percentile for that individual, based on height percentile, age, and gender, on at least 3 separate occasions. Extreme elevation in BP may prompt more aggressive assessment and management but, unfortunately, there are no clear guidelines to aid the physician as to the exact level of BP that requires immediate attention. This is discussed further in the section on the approach to acute HT. Excellent reviews are available on the methodology for BP measurement and the percentile-based normal values for each gender, age, and height percentile.[1-3] The normative data tables and recommendations for the evaluation and treatment of high BP were recently updated by the National High Blood Pressure Education Program Working Group on High Blood Pressure in Children and Adolescents. Please refer to this comprehensive and updated discussion for further information.[2]

The first requirement for measurement of BP in children is the proper equipment to ensure that accurate measurements are obtained. The preferred method is auscultation—using either a mercury sphygmomanometer or aneroid device. However, this may not be practical. Therefore, oscillometric devices have assumed a much more prominent place in modern pediatric clinics. Use of the appropriate-sized cuff is essential. Often the cuff labeled "child-size" is more appropriate for toddlers, and the small adult cuff is appropriate for children. Adult and large adult cuffs are required for measurement in older children and adolescents, and with the alarming emergence of extreme obesity among adolescents, even a thigh cuff may be needed. One practical rule is that the largest cuff that will comfortably fit on the upper arm is the most appropriate size. If BP is elevated, obtain repeat measurements, preferably with an auscultatory method. If that is not practical, then repeat oscillometric measurement with attention to technique, including cuff size. This is particularly challenging for infants and toddlers for whom auscultation may prove difficult, especially when cooperation is less than optimal. It may be necessary to place a BP cuff on the arm and wait for the child to become calm or fall asleep before a reliable BP measurement may be obtained.

Common errors in BP measurement may be related to equipment, patient factors, or observer-related factors.[4] Equipment used to measure BP must be properly maintained and calibrated. The most frequently observed error in BP measurement in children is use of the incorrect cuff size; usually the selected cuff is too small for the patient's arm. Guidelines for cuff size are often confusing or conflicting. In addition, the manufacturers' cuff and internal bladder sizes for each category of size (ie, child-size, small adult) vary. Patient-related factors that may introduce error include not resting for at least 5 minutes before measurement. This may apply to the clinic in which the patient is rushed into the triage room for vital signs. Improper position of the cuff or intake of substances that cause transient increases in BP (caffeine, tobacco, decongestants, and stimulants) may also result in erroneous measurement. The medical personnel responsible for obtaining BP measurements must be properly trained and able to ascertain when measurements may be invalid. Blood pressure measurement by auscultation requires a quiet room and sufficient auditory skills.

All children older than 3 years should have BP measurements taken when they are evaluated in a medical setting. Blood pressure should be measured in children younger than 3 years in certain conditions, such as when there is a history of premature birth, congenital heart disease, kidney disease, treatment with medications associated with increased BP, or a previous transplant.

Confirmation of increased BP on subsequent occasions is required to avoid overdiagnosis of HT, particularly because BP tends to go down with repeated measurement. Based on the level of BP, an individual may be classified as having normal BP, pre-HT, or HT. Hypertension is defined as having an average SBP and/or DBP at or greater than the 95th percentile on at least 3 occasions (Tables 15-1 and 15-2). Pre-HT is defined as having an average SBP and/or DBP at or greater than the 90th but less than the 95th percentile on at least 3 occasions with the caveat that any level of BP at least 120/80, even if the 90th percentile is greater than this, is considered to be pre-HT. This principle has been adopted from the seventh report by the Joint National Committee by the Pediatric Working Group in its recent update.[5]

❧ Pearl

Hypertension in children and adolescents is defined as BP levels persistently greater than the 95th percentile for that individual, based on height percentile, age, and gender, on at least 3 separate occasions.

Hypertension has been further subdivided into 2 stages according to the degree of BP elevation: stage 1 refers to mean SBP and/or DBP from the 95th percentile to the 99th percentile plus 5 mm Hg, and stage 2 refers to mean SBP and/or DBP greater than the 99th percentile plus 5 mm Hg. Staging of HT by the Working Group provides an objective indication for initiation of antihypertensive therapy.

Epidemiology

During childhood and adolescence, both SBP and DBP levels increase with age and body size. Gender and ethnicity also affect BP levels. Blood pressure increases at a steeper rate among girls 6 to 11 years of age compared with boys of the same age, but the rate of increase is steeper among 12- to 17-year-old males than among females of the same age. Blood pressure levels tend to be higher in black children compared with gender-matched white children. Therefore, useful normative data must be derived from multiethnic populations. Blood pressure has been observed to "track" over time, mean-

Table 15-1. BP Levels for Boys by Age and Height Percentile[2,a]

Age, y	BP Percentile	SBP, mm Hg							DBP, mm Hg						
		Percentile of Height							Percentile of Height						
		5th	10th	25th	50th	75th	90th	95th	5th	10th	25th	50th	75th	90th	95th
1	50th	80	81	83	85	87	88	89	34	35	36	37	38	39	39
	90th	94	95	97	99	100	102	103	49	50	51	52	53	53	54
	95th	98	99	101	103	104	106	106	54	54	55	56	57	58	58
	99th	105	106	108	110	112	113	114	61	62	63	64	65	66	66
2	50th	84	85	87	88	90	92	92	39	40	41	42	43	44	44
	90th	97	99	100	102	104	105	106	54	55	56	57	58	58	59
	95th	101	102	104	106	108	109	110	59	59	60	61	62	63	63
	99th	109	110	111	113	115	117	117	66	67	68	69	70	71	71
3	50th	86	87	89	91	93	94	95	44	44	45	46	47	48	48
	90th	100	101	103	105	107	108	109	59	59	60	61	62	63	63
	95th	104	105	107	109	110	112	113	63	63	64	65	66	67	67
	99th	111	112	114	116	118	119	120	71	71	72	73	74	75	75
4	50th	88	89	91	93	95	96	97	47	48	49	50	51	51	52
	90th	102	103	105	107	109	110	111	62	63	64	65	66	66	67
	95th	106	107	109	111	112	114	115	66	67	68	69	70	71	71
	99th	113	114	116	118	120	121	122	74	75	76	77	78	78	79
5	50th	90	91	93	95	96	98	98	50	51	52	53	54	55	55
	90th	104	105	106	108	110	111	112	65	66	67	68	69	69	70
	95th	108	109	110	112	114	115	116	69	70	71	72	73	74	74
	99th	115	116	118	120	121	123	123	77	78	79	80	81	81	82

Table 15-1. BP Levels for Boys by Age and Height Percentile[2,a], continued

Age, y	BP Percentile	SBP, mm Hg							DBP, mm Hg						
		Percentile of Height							Percentile of Height						
		5th	10th	25th	50th	75th	90th	95th	5th	10th	25th	50th	75th	90th	95th
6	50th	91	92	94	96	98	99	100	53	53	54	55	56	57	57
	90th	105	106	108	110	111	113	113	68	68	69	70	71	72	72
	95th	109	110	112	114	115	117	117	72	72	73	74	75	76	76
	99th	116	117	119	121	123	124	125	80	80	81	82	83	84	84
7	50th	92	94	95	97	99	100	101	55	55	56	57	58	59	59
	90th	106	107	109	111	113	114	115	70	70	71	72	73	74	74
	95th	110	111	113	115	117	118	119	74	74	75	76	77	78	78
	99th	117	118	120	122	124	125	126	82	82	83	84	85	86	86
8	50th	94	95	97	99	100	102	102	56	57	58	59	60	60	61
	90th	107	109	110	112	114	115	116	71	72	72	73	74	75	76
	95th	111	112	114	116	118	119	120	75	76	77	78	79	79	80
	99th	119	120	122	123	125	127	127	83	84	85	86	87	87	88
9	50th	95	96	98	100	102	103	104	57	58	59	60	61	61	62
	90th	109	110	112	114	115	117	118	72	73	74	75	76	76	77
	95th	113	114	116	118	119	121	121	76	77	78	79	80	81	81
	99th	120	121	123	125	127	128	129	84	85	86	87	88	88	89
10	50th	97	98	100	102	103	105	106	58	59	60	61	61	62	63
	90th	111	112	114	115	117	119	119	73	73	74	75	76	77	78
	95th	115	116	117	119	121	122	123	77	78	79	80	81	81	82
	99th	122	123	125	127	128	130	130	85	86	86	87	88	89	90

Table 15-1. BP Levels for Boys by Age and Height Percentile[2,a], continued

Age, y	BP Percentile	SBP, mm Hg							DBP, mm Hg						
		Percentile of Height							Percentile of Height						
		5th	10th	25th	50th	75th	90th	95th	5th	10th	25th	50th	75th	90th	95th
11	50th	99	100	102	104	105	107	107	59	59	60	61	62	63	63
	90th	113	114	115	117	119	120	121	74	74	75	76	77	78	78
	95th	117	118	119	121	123	124	125	78	78	79	80	81	82	82
	99th	124	125	127	129	130	132	132	86	86	87	88	89	90	90
12	50th	101	102	104	106	108	109	110	59	60	61	62	63	63	64
	90th	115	116	118	120	121	123	123	74	75	75	76	77	78	79
	95th	119	120	122	123	125	127	127	78	79	79	81	82	82	83
	99th	126	127	129	131	133	134	135	86	87	88	89	90	90	91
13	50th	104	105	106	108	110	111	112	60	60	61	62	63	64	64
	90th	117	118	120	122	124	125	126	75	75	76	77	78	79	79
	95th	121	122	124	126	128	129	130	79	79	80	81	82	83	83
	99th	128	130	131	133	135	136	137	87	87	88	89	90	91	91
14	50th	106	107	109	111	113	114	115	60	61	62	63	64	65	65
	90th	120	121	123	125	126	128	128	75	76	77	78	79	79	80
	95th	124	125	127	128	130	132	132	80	80	81	82	83	84	84
	99th	131	132	134	136	138	139	140	87	88	89	90	91	92	92
15	50th	109	110	112	113	115	117	117	61	62	63	64	65	66	66
	90th	122	124	125	127	129	130	131	76	77	78	79	80	80	81
	95th	126	127	129	131	133	134	135	81	81	82	83	84	85	85
	99th	134	135	136	138	140	142	142	88	89	90	91	92	93	93

Table 15-1. BP Levels for Boys by Age and Height Percentile[2,a], continued

Age, y	BP Percentile	SBP, mm Hg							DBP, mm Hg						
		Percentile of Height							Percentile of Height						
		5th	10th	25th	50th	75th	90th	95th	5th	10th	25th	50th	75th	90th	95th
16	50th	111	112	114	116	118	119	120	63	63	64	65	66	67	67
	90th	125	126	128	130	131	133	134	78	78	79	80	81	82	82
	95th	129	130	132	134	135	137	137	82	83	83	84	85	86	87
	99th	136	137	139	141	143	144	145	90	90	91	92	93	94	94
17	50th	114	115	116	118	120	121	122	65	65	66	67	68	69	70
	90th	127	128	130	132	134	135	136	80	80	81	82	83	84	84
	95th	131	132	134	136	138	139	140	84	85	86	87	87	88	89
	99th	139	140	141	143	145	146	147	92	93	93	94	95	96	97

Abbreviations: BP, blood pressure; SBP, systolic blood pressure; DBP, diastolic blood pressure.

[a] *From Fourth Report on the Diagnosis, Evaluation and Treatment of High Blood Pressure in Children and Adolescents*, National Institutes of Health, 2004.

Table 15-2. BP Levels for Girls by Age and Height Percentile[2,a]

Age, y	BP Percentile	SBP, mm Hg							DBP, mm Hg						
		Percentile of Height							Percentile of Height						
		5th	10th	25th	50th	75th	90th	95th	5th	10th	25th	50th	75th	90th	95th
1	50th	83	84	85	86	88	89	90	38	39	39	40	41	41	42
	90th	97	97	98	100	101	102	103	52	53	53	54	55	55	56
	95th	100	101	102	104	105	106	107	56	57	57	58	59	59	60
	99th	108	108	109	111	112	113	114	64	64	65	65	66	67	67
2	50th	85	85	87	88	89	91	91	43	44	44	45	46	46	47
	90th	98	99	100	101	103	104	105	57	58	58	59	60	61	61
	95th	102	103	104	105	107	108	109	61	62	62	63	64	65	65
	99th	109	110	111	112	114	115	116	69	69	70	70	71	72	72
3	50th	86	87	88	89	91	92	93	47	48	48	49	50	50	51
	90th	100	100	102	103	104	106	106	61	62	62	63	64	64	65
	95th	104	104	105	107	108	109	110	65	66	66	67	68	68	69
	99th	111	111	113	114	115	116	117	73	73	74	74	75	76	76
4	50th	88	88	90	91	92	94	94	50	50	51	52	52	53	54
	90th	101	102	103	104	106	107	108	64	64	65	66	67	67	68
	95th	105	106	107	108	110	111	112	68	68	69	70	71	71	72
	99th	112	113	114	115	117	118	119	76	76	76	77	78	79	79
5	50th	89	90	91	93	94	95	96	52	53	53	54	55	55	56
	90th	103	103	105	106	107	109	109	66	67	67	68	69	69	70
	95th	107	107	108	110	111	112	113	70	71	71	72	73	73	74
	99th	114	114	116	117	118	120	120	78	78	79	79	80	81	81

Table 15-2. BP Levels for Girls by Age and Height Percentile[2,a], continued

Age, y	BP Percentile	SBP, mm Hg							DBP, mm Hg						
		Percentile of Height							Percentile of Height						
		5th	10th	25th	50th	75th	90th	95th	5th	10th	25th	50th	75th	90th	95th
6	50th	91	92	93	94	96	97	98	54	54	55	56	56	57	58
	90th	104	105	106	108	109	110	111	68	68	69	70	70	71	72
	95th	108	109	110	111	113	114	115	72	72	73	74	74	75	76
	99th	115	116	117	119	120	121	122	80	80	80	81	82	83	83
7	50th	93	93	95	96	97	99	99	55	56	56	57	58	58	59
	90th	106	107	108	109	111	112	113	69	70	70	71	72	72	73
	95th	110	111	112	113	115	116	116	73	74	74	75	76	76	77
	99th	117	118	119	120	122	123	124	81	81	82	82	83	84	84
8	50th	95	95	96	98	99	100	101	57	57	57	58	59	60	60
	90th	108	109	110	111	113	114	114	71	71	71	72	73	74	74
	95th	112	112	114	115	116	118	118	75	75	75	76	77	78	78
	99th	119	120	121	122	123	125	125	82	82	83	83	84	86	86
9	50th	96	97	98	100	101	102	103	58	58	58	59	60	61	61
	90th	110	110	112	113	114	116	116	72	72	72	73	74	75	75
	95th	114	114	115	117	118	119	120	76	76	76	77	78	79	79
	99th	121	121	123	124	125	127	127	83	83	84	84	85	86	87
10	50th	98	99	100	102	103	104	105	59	59	59	60	61	62	62
	90th	112	112	114	115	116	118	118	73	73	73	74	75	76	76
	95th	116	116	117	119	120	121	122	77	77	77	78	79	80	80
	99th	123	123	125	126	127	129	129	84	84	85	86	86	87	88

Table 15-2. BP Levels for Girls by Age and Height Percentile[2,a], continued

Age, y	BP Percentile	SBP, mm Hg Percentile of Height							DBP, mm Hg Percentile of Height						
		5th	10th	25th	50th	75th	90th	95th	5th	10th	25th	50th	75th	90th	95th
11	50th	100	101	102	103	105	106	107	60	60	60	61	62	63	63
	90th	114	114	116	117	118	119	120	74	74	74	75	76	77	77
	95th	118	118	119	121	122	123	124	78	78	78	79	80	81	81
	99th	125	125	126	128	129	130	131	85	85	86	87	87	88	89
12	50th	102	103	104	105	107	108	109	61	61	61	62	63	64	64
	90th	116	116	117	119	120	121	122	75	75	75	76	77	78	78
	95th	119	120	121	123	124	125	126	79	79	79	80	81	82	82
	99th	127	127	128	130	131	132	133	86	86	87	88	88	89	90
13	50th	104	105	106	107	109	110	110	62	62	62	63	64	65	65
	90th	117	118	119	121	122	123	124	76	76	76	77	78	79	79
	95th	121	122	123	124	126	127	128	80	80	80	81	82	83	83
	99th	128	129	130	132	133	134	135	87	87	88	89	89	90	91
14	50th	106	106	107	109	110	111	112	63	63	63	64	65	66	66
	90th	119	120	121	122	124	125	125	77	77	77	78	79	80	80
	95th	123	123	125	126	127	129	129	81	81	81	82	83	84	84
	99th	130	131	132	133	135	136	136	88	88	89	90	90	92	92
15	50th	107	108	109	110	111	113	113	64	64	64	65	66	67	67
	90th	120	121	122	123	125	126	127	78	78	78	79	80	81	81
	95th	124	125	126	127	129	130	131	82	82	82	83	84	85	85
	99th	131	132	133	134	136	137	138	89	89	90	91	91	92	93

Table 15-2. BP Levels for Girls by Age and Height Percentile[2,a], continued

Age, y	BP Percentile	SBP, mm Hg							DBP, mm Hg						
		Percentile of Height							Percentile of Height						
		5th	10th	25th	50th	75th	90th	95th	5th	10th	25th	50th	75th	90th	95th
16	50th	108	108	110	111	112	114	114	64	64	65	66	66	67	68
	90th	121	122	123	124	126	127	128	78	78	79	80	81	81	82
	95th	125	126	127	128	130	131	132	82	82	83	84	85	85	86
	99th	132	133	134	135	137	138	139	90	90	90	91	92	93	93
17	50th	108	109	110	111	113	114	115	64	65	65	66	67	67	68
	90th	122	122	123	125	126	127	128	78	79	79	80	81	81	82
	95th	125	126	127	129	130	131	132	82	83	83	84	85	85	86
	99th	133	133	134	136	137	138	139	90	90	91	91	92	93	93

Abbreviations: BP, blood pressure; SBP, systolic blood pressure; DBP, diastolic blood pressure.

[a]From *Fourth Report on the Diagnosis, Evaluation and Treatment of High Blood Pressure in Children and Adolescents*, National Institutes of Health, 2004.

ing that if an individual's BP level is in the highest quintile, it tends to remain in that quintile.

Prediction of adult cardiovascular disease among youth based on cardiovascular risk factors, including HT, has been demonstrated by epidemiologic studies. Based on autopsy findings in asymptomatic children and young adults who were participants in the Bogalusa heart study, as the number of cardiovascular risk factors increases, the severity of coronary artery atherosclerotic lesions increases.[6] The risk for adult HT is increased if childhood BP levels are in the highest quintile. In addition, boys 5 to 18 years of age and girls 8 to 18 years of age (data from the Fels Longitudinal study) whose SBP levels were higher than acceptable levels were at significantly greater risk for developing adult HT compared with individuals whose BP was rarely found to be above normal.[7] Also, childhood SBP was predictive of adult metabolic syndrome (abdominal obesity, dyslipidemia, elevated BP, and insulin resistance).

The prevalence of HT appears to be increasing as the BP among normal children is also showing an upward trend.[8] The increased prevalence of HT is associated with increased BMI and increasing age.[9] In a school-based BP screening program in Houston, TX, which enrolled more than 5,000 children aged 10 to 19 years, HT was found in 4.5%.[10] As BMI percentile increased, the prevalence of elevated BP increased. The relative risk for HT was 3.26 for children identified as overweight compared with children with normal weight (based on BMI percentile) after controlling for gender, ethnicity, and age.

Factors that affect the likelihood for HT include family history, ponderosity, dietary salt intake, exercise, birth weight, ethnicity, insulin resistance, and stress and sympathetic nervous system activation. The tendency for several cardiovascular risk factors to cluster has been recognized: these include obesity, dyslipidemia, hyperinsulinemia, and altered glucose tolerance.

> **꘎ Pearl**
>
> As BMI percentile increases, the prevalence of elevated BP increases.

Etiology

Children are more likely to have an identifiable cause for HT compared with adults. However, adult essential HT clearly originates during youth. As one moves into the second decade of life, essential HT becomes increasingly prevalent. Essential HT is characterized by mild-to-moderate, often asymptomatic, elevation of BP in the presence of a positive family history or other comorbid conditions such as obesity, insulin resistance, or metabolic syndrome.

Identification of primary HT implies that the search for a cause for HT has been unsuccessful. Because not all hypertensive children are submitted to an exhaustive diagnostic evaluation, the confidence of this diagnosis is variable. There is debate among experts as to how extensive a workup is required for mild HT in a child with obesity and/or a strong family history of HT.

Secondary HT may be transient or chronic. Distinguishing between these 2 possibilities is one goal of the initial evaluation. Common causes of acute, transient HT are listed in Box 15-1, and a list of the most common causes of chronic HT is provided in Box 15-2.[11] In general, secondary HT is caused by renal, cardiac, or neuroendocrine abnormalities. Renal causes, including renal parenchymal disease, renovascular disease, reflux nephropathy, renal scarring, congenital renal diseases, acute renal failure, chronic renal insufficiency, and urinary tract obstruction, comprise the most common forms of secondary HT. The primary cardiac cause of HT is coarctation of the aorta. Neuroendocrine causes are rare but important, and include neuroblastoma, pheochromocytoma, and mineralocorticoid excess states. There are also important causes of transient HT, the most common of which are pain, stress, medication, or neurologic diseases such as increased intracranial pressure, seizures, or Guillain-Barré syndrome.

It is difficult to estimate the frequency of the various causes of HT among children and adolescents. The distribution of causes is likely to vary depending on whether they are reported from a primary care or a tertiary care center. The overall frequency of major causes of HT in the primary care setting is presented in Table 15-3.[11] Secondary HT reported from a tertiary care center comprised 84% of the total, with renal parenchymal disease accounting for 70% within this category. The most common causes of HT occurring in various age groups are shown in Box 15-3.[6]

One may be able to predict whether children in the second decade of life are likely to have primary or secondary HT by use of ambulatory BP monitoring. Ambulatory BP monitoring has gained use as a clinical tool by allowing the assessment of BP during a 24-hour period in a nonmedical set-

Box 15-1. Causes of Acute Hypertension

Renal parenchymal disease
  Postinfectious GN
  Henoch-Schönlein GN
  Hemolytic uremic syndrome
  Acute tubulointerstitial nephritis
  Nephrotic syndrome
  Acute kidney injury
Traumatic injury
  Kidney trauma, particularly to
    vasculature
  Orthopedic trauma requiring
    traction
Acute urinary tract obstruction

Vascular disease
  Renal vein and renal artery
    thrombosis
  Embolic disease to renal vasculature
    (bacterial endocarditis)
  Vasculitis
Neurologic causes
  Increased intracranial pressure
  Seizures
  Guillain-Barré syndrome
  Spinal cord injury
Drug mediated (most common)
  Cocaine/amphetamines, sympath-
    omimetic drugs, corticosteroids,
    oral contraceptives

Abbreviation: GN, glomerulonephritis.

Box 15-2. Causes of Chronic Hypertension

Coarctation of the aorta
Associated with chronic kidney disease
  and ESRD
Parenchymal renal diseases
  Reflux nephropathy
  Chronic glomerular disease
  Congenital renal disease (hypoplasia/
    dysplasia, obstructive uropathy)
  Inherited renal disease (polycystic
    kidney disease, Alport hereditary
    nephritis)
  Acute kidney injury (hemolytic
    uremic syndrome, acute tubular
    necrosis)
Renovascular HT
  Renal artery stenosis
  Takayasu arteritis
  Congenital syndromes (neurofibro-
    matosis, William syndrome)
  External compression

Renal tumor–associated HT
  Wilms tumor
  Hemangiopericytoma
Catecholamine excess
  Pheochromocytoma
  Neuroblastoma
  Paraganglioma
Corticosteroid excess states/low
  renin HT
  Cushing disease
  Conn syndrome
  Liddle syndrome
  Mineralocorticoid excess
  Gordon syndrome

Abbreviations: ESRD, end-stage renal disease; HT, hypertension.

Box 15-3. Common Causes of Hypertension by Age[6]

Newborn
  Vascular disease (thrombosis, renal
  artery stenosis)
  Congenital renal disease
  Coarctation of the aorta
First year of life
  Coarctation of the aorta
  Renovascular disease
  Renal parenchymal disease
Age 1–6 years
  Renal parenchymal disease
  Renovascular disease
  Coarctation of the aorta

Age 6–12 years
  Renal parenchymal disease
  Renovascular disease
  Essential HT
  Coarctation of the aorta
Older than 12 years
  Essential HT
  Renal parenchymal disease
  Iatrogenic HT

Abbreviation: HT, hypertension.

Table 15-3. Frequency of Major Causes of Hypertension in Primary Care Settings[11]

Essential	27%
Obesity-associated	45%
Secondary	28%
Renal parenchymal disease	34%
Coarctation of the aorta	35%
Renovascular	17%
Endocrinopathy	7%
Other	7%

ting. Daytime DBP "load" (which refers to the percent of readings that are greater than normal) and nighttime SBP load were significantly greater in subjects with secondary HT compared with those with suspected primary HT.[12] When daytime DBP load was 25% or higher and nighttime SBP load was 50% or higher, children were more likely to have secondary HT. Normally, BP decreases during sleep; this is known as nocturnal decline. Reduced nocturnal decline in BP was associated with secondary HT, as were increased nighttime SBP and DBP loads.[13]

ᕷ Pearl

Children are more likely to have an identifiable cause for HT than adults.

In contrast to primary HT, secondary HT exhibits more severe BP elevation, which is sustained throughout sleep.

Presenting Symptoms

Hypertension is often silent. Many children exhibit no symptoms in the face of extreme, usually chronic, BP elevation. Acute increases in BP are more likely to be symptomatic. For example, children with acute postinfectious GN may present with acute hypertensive encephalopathy with seizures, visual changes, and mental status alterations, even before the underlying renal involvement is appreciated. Transient blindness and Bell palsy (facial weakness caused by 7th nerve involvement) are rare but important signs of acute, severe HT.

Among children with chronic HT, the most common symptoms reported include headache (42%), trouble falling asleep (27%), fatigue (26%), chest pain (14%), abdominal pain (10%), poor school performance (10%), and trouble concentrating (10%).[14] Most symptoms (except school performance) were found to improve after treatment of HT. Infants and toddlers with HT may present with nonspecific symptoms such as poor growth, general lassitude, tachypnea or tachycardia, feeding intolerance, and irritability. In addition, young children with severe HT may present with signs consistent with congestive heart failure.

Sometimes the presenting symptoms are related to the underlying cause of HT and not to the HT per se. For example, urinary tract complaints such as enuresis, polyuria, or dysuria may indicate congenital urinary tract disease, urinary tract infection, or reflux nephropathy. Edema may be a presenting complaint in acute GN or CKD. Gross hematuria is often the first complaint in both acute and chronic forms of GN. The combination of fatigue, anemia, abnormal urinalysis, and HT may be seen with late presentation of advanced renal insufficiency.

৯ *Pearl*

The most common symptoms of chronic HT include headache, trouble falling asleep, and fatigue.

History and Physical Examination

The patient history should be focused on assessing any symptoms related to HT or to the underlying cause of HT.[15] In addition to those potential symptoms already listed, the following information should be obtained: (1) birth history, including preterm birth, low birth weight, and use of an umbilical artery catheter, along with the history of an abnormal prenatal ultrasound; (2) family history of HT, heart disease, stroke, kidney disease, and diabetes; (3) dietary and medication history, including use of alcohol, illicit drugs, herbal supplements, and nutritional supplements used to enhance athletic performance; and (4) sleep history, especially obstructive sleep apnea.[2] Early onset of HT in multiple family members suggests rare, monogenic forms of HT, such as glucocorticoid remediable aldosteronism, apparent mineralocorticoid excess, Liddle syndrome, and Gordon syndrome.

Physical examination should include vital signs (tachycardia may be a clue) along with height and weight percentiles.[15] Body mass index is helpful in indicating the degree of obesity. Poor growth may be an important clue to underlying chronic disease. Blood pressure should be measured in both upper extremities and at least one lower extremity. Peripheral pulses and femoral pulses should be palpated. Blood pressure levels that are lower in the legs together with weak lower extremity pulses should prompt a physician to look for coarctation of the aorta.

Retinal changes support a diagnosis of severe HT. The finding of café-au-lait spots is an important clue to the underlying diagnosis of neurofibromatosis, which is associated with renovascular HT and pheochromocytoma. In addition, skin rashes may indicate systemic inflammatory diseases such as systemic lupus erythematosus, GN, or vasculitis. Adenoma sebaceum are a characteristic finding in individuals with tuberous sclerosis, which may cause HT from renal cysts or angiomyolipoma. Cushingoid features such a moon facies, acne, and a buffalo hump may support corticosteroid excess—either iatrogenic or endogenous. Acanthosis nigricans is commonly seen in the metabolic syndrome or insulin excess states. The finding of a murmur on cardiac examination may support the diagnosis of coarctation of the aorta. Although not consistently present, abdominal bruits are a classic finding in renal artery stenosis. Abdominal or flank masses would prompt imaging aimed at finding renal or other tumors. Abnormal genitalia may be associated with other developmental abnormalities of the urinary tract: ambiguous genitalia or virilization may be a clue to undiagnosed adrenal hyperplasia. Any clinical clues allow one to narrow the list of potential diagnoses.

Diagnosis

Once the diagnosis of HT is confirmed, and after a comprehensive history and physical examination are completed, a physician may have gained important clues as to the cause of the HT. Laboratory testing and radiographic imaging may follow a logical course if there is a working diagnosis (Box 15-4). Unfortunately, the appropriate diagnostic evaluation for children and adolescents with stage 1 and stage 2 HT is not evidence based. Rather, it follows good clinical judgment. Most experts recommend starting the evaluation with a renal profile: electrolytes, creatinine, BUN, complete blood count, and urinalysis. Hypokalemia may be associated with renal vascular disease, mineralocorticoid excess states, and Liddle syndrome. Hyperkalemia and/or metabolic acidosis may be found in children with chronic renal insufficiency, obstructive uropathy, or Gordon syndrome (distal tubular disorder with HT and hyperkalemic metabolic acidosis). Abnormal elevations of creatinine provide an important clue as to underlying renal insufficiency. In general, abnormal levels of electrolytes, BUN, or creatinine indicate underlying renal disease. The abnormality should be confirmed by repeat testing and requires prompt referral to a pediatric nephrologist.

Examination of the urine is helpful in the evaluation of possible renal causes of HT (see Chapter 3). The finding of hematuria and proteinuria in the presence of HT indicates a strong possibility for underlying GN, which may be acute or chronic (see Chapters 7 and 8). Isolated, heavy proteinuria in a child with elevated BP is also a common presentation for glomerular disease or scarring related to VUR. Renal parenchymal disease becomes a less likely cause of HT if the urinalysis is normal; however, renal vascular disease, scarring related to VUR, cystic kidney disease, and even congenital renal disease are not ruled out by a normal urinalysis. Extremely dilute urine (as seen in obstructive uropathy or congenital renal disease) may be

Box 15-4. Workup of Children With Hypertension

Phase 1

CBC, urinalysis, electrolytes, BUN, creatinine, calcium, uric acid, lipid profile

Renal ultrasound with Doppler

Echocardiogram

Phase 2[a] (may not be required if essential or obesity-related HT is suspected)

Plasma renin activity

Plasma aldosterone

Captopril radionuclide scan

Catecholamine levels in plasma/urine

Angiography +/– renal vein renin sampling

Renal biopsy

MIBG scan

Abbreviations: CBC, complete blood count; BUN, blood urea nitrogen; HT, hypertension; MIBG, metaiodobenzylguanidine.

[a]*Some studies may be included in Phase 1 evaluation depending on symptoms and examination findings.*

misleading, because protein and cellular elements may be negative on the dipstick of dilute urine while their excretion is greater than normal. Urine culture is indicated for children with abnormal urinalysis (pyuria, hematuria) or when lower urinary tract symptoms are present.

Other diagnostic studies may be warranted and are recommended by the Working Group in some cases. Fasting lipid profile and fasting glucose along with a urine drug screen are recommended for adolescents with HT. Plasma renin and aldosterone levels may also be helpful in the diagnostic evaluation of unexplained HT, and they should be obtained before pharmacologic treatment. Low-renin HT may be caused by excessive dietary salt, excess mineralocorticoids or underlying genetic abnormalities of the renal sodium channel, and the condition known as Liddle syndrome. High renin levels increase the suspicion of renal vascular disease. However, treatment of HT with diuretics, vasodilators, and ACE inhibitors may stimulate an increased plasma renin. There may be some use for serum uric acid level because it appears to be a surrogate marker for vascular disease in adults; however, routine measurement of uric acid in children is not recommended.

In younger children, renal ultrasound is indicated to look for congenital renal disease or disparate renal size related to renal scarring. However, a normal renal ultrasound does not eliminate the possibility of renal scarring. Renal imaging may not be indicated in adolescents with metabolic syndrome or suspected obesity-related HT. However, this has not been systematically studied. More detailed renal imaging studies, and especially invasive studies such as angiography, should be performed at tertiary care centers experienced in the evaluation of complicated HT. The use of less invasive renal vascular imaging such as magnetic resonance angiography or computed tomography scan to screen for renal artery stenosis has not been validated in children (see Chapter 5).

Echocardiography has been recommended for children with pre-HT and comorbid conditions (diabetes and renal disease) and for all children with HT.[2] The presence of LV hypertrophy is a clear indication for more aggressive BP-lowering therapy. Again, this is based on sound clinical indications and has not been supported by clinical trials in children and adolescents. One challenge to the reliability of echocardiograms is the variability in their interpretation. The best available method to assess LV mass has been standardized by the American Society for Echocardiography. After careful measurement of LV dimensions, a formula is used to estimate LV mass in grams, which is then standardized to patient height and interpreted according to published normal values.[16]

> ### ⁊❥ Pearl
>
> The presence of LV hypertrophy is a clear indication for more aggressive BP-lowering therapy.

Treatment

Treatment options for children or adolescents with HT include both pharmacologic and nonpharmacologic therapies. Lifestyle changes that may prove beneficial in individuals with pre-HT, or any stage of HT, include weight reduction for those who are overweight, regular physical exercise, and a healthy diet. Initiation of antihypertensive drug therapy is recommended for children with secondary forms of HT and those with primary HT who persist with elevated BP despite attempts at lifestyle change. Individuals with stage 2 HT should start medication after they are identified as such. They should make lifestyle changes and start medication. Individuals with stage 1 HT who have other comorbid conditions, who are symptomatic, who have LV hypertrophy, or who do not respond to lifestyle modification, should start taking an antihypertensive medication.

There are no randomized clinical trials comparing antihypertensive agents in children or adolescents. Certain drugs have been submitted to safety and efficacy trials, yet the specific indication of one class of drugs over another is left to the sound clinical judgment of the physician. The underlying cause of HT may provide a compelling argument for choice of agent: ACE inhibitors (or alternatively, ARBs) are the drugs of choice for hypertensive youth with underlying renal disease or diabetes.[17] In addition to these 2 indications, they also provide a potential benefit in obese patients because they prevent the development of diabetes, a positive effect noted from clinical trials in adults with HT.[18] For children with primary HT, the first choices among pediatric nephrologists are ACE inhibitors (47%) or CCBs (37%), followed by diuretics and beta-blockers. In contrast to treatment of adults with HT, diuretics are rarely the first choice among pediatric nephrologists who treat childhood HT. They are used in combination with other classes of drugs. The most commonly used second-line agents are CCBs (39%) and ACE inhibitors (33%).[17] Both ACE inhibitors and CCBs appear to be well tolerated and may be formulated in a liquid preparation if needed. Beta-blockers have been used to treat pediatric HT for decades and have also undergone safety and efficacy testing. They are well tolerated and may have a specific indication for patients with HT who also have migraine headaches. Beta-blockers are contraindicated in patients with asthma and type 1 diabetes mellitus.

In general, a single agent is started and the dose is increased according to the BP response while the patient is monitored for drug-related side effects. The goal of therapy is to lower BP to a level less than the 95th percentile; however, in individuals with comorbid conditions such as renal disease, diabetes, or cardiac dysfunction, the goal is to lower BP to less than the 90th percentile. An abbreviated list of maintenance antihypertensive drugs is presented in Table 15-4.

ᴆᴄ *Pearl*

The first choices among pediatric nephrologists for the treatment of primary HT in children are ACE inhibitors and CCBs, followed by diuretics and beta-blockers.

Table 15-4. Maintenance Antihypertensive Drugs[2,19] (abbreviated list)	
Drug	Dose
ACE Inhibitors	
Enalapril	Initial: 0.08 mg/kg/d up to 5 mg/day (QD–BID) Maximum: 0.6 mg/kg/d up to 40 mg/d
Lisinopril	Initial: 0.08 mg/kg/d up to 5 mg/d (QD) Maximum: 0.6 mg/kg/d up to 80 mg/d
Angiotensin-Receptor Blocker	
Losartan	Initial: 0.7 mg/kg/d up to 50 mg/d (QD–BID) Maximum: 1.4 mg/kg/d up to 100 mg/d
Beta-Blocker	
Atenolol	Initial: 0.5–1 mg/kg/d (QD–BID) Maximum: 2 mg/kg/d up to 100 mg/d
Calcium Channel Blockers	
Amlodipine	Initial: 0.1–0.2 mg/kg/d (QD) Maximum: 0.6 mg/kg/d up to 10 mg/d
Nifedipine XR	Initial: 0.25–0.5 mg/kg/d Maximum: 3 mg/kg/d up to 120 mg/d
Diuretic	
Hydrochlorothiazide	Initial: 1 mg/kg/d Maximum: 3 mg/kg/d

Abbreviations: ACE, angiotensin-converting enzyme; QD, every day; BID, twice a day.

Emergency Management

It is very difficult to arrive at exact threshold BP levels that define hypertensive emergency (severe HT with acute target organ damage) or hypertensive urgency (severe HT in the absence of noted changes). Children described in early reports of malignant HT had DBP in excess of 120 mm Hg, a level far greater than the 99th percentile for any age. Some experts have defined severe HT as greater than the 99th percentile: the most recent update defines stage 2 HT as a BP level greater than the 99th percentile plus 5 mm Hg. Although more aggressive treatment is recommended for children with stage 2 HT, most do not receive intravenous therapy. Therefore, definition of an exact level of BP that requires intravenous antihypertensive therapy is difficult. The presence of symptoms suggesting hypertensive encephalopathy along with extreme BP elevation (usually ≥99th percentile) would prompt aggressive intravenous therapy, specifically continuous infusion in a critical care setting. There is a potential risk for neurologic sequelae if BP is rapidly lowered during an acute hypertensive crisis. Therefore, BP should be gradually lowered over several days. One recommendation is to reduce BP by one-third of the eventual goal in the first 6 hours, followed by another one-third reduction over the next 24 hours, with a final correction to goal BP in the next 2 to 3 days.[20] The use of agents such as sublingual nifedipine for acute HT is discouraged because they can cause an abrupt drop in BP (often 30 mm Hg).

Agents recommended for children with hypertensive emergency or hypertensive urgency are found in Table 15-5. For a more comprehensive list, refer to one of several excellent resources.[2,19,20] After stabilization of BP, maintenance medications should be started and diagnostic evaluation should follow.

ॐ *Pearl*

During a hypertensive crisis, BP should be lowered gradually over several days.

Table 15-5. Drugs for Management of Hypertensive Emergencies[22,20]	
Drug	**Dose**
Labetalol	Bolus IV: 0.2–1.0 mg/kg/dose up to 40 mg per dose q 4 h Infusion IV: 0.25–3 mg/kg/h
Nicardipine	Infusion IV: 1–3 µg/kg/min
Nitroprusside	Infusion IV: 0.5–10 ug/kg/min
Hydralazine	Bolus IV: 0.2–0.6 mg/kg/dose q 4 h
Enalaprilat	Bolus IV: 0.05–0.1 mg/kg/dose up to 1.25 mg q 6–8 h
Clonidine	PO: 0.05–0.1 mg/dose, may be repeated
Minoxidil	PO: 0.1–0.2 mg/kg/dose

Abbreviations: IV intravenous; q, every; PO, by mouth.

Summary

The prevalence of HT among children and adolescents appears to be increasing. This is largely attributed to the increasing prevalence of obesity in today's youth. However, over the past 2 decades, children have been more likely to have their BP measured and the upper limits of normal have been more precisely defined. These factors may also increase the likelihood that children with increased BP will be detected. Because prevention of future cardiovascular disease is a primary goal of the pediatric medical community, early detection of risk factors such as HT is essential. However, the diagnosis of primary HT during youth is accompanied by many unanswered questions: Will children continue to have HT throughout life? Will they be able to discontinue use of antihypertensive medications? Which children stand to benefit the most from drug therapy? At what BP levels should therapy be initiated? Future studies will be aimed at refining treatment strategies and enabling early detection of vascular disease.

For children with HT who are identified with underlying disease, treatment of that disease in addition to HT undoubtedly provides health benefits. Both aggressive control of HT and use of renoprotective drugs such as ACE inhibitors and ARBs have proven positive effects on the health of children with CKD.

References

1. Bartosh SM, Aronson AJ. Childhood hypertension. An update on etiology, diagnosis, and treatment. *Pediatr Clin North Am.* 1999;46:235–252

2. National High Blood Pressure Education Program Working Group on High Blood Pressure in Children and Adolescents. The fourth report on the diagnosis, evaluation, and treatment of high blood pressure in children and adolescents. *Pediatrics.* 2004;114 (2 suppl 4th Report):555–576

3. Mitsnefes MM. Hypertension in children and adolescents. *Pediatr Clin North Am.* 2006;53:493–512, viii

4. Bruce Z. Morgenstern LB. Casual BP measurement methodology. In: Portman RJ, Sorof JM, Ingelfinger JR eds. *Pediatric Hypertension.* Totowa, NJ: Humana Press; 2004:77–96

5. Chobanian AV, Bakris GL, Black HR, et al. The seventh report of the Joint National Committee on prevention, detection, evaluation, and treatment of high blood pressure: the JNC 7 report. *JAMA.* 2003;289:2560–2572

6. Berenson GS, Srinivasan SR, Bao W, Newman WP III, Tracy RE, Wattigney WA. Association between multiple cardiovascular risk factors and atherosclerosis in children and young adults. The Bogalusa Heart Study. *N Engl J Med.* 1998;338:1650–1656

7. Sun SS, Grave GD, Siervogel RM, Pickoff AA, Arslanian SS, Daniels SR. Systolic blood pressure in childhood predicts hypertension and metabolic syndrome later in life. *Pediatrics.* 2007;119:237–246

8. Luepker RV, Jacobs DR, Prineas RJ, Sinaiko AR. Secular trends of blood pressure and body size in a multi-ethnic adolescent population: 1986 to 1996. *J Pediatr.* 1999;134:668–674

9. Falkner B, Gidding SS, Ramirez-Garnica G, Wiltrout SA, West D, Rappaport EB. The relationship of body mass index and blood pressure in primary care pediatric patients. *J Pediatr.* 2006;148:195–200

10. Sorof JM, Lai D, Turner J, Poffenbarger T, Portman RJ. Overweight, ethnicity, and the prevalence of hypertension in school-aged children. *Pediatrics.* 2004;113:475–482

11. Dillon MJ. Secondary forms of hypertension in children. In: Portman RJ, Sorof JM, Ingelfinger JR, ed. *Pediatric Hypertension.* Totowa, NJ: Humana Press; 2004:159–179

12. Flynn JT. Differentiation between primary and secondary hypertension in children using ambulatory blood pressure monitoring. *Pediatrics.* 2002;110:89–93

13. Seeman T, Palyzova D, Dusek J, Janda J. Reduced nocturnal blood pressure dip and sustained nighttime hypertension are specific markers of secondary hypertension. *J Pediatr.* 2005;147:366–371

14. Croix B, Feig DI. Childhood hypertension is not a silent disease. *Pediatr Nephrol.* 2006;21:527–532

15. Brewer ED. Evaluation of hypertension in childhood diseases. In: Avner ED, Harmon WE, Niaudet P, ed. *Pediatric Nephrology.* 5th ed. Philadelphia, PA: Lippincott, Williams & Wilkins; 2004:1179–1197

16. Daniels SR, Meyer RA, Strife CF, Lipman M, Loggie JM. Distribution of target-organ abnormalities by race and sex in children with essential hypertension. *J Hum Hypertens.* 1990;4:103–104

17. Woroniecki RP, Flynn JT. How are hypertensive children evaluated and managed? A survey of North American pediatric nephrologists. *Pediatr Nephrol.* 2005;20:791–797

18. Jandeleit-Dahm KA, Tikellis C, Reid CM, Johnston CI, Cooper ME. Why blockade of the renin-angiotensin system reduces the incidence of new-onset diabetes. *J Hypertens.* 2005;23:463–473

19. Blowey DL. Approach to the pharmacologic treatment of pediatric hypertension. In: Portman RJ, Sorof, JM, Ingelfinger RJ, ed. *Pediatric Hypertension.* Totowa, NJ: Humana Press; 2004:429–442

20. Adelman RD, Coppo R, Dillon MJ. The emergency management of severe hypertension. *Pediatr Nephrol.* 2000;14:422–427

Chapter 16

Genetic Diseases of the Kidney

John Foreman

Introduction

The number of genes associated with renal disease is increasing every day. The discovery of new genes has led to a clearer understanding of renal disease pathophysiology in many disorders. It is now known that many genetic renal syndromes are caused by a mutation in a number of genes. Genetic testing also has made possible the identification of some renal diseases without the need for invasive procedures. Genetic testing allows the prenatal diagnosis of certain renal diseases in a fetus at risk or identification of a potential problem before it has become manifest. Finally, identification of a specific gene mutation holds the possibility of correction through gene therapy, although gene therapy remains only a promise at this point in time.

The first step in identifying a genetic renal disorder is to consider it. A gene mutation should be thought of if another family member is affected, if there are other malformations in addition to the renal disease, or if the clinical course is different from that of the typical patient with the disorder. A primary care pediatrician can play an important role in this regard.

However, there are a number of problems associated with genetic testing that primary care pediatricians must keep in mind. First, the identification of a gene mutation for many renal diseases remains a research procedure that requires informed consent, and often this information cannot be used for making clinical decisions. Furthermore, most genetic disorders are caused by many gene mutations in multiple genes, making it difficult to identify the precise mutation in the right gene in a given patient. Most commercial genetic testing laboratories can only identify the common mutations, thereby missing some patients. Finally, patients and/or their parents need to understand that the genetic test itself carries the risk of labeling someone as a carrier or a potential victim of a particular disease, which may have implications for future insurability or employment. Some genetic disorders with a known gene defect are presented in Table 16-1.

> ### ⧉ Pearl
>
> A gene mutation should be thought of if another family member is affected, if there are other malformations, or if the clinical course is atypical.

Alport Syndrome

Hereditary nephritis, or Alport syndrome, is a progressive form of glomerular disease often associated with neural deafness and eye abnormalities.[1] It occurs in approximately 1 in 5,000 live births and accounts for 2% of the new cases of ESRD.

Alport syndrome occurs from a mutation in the genes coding for the alpha-3, -4, or -5 chains of type IV collagen.[2] These 3 chains in concert make up type IV collagen, which is found in the basement membrane of the glomerulus, cochlea, and eye. The most common form of Alport syndrome is a mutation in COL4A5 located on the X chromosome coding for the alpha-5 (IV) chain and accounts for about 80% of patients with Alport syndrome. Males are severely affected, whereas most females have only hematuria; however, some female carriers do develop renal failure. Approximately 15% of patients with Alport syndrome have an autosomal recessive inheritance pattern and the mutation is in both the COL4A3 or COL4A4 genes carried on chromosome 2. The remaining patients are heterozygous for a mutation

Table 16-1. Some Genetic Disorders Associated With Renal Disease

Disorder	Inheritance	Gene Defect	Genetic Test	Manifestation/ Outcome
Glomerular Disorders				
Alport syndrome	XL	COL4A5	Y	Hematuria, eventually ESRD
	AR	COL4A3 or COL4A4	Y	Hematuria, eventually ESRD
Thin basement membrane	AD	COL4A3 or COL4A4	Y	Hematuria
Atypical HUS	AR	CHF	Y	HUS
	AR	IF	Y	HUS
	AR	MCP	Y	HUS
	AR	ADAMTS13	N	HUS
Glomerular Disorders—Steroid-Resistant Nephrotic Syndrome				
Finnish CNS	AR	NPHS1	Y	Neonatal NS
SRNS	AR	NPHS2	Y	Early-onset NS
SRNS	AD	ACTN4	N	Teen-to-adult–onset NS
SRNS	AD	TRPC6	N	Teen-to-adult–onset NS
Nail–patella syndrome	AD	LMX1B	Y	Dysplastic nails and patellae, proteinuria
Denys-Drash syndrome	Sporadic	WT1	Y	Male pseudohermaphroditism, NS, Wilms tumor
Cystic Disorders				
Juvenile nephronophthisis	AR	NPHP1	Y	Interstitial fibrosis, microcysts, ESRD
Infantile nephronophthisis	AR	NPHP2	N	Interstitial fibrosis, microcysts, situs inversus, ESRD
Adolescent nephronophthisis	AR	NPHP3	N	Interstitial fibrosis, microcysts, ESRD
Type IV nephronophthisis	AR	NPHP4	N	Interstitial fibrosis, microcysts, ESRD
Medullary cystic disease 1	AD	Unknown	N	Interstitial fibrosis, microcysts, ESRD
Medullary cystic disease 2	AD	UMOD	Y	Interstitial fibrosis, microcysts, hyperuricemia, ESRD
ARPKD	AR	PKHD1	Y	Nephromegaly, microcysts, hypertension, ESRD

Table 16-1. Some Genetic Disorders Associated With Renal Disease, continued

Disorder	Inheritance	Gene Defect	Genetic Test	Manifestation/ Outcome
Cystic Disorders, continued				
ADPKD	AD	PKD1	Y	Nephromegaly, macrocysts, hypertension, ESRD
ADPKD	AD	PKD2	Y	Nephromegaly, macrocysts, hypertension, ESRD
Tuberous sclerosis	AD	TSC1, TSC2	Y	MR, seizures, facial angioma, renal cysts, renal angiomyo-lipoma
Tubular Disorders				
Renal glucosuria	AR	SLC5A2	Y	Renal glucosuria
Cystinuria type A	AR	SLC3A1	Y	Cystinuria, stones
Cystinuria type B	AR	SLC7A9	Y	Cystinuria, stones
Hypophos-phatemic rickets	XL	PHEX	Y	Hypophosphatemia, rickets
Tubular Disorders—RTA				
Proximal RTA	AR	SLC4A4	N	MR, acidosis, eye disorders
Proximal RTA	AD	Unknown	N	Acidosis
Distal RTA	AD	SLC4A1	Y	Acidosis, stones, nephrocal-cinosis
Distal RTA	AR	ATP6V1B1	Y	Deafness, acidosis, stones, nephrocalcinosis
Distal RTA	AR	ATP6V0A4	Y	Acidosis, stones, nephrocal-cinosis
Tubular Disorders—Metabolic Alkalosis				
Bartter syndrome type 1	AR	SLC12A1	N	Neonatal onset of hypokale-mia, metabolic alkalosis
Bartter syndrome type 2	AR	KCNJ1	N	Neonatal onset of hypokale-mia, metabolic alkalosis
Bartter syndrome type 4	AR	BSND	N	Deafness, neonatal onset of hypokalemia, metabolic alkalosis
Bartter syndrome type 3	AR	CLCNKB	N	Hypokalemia, metabolic alkalosis
Gitelman syn-drome	AR	SLC12A3	Y	Hypomagnesemia, hypocalce-mia, hypokalemia, metabolic alkalosis, tetany

Table 16-1. Some Genetic Disorders Associated With Renal Disease, continued

Disorder	Inheritance	Gene Defect	Genetic Test	Manifestation/ Outcome
Tubular Disorders—Diabetes Insipidus				
Nephrogenic diabetes insipidus	XL	AVPR2	Y	Hypernatremia, polyuria, polydipsia
Nephrogenic diabetes insipidus	AR	AQP2	N	Hypernatremia, polyuria, polydipsia
Structural Disorders				
Barakat syndrome	AR	GATA3	Y	Hypoparathyroidism, deafness, renal disease
Bardet-Biedl syndrome	AR	Multiple BBS genes, MKKS	Y	Renal dysplasia, obesity, MR, polysyndactyly, retinopathy, hypogonadism
Brachio-oto-renal syndrome	AD	EYA1	Y	Branchial cleft remnant, deafness, renal dysplasia
Vesicoureteral reflux	AD	Unknown	N	Vesicoureteral reflux

Abbreviations: XL, X-linked; AR, autosomal recessive; Y, yes; ESRD, end-stage renal disease; HUS, hemolytic uremic syndrome; AD, autosomal dominant; N, no; NS, nephrotic syndrome; CNS, congenital nephrotic syndrome; SRNS, steroid-resistant nephrotic syndrome; ARPKD, autosomal recessive polycystic kidney disease; ADPKD, autosomal dominant polycystic kidney disease; RTA, renal tubular acidosis; MR, mental retardation.

in the COL4A3 or COL4A4 gene, yet have progressive renal disease, albeit more slowly progressive than males with X-linked disease.

The initial manifestation in patients with Alport syndrome is microhematuria that is present early in life. In time these patients develop hypertension, proteinuria, and progressive renal insufficiency. End-stage renal disease usually occurs in males by the end of adolescence or early adulthood. The most common extrarenal manifestation of Alport syndrome is progressive sensorineural hearing loss that can be detected in childhood. Female heterozygotes of X-linked Alport syndrome can also develop sensorineural deafness, but it appears much later in life. Anterior lenticonus of the cornea occurs in 20% to 30% of males with X-linked Alport syndrome and is diagnostic. Rarely, males with X-linked Alport syndrome and female carriers can develop leiomyomas of the esophagus, and female carriers can develop leiomyomas of the genitalia.

The diagnosis of Alport syndrome is usually indicated by the presence of hematuria in a patient with family history of renal failure and deafness, especially if it affects the mother's male relatives. In about 15% of cases there is no family history because the case represents a new COL4A5 mutation or is an autosomal recessive form of Alport syndrome. The diagnosis is usually made by a renal biopsy showing thin GBMs with a laminated appearance. This can be confirmed by staining the GBM for the components of type IV collagen. The alpha-5 (IV) chain is also present in the epidermal basement membrane. Its absence in a skin biopsy from a male or a mosaic expression in a female by immunostaining with an antibody against the alpha-5 (IV) chain is also diagnostic of X-linked Alport syndrome. However, 20% of affected males have positive staining, so a positive result does not exclude the diagnosis of Alport syndrome. Genetic testing for Alport syndrome is difficult and not currently commercially available. The presence of sensorineural hearing loss is another diagnostic clue for Alport syndrome.

Included in the differential diagnosis for Alport syndrome in young children are the other causes of microhematuria (see Chapter 7). A family history of microhematuria indicates the possibility of Alport syndrome or another GBM disorder, such as thin basement membrane disease. The history of ESRD in other family members, especially maternal male family members, is an important diagnostic clue for Alport syndrome. Early onset of deafness in male family members is another useful diagnostic symptom.

There is no specific treatment for Alport syndrome, and children suspected of having this disorder should be referred early to a pediatric nephrologist who will assist in making the diagnosis and monitoring for the complications of the syndrome. However, regular pediatric care should be given by a primary care physician because most of these children have normal renal function throughout childhood. Angiotensin-converting enzyme inhibitors may be useful in preserving renal function in patients with hypertension and/or proteinuria. Alport syndrome does not occur in a renal transplant, but 3% to 4% of patients with Alport syndrome who have received transplants develop anti-GBM antibodies and a crescentic glomerulonephritis.

♔ Pearl

Alport syndrome is suspected in a patient with hematuria and family history of renal failure or deafness.

Thin Basement Membrane Disease
(Benign Familial Hematuria)

Thin basement membrane disease is a relatively common familial disorder.[3] It also has been called *benign familial hematuria* because this is the only symptom in most affected individuals. The hallmark is thin GBMs detected by a renal biopsy. It is inherited in an autosomal dominant pattern and in most families the defect is a mutation in either COL4A3 or COL4A4, the genes coding for alpha-3 and alpha-4 chains of type IV collagen.[2] These are the same genes associated with autosomal recessive Alport syndrome. Patients with thin basement membrane disease are carriers of autosomal recessive Alport syndrome, but they rarely have significant proteinuria or progress to renal failure. They also do not develop hearing loss or eye changes. They can have gross hematuria and occasionally flank pain. A few families have also had hypercalciuria and/or hyperuricosuria.

The diagnosis of thin basement membrane disease can only be made with certainty by a renal biopsy demonstrating thin GBMs. In young children the biopsy can be difficult to interpret because they have thinner basement membranes than adults, so it is not easy to differentiate normal thickness from abnormal in young children. Furthermore, it is sometimes difficult to distinguish Alport syndrome from thin basement membrane disease in the young child because the renal biopsy findings in young children with these 2 disorders are quite similar. However, patients with thin basement membrane disease rarely have a family history of ESRD compared with families with Alport syndrome. The differential diagnosis would include other causes of asymptomatic microscopic hematuria, including immunoglobulin A nephropathy, hypercalciuria, and early stages of Alport syndrome (see Chapter 7).

Children with suspected thin basement membrane disease should be referred early to a pediatric nephrologist who will aid in the diagnosis, especially if a renal biopsy is needed to confirm the diagnosis. However, not all children with thin basement membrane disease need a renal biopsy, particularly if the family history is consistent with this disorder and there are no other abnormalities aside from hematuria. Testing a patient's parents and sometimes other family members for the presence of microhematuria can aid in the diagnosis of thin basement membrane disease in an otherwise asymptomatic child with microhematuria.

There is no specific treatment for thin basement membrane disease. Although most patients have only asymptomatic microhematuria, patients with thin basement membrane disease should get regular follow-up care, usually through the primary care physician, to look for signs suggestive of the onset of more worrisome renal disease such as hypertension and/or proteinuria.

Genetic Atypical Hemolytic Uremic Syndrome

Several rare gene mutations can lead to atypical HUS. These patients usually present with typical HUS—with microangiopathic anemia, thrombocytopenia, and renal insufficiency—except they do not have a diarrheal prodrome.[4] Patients with these disorders usually have a more insidious onset, often in association with an upper respiratory disease. They also usually have evidence of complement activation with a low C3 complement level. They typically have a relapsing course, often resulting in irreversible renal failure and sometimes death.

The most common genetic defect in atypical HUS is a defect in factor H, coded for on the short arm of chromosome 1.[5] Like factor H, genetic defects in other complement regulatory proteins, membrane complement protein and factor I, can also cause atypical HUS. Mutations in any of these proteins, even a heterozygous mutation, can lead to unregulated complement activation, endothelial cell injury, activation of the clotting system, and the development of HUS. A few patients have been described with genetic defects in the von Willebrand cleavage factor that allow the circulation of abnormally large multimers of von Willebrand factor, leading to platelet activation and HUS.

The diagnosis of these genetic forms of HUS is difficult. Features that suggest a genetic form of HUS include lack of a diarrheal prodrome, recurrent disease, family history of HUS, and evidence of complement activation. Most forms require identification of the mutated gene for definitive diagnosis, yet for all of these diseases, genetic testing is only available in research laboratories at present. The differential diagnosis for atypical HUS includes genetic disorders, certain malignancies, *Streptococcus pneumoniae* infections, human immunodeficiency virus, bone marrow transplantation, and association with a number of medications.

Management of these patients requires several specialists, and these children should be referred early to a center experienced in caring for them. Aside from supportive measures, the mainstay of therapy is replacement of the missing plasma factor, which requires plasmapheresis. In spite of therapy, there is a high likelihood of ESRD and death. There is also a high likelihood of recurrence of the disease in a renal transplant.

¿● Pearl

Lack of a diarrheal prodrome, recurrent disease, family history of HUS, and evidence of complement activation suggest a genetic form of HUS.

Finnish-Type Congenital Nephrotic Syndrome

Congenital NS of the Finnish type is a rare autosomal recessive disorder. The highest incidence is in Finland, where it occurs with an incidence of 1 in 10,000 newborns.[6] It is much rarer in other countries. It is caused by a defect in the gene NPHS1, which codes for the protein nephrin, found in the slit diaphragm between podocytes. The podocyte is the epithelial cell on top of the glomerular capillary basement membrane and is the final barrier to proteins moving from the capillary to the urine. The NPHS1 gene is found on the long arm of chromosome 19.

Infants with Finnish-type congenital NS have massive proteinuria that begins in utero. Most of these infants are born prematurely and often have large placentas that weigh more than 25% of their birth weight. Edema is either present at birth or appears shortly afterward. The heavy proteinuria causes very low serum albumin levels, often less than 1 g/dL, along with low immunoglobulin G vitamin D, thyroglobulin-binding proteins, antithrombin III, and transferrin levels. The urinary protein losses and anorexia lead to malnutrition and poor somatic growth. Infants with this disorder are highly susceptible to bacterial infections, including peritonitis, cellulitis, and pneumonia. The loss of thyroglobulin and vitamin D–binding proteins leads to hypothyroidism and vitamin D deficiency. Thromboembolic complications are also common. Initially, the renal function is normal, but it declines after the first year of life. Until recently, most of these children died in the first year of life because of infection and inanition.

A renal biopsy is helpful in making the diagnosis, but there are no pathognomonic features specific to Finnish-type congenital NS. Irregular dilation of the proximal convoluted tubules is the most characteristic feature, with some increase in mesangial matrix and cellularity. With time the glomeruli become sclerotic with increasing interstitial fibrosis.

The diagnosis is suspected in any infant with the onset of nephrotic syndrome early in life. Genetic testing is available for the common mutations of the NPHS1 gene and can obviate the need for a renal biopsy. A prenatal diagnosis can be made by demonstrating high levels of alphafetoprotein in the amniotic fluid. Other diseases presenting in the first weeks of life with NS include idiopathic NS, congenital infections (especially syphilis, toxoplasmosis, and cytomegalovirus), diffuse mesangial sclerosis, and podocin mutations.

Finnish-type congenital NS is very challenging to manage, and patients should be referred early to a center experienced in the care of these infants. The NS is resistant to corticosteroids, and corticosteroids increase the risk of infection in an infant already immunocompromised from immunoglobulin losses. Daily infusions of albumin and diuretics are used to manage the edema. Gamma globulin infusions are helpful in preventing infections. Often these infants require tube feeding to maintain adequate calories. Angiotensin-converting enzyme inhibitors and indomethacin are helpful in reducing the proteinuria, but many infants require bilateral nephrectomy and dialysis to stop the massive protein loss and malnutrition. Renal transplants can be successful if the affected infant can reach a size that will allow a transplant kidney to be placed, which is usually 8 to 10 kg.

Steroid-Resistant Nephrotic Syndrome

Although most pediatric patients with NS respond to steroids, approximately 20% to 40% do not (see Chapter 9). Of those who do not, it is estimated that 10% to 20% have a genetic disorder that causes NS.[7] A number of gene mutations have been described in this subset of patients with SRNS. Besides a defect in the gene NPHS1, which codes for nephrin, the most common genetic cause of SRNS is a defect in the gene NPHS2, which encodes for the protein podocin and is located on the short arm of chromosome 1.[8] It is inherited in an autosomal recessive manner. Genetic testing for podocin mutations is commercially available. The onset of this disorder occurs between 3 months and 5 years of age, with rapid progression to renal failure. There is a wide range of renal pathologic findings varying from virtually no abnormalities to focal segmental sclerosis. Podocin appears to help form and align nephrin in the slit diaphragm and connect it to the CD2 adapter protein on the podocyte. There is no specific therapy for this disorder, but most patients do not have a recurrence after a transplant.

Two autosomal dominantly inherited forms of SRNS have been described. The first described was a mutation in the gene coding for alpha-actinin-4 protein, located on the short arm of chromosome 19.[9] Alpha-actinin-4 plays an important role in maintaining the cytoskeleton of the podocyte. This NS typically appears in adults, with variable age of onset and rate of progression to renal failure.

The second autosomal dominant form of SRNS is caused by a mutation in the gene coding for the transient receptor potential cation calcium 6 (TRPC6) protein, located on the short arm of chromosome 11.[10] This is the first ion channel to be associated with NS, and the mutation in this channel leads to increased intracellular calcium in the podocyte, which seems to interfere with cell function or increased apoptosis of the podocyte, leading to proteinuria and NS. The onset of NS in most patients with this defect has been in the third or fourth decade of life.

Denys-Drash, Frasier, and WAGR Syndromes

Denys-Drash, Frasier, and WAGR (Wilms tumor, aniridia, genitourinary anomalies, and mental retardation) syndromes have in common a mutation in the WT1 gene located on the long arm of chromosome 11. These are rare disorders and are usually associated with spontaneous germline mutations. In most cases, there is no family history to suggest a genetic disease. Management of these syndromes is complicated, and affected patients should be referred early to a specialized center.

Denys-Drash syndrome presents in infancy with NS and ambiguous genitalia. These patients have diffuse mesangial glomerulosclerosis on kidney biopsy.[11] They also often develop Wilms tumor. Nephrotic syndrome is refractory to immunosuppressive therapy, and patients who have it usually progress to renal failure by 3 years of age. Frasier syndrome is similar, but the renal disease consists of focal and segmental glomerulosclerosis, it presents later in childhood, and it is not associated with Wilms tumor. There is no specific therapy for either syndrome, and renal disease in both syndromes is unresponsive to immunosuppression.

The differential diagnosis for Denys-Drash syndrome is the same as for causes of infantile NS, such as congenital nephrotic syndrome of the Finnish type. Frasier syndrome should be suspected in any child with SRNS and ambiguous genitalia and in females with NS and primary amenorrhea.[12] Genetic testing is only available in a research laboratory.

WAGR syndrome includes Wilms tumor, aniridia, genitourinary malformations, and mental retardation.[13] It is caused by a deletion of a band of chromosome 11p13 that includes the WT1 gene and PAX6 gene necessary for normal eye development. Patients with WAGR syndrome present at birth with aniridia and various genitourinary malformations. They are at high risk for the later development of Wilms tumor. This syndrome should be suspected in any baby with aniridia, especially in association with genitourinary abnormalities. Patients should be referred early to a tertiary care facility because they will require the services of subspecialists. Many patients with this syndrome eventually develop renal failure. The diagnosis can be made by fluorescent in situ hybridization demonstrating the deletion on chromosome 11.

Nephronophthisis

Nephronophthisis is a group of rare autosomal recessive disorders characterized by progressive renal failure associated with tubulointerstitial fibrosis.[14] It is probably the most common genetic cause of renal failure in the first 3 decades of life, accounting for 2% to 10% of ESRD in children. The symptoms of nephronophthisis are insidious. Patients initially present with polyuria and polydipsia and may have recurrent episodes of dehydration, usually after the first years of life. Later, as renal failure ensues, they develop anemia and growth failure. The renal failure is progressive, and most patients develop ESRD in their teenage years. Kidneys from patients with nephronophthisis show tubulointerstitial fibrosis, disruption of the tubular basement membrane, and small cysts at the corticomedullary junction.

The most common form of nephronophthisis is caused by a mutation in NPHP1, which maps to chromosome 2q12 and codes for nephrocystin.[15] Another form of nephronophthisis is caused by a mutation in NPHP2, located on chromosome 9q21-22, which encodes for the protein inversin.[16]

Patients with this form of nephronophthisis present with ESRD before age 5 and may have situs inversus. Mutations in the NPHP3 gene on chromosome 3q22 cause an adolescent form of nephronophthisis with progression to ESRD at a median age of 19 years.[17] In some families, the renal disease has been associated with hepatic fibrosis or tapetoretinal degeneration. The proteins from the genes associated with nephronophthisis localize to primary cilia, centrosomes, and the connections between renal tubular cells and play a role in cell-cell and cell-matrix signaling.

The differential diagnosis of nephronophthisis includes other forms of insidious but progressive renal disease, such as renal hypoplasia or dysplasia, obstructive uropathy, and reflux nephropathy. The diagnosis is suggested by the clinical picture and the renal biopsy, although there is nothing pathognomonic on the biopsy. Genetic testing demonstrating a homozygous mutation is definitive, and tests are commercially available for NPHP1, the most common form of nephronophthisis. As soon as this disorder is suspected, refer patients to a pediatric nephrologist who will aid in diagnosing and managing them. Aside from treating the complications of renal insufficiency and the inability to conserve salt and water, there is no specific therapy.

Polycystic Kidney Disease

There are many renal diseases, both genetic and congenital, that are associated with multiple cysts of one or both kidneys. However, the term *polycystic kidney disease* is reserved for 2 specific hereditary kidney diseases: ADPKD and ARPKD. The most common form of polycystic kidney disease in children is ARPKD.[18] Autosomal recessive polycystic kidney disease, previously called infantile polycystic kidney disease, typically presents in infancy, although there are childhood and adolescent forms that are generally less severe. The estimated incidence is 1 in 10,000 to 1 in 40,000 children. Autosomal recessive polycystic kidney disease is always associated with hepatic involvement, which is characterized by cysts, fibrosis, and portal hypertension. The presentation can be quite variable even within a family.[19] About one-third of affected infants present in the neonatal period with marked nephromegaly, poor renal function, and oligohydramnios with pulmonary hypoplasia. Such infants can be detected by a fetal ultrasound showing large echogenic kidneys. The cysts are microscopic in size and not detected by ultrasonography. Many of these infants die of respiratory failure in the first few days of life. If they survive the first few days of life, renal function often improves, but infants presenting in the first year of life develop ESRD, usually by late childhood. Hypertension is common and often severe. All patients with an infantile presentation will have a urinary concentrating defect and can have a defect in renal acidification.

Another third of patients with ARPKD present after infancy, either with hypertension as the initial symptom or hematemesis from esophageal varices.[20] Often, in this group, hepatic fibrosis with subsequent portal hypertension, hypersplenism, and esophageal varices is the major initial problem. Later, these children develop chronic renal failure, although this may not occur until adulthood. Another third may not present until they are older than 20 years.

Kidneys of patients with ARPKD are enlarged and show microcysts, usually only a few millimeters in diameter as a result of ectasia of the collecting ducts (Figure 16-1). The liver shows enlargement of the portal spaces because of fibrosis and bile duct proliferation and dilation. Autosomal recessive polycystic kidney disease is caused by a mutation in the very large gene

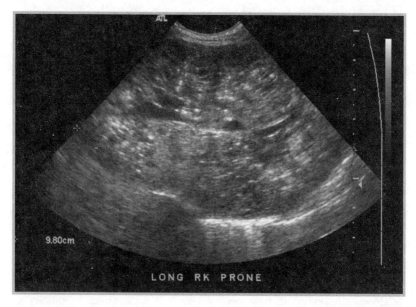

Figure 16-1.
Sonogram of an infant with autosomal recessive polycystic kidney disease. The kidney is enlarged and echogenic.

PHKD1, which codes for the protein fibrocystin and is localized to the long arm of chromosome 6.

The differential diagnosis of typical ARPKD is quite limited because most infants with large, echogenic kidneys on renal ultrasound have ARPKD. Renal pathology demonstrating tubular ectasia is usually not necessary. Genetic testing is not commercially available yet. Refer patients to a center experienced with these children as soon as the diagnosis is suspected, especially if detected on a prenatal ultrasound because the initial management is quite complicated. There is no specific therapy.

Autosomal dominant polycystic kidney disease usually presents in adults, but can be seen in children and, rarely, even in neonates.[21] It occurs in 1 out of 400 to 2,000 live births, although it is estimated that only half of affected patients are diagnosed because many patients have clinically silent disease. Approximately 86% of affected families have an abnormality on chromosome 16 (PKD1 gene). Most of the remaining families have a mutation on chromosome 4 (PKD2 gene), and the location of the mutation in a few families remains to be identified.[22] Patients are usually found because of a positive family history, which is the most common way for pediatric patients to be identified. Other presenting complaints include flank pain, gross hematuria from cyst rupture, and renal insufficiency. The diagnosis is made by the presence of at least 2 renal cysts, especially if they are bilateral, in patients younger than 30 years, because simple renal cysts are uncommon in this age group. In patients older than 30 years, more than 2 cysts and bilateral involvement are necessary for the diagnosis. In a study of more than 100 potentially affected children, more than 60% of children with a PKD1 mutation had ultrasonically detectable cysts. Other studies have shown a much lower rate, so children of affected parents cannot be said to be free of the disease unless they have no cysts in either the liver or kidneys visible by computed tomography scanning and are older than 25 years. Genetic testing for PKD1 and PKD2 genes is commercially available.

The natural history of ADPKD is to develop cysts of increasing size and numbers, leading to massive nephromegaly and renal failure (Figure 16-2). Although ADPKD can lead to renal failure in childhood, it commonly does not occur until middle age.[23] Negative prognostic factors include early age at diagnosis, male gender, hypertension, proteinuria, rapid increase in cyst growth, and the PKD1 as opposed to the PKD2 genotype. Although there

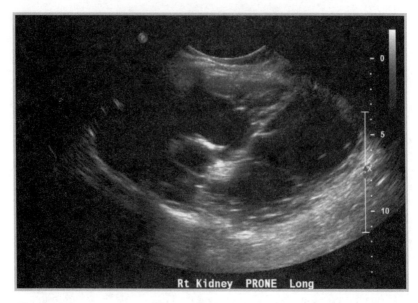

Figure 16-2.
Sonogram of a child with autosomal dominant polycystic kidney disease. The kidney is enlarged with large cysts.

is some difference between families with the PKD1 mutation and the PKD2 mutation, there is considerable variability within a family with regard to the onset of disease manifestations related to other modifier genes.

There is no specific therapy for ADPKD. Early treatment of hypertension, especially with an angiotensin-converting enzyme inhibitor, slows the progression of the renal failure. Children with ADPKD usually have few symptoms and problems until adulthood and can be managed by the general pediatrician, although referral to a pediatric nephrologist is helpful in making the diagnosis and with management.

There are a number of extrarenal manifestations of ADPKD.[24] Hepatic cysts are common, especially in women. Typically they are asymptomatic, but occasionally they can become quite large and cause pain. They occasionally can become infected. Mild cardiac valvular lesions can occur in 25% to 30% of patients with ADPKD. The most worrisome extrarenal manifestation is cerebral aneurysm. The risk in young adults is 4%, rising to as high as 10% in older patients. The risk

> 🐚 *Pearl*
>
> The most common form of polycystic kidney disease presenting during childhood is ARPKD.

is increased in families with a history of aneurysms or cerebral bleeding. The role of screening is unclear because the risk is low and the complications associated with the treatment of asymptomatic aneurysms are many. Routine screening is recommended for high-risk patients only, such as patients with a family history of aneurysms or intracerebral bleeding or patients with symptoms suggestive of an aneurysm.

Vesicoureteral Reflux

Family studies have shown that VUR is a heritable disorder. The gene responsible for VUR has not been identified yet, although approximately 30% of the siblings of index cases of VUR also have VUR.[25] The inheritance pattern is thought to be autosomal dominant with incomplete penetrance. Therefore, siblings of index cases, especially younger siblings, should be screened for VUR. The management and natural history of VUR is discussed in Chapters 6 and 18.

> **Pearl**
>
> Thirty percent of siblings of index cases of VUR have VUR.

Renal Disorders in Other Syndromes and Chromosomal Abnormalities

A number of syndromes and chromosomal abnormalities are associated with renal disorders. Most are associated with renal malformations such as hypoplasia or dysplasia, cysts, obstruction, and reflux. Therefore, children with renal malformations should be examined for other malformations that could lead to a unifying diagnosis. Correctly identifying a syndrome or chromosome abnormality aids in looking for other anomalies, helps direct these children to the proper services and specialists for care, and aids in assessing the future. This is an important role for the primary care pediatrician. Appendix IV lists many of these syndromes and chromosomal malformations. Common syndromes in which renal abnormalities are seen include VATER syndrome (verte-

> **Pearl**
>
> Children with renal malformations should be examined for other malformations that could lead to a unifying diagnosis.

bral defects, anal atresia, tracheoesophageal fistula, esophageal atresia, and radial dysplasia); VACTERAL, which is an expanded listing of the VATER syndrome that includes cardiac and limb abnormalities; and CHARGE syndrome (coloboma, heart defects, atresia choanae, retarded growth and development, genitourinary abnormalities, and ear anomalies or deafness). Trisomy 8, 13, and 18 are commonly associated with renal abnormalities, whereas the most common trisomy syndrome, trisomy 21, is infrequently associated with renal disorders. Some of the chromosome deletion syndromes are also associated with renal abnormalities. The most common is Turner syndrome (XO), in which the most common renal malformation is a horseshoe kidney. Other chromosome deletion and monosomies are listed in Appendix IV.

References

1. Kashtan CE. Familial hematuria due to type IV collagen mutations: Alport syndrome and thin basement membrane nephropathy. *Curr Opin Pediatr.* 2004;16:177–181

2. Torra R, Tazon-Vega B, Ars E, Balarin J. Collagen type IV (alpha3-alpha4) nephropathy: from isolated haematuria to renal failure. *Nephrol Dial Transplant.* 2004;19:2429–2432

3. Rana K, Wang YY, Powell H, et al. Persistent familial hematuria in children and the locus for thin basement membrane nephropathy. *Pediatr Nephrol.* 2005;20:1729–1737

4. Noris M, Remuzzi G. Hemolytic uremic syndrome. *J Am Soc Nephrol.* 2005;16:1035–1050

5. Warwicker P, Goodship THJ, Donne RL, et al. Genetic studies into inherited and sporadic hemolytic uremic syndrome. *Kidney Int.* 1998;53:836–844

6. Papez KE, Smoyer WE. Recent advances in congenital nephrotic syndrome. *Curr Opin Pediatr.* 2004;16:165–170

7. Boute N, Gribouval O, Roselli S, et al. NPHS2, encoding the glomerular protein podocin, is mutated in autosomal recessive steroid-resistant nephrotic syndrome. *Nat Genet.* 2000;24:349–354

8. Schultheiss M, Ruf MG, Mucha BE, et al. No evidence for genotype/phenotype correlation in NPHS1 and NPHS2 mutations. *Pediatr Nephrol.* 2004;19:1340–1348

9. Kaplan JM, Kim SH, North KN, Renneke H,et al. Mutations in ACTN4, encoding alpha-actinin-4, cause familial focal segmental glomerulosclerosis. *Nat Genet.* 2000;24:251–256

10. Winn MP, Conlon PJ, Lynn KL, et al. A mutation in the TRPC6 cation channel causes familial focal segmental glomerulosclerosis. *Science.* 2005;308:1801–1804

11. Drash A, Sherman F, Hartmann WH, Blizzard RM. A syndrome of pseudohermaphroditism and Wilms' tumor, hypertension, and degenerative renal disease. *J Pediatr.* 1970;76:585–593

12. Moorthy AV, Chesney RW, Lubinsky M. Chronic renal failure and XY gonadal dysgenesis: "Frasier" syndrome—a commentary on reported cases. *Am J Med Genet Suppl.* 1987;3:297–302

13. Fishbach BV, Trout KL, Lewis J, Luis CA, Sika M. WAGR syndrome: a clinical review of 54 cases. *Pediatrics.* 2005;116:984–988

14. Watnick T, Germino G. From cilia to cyst. *Nat Genet.* 2003;34:355–356

15. Hildebrandt F, Otto E, Rensing C, et al. A novel gene encoding an SH3 domain protein is mutated in nephronophthisis type 1. *Nat Genet.* 1997;17:149–153

16. Otto EA, Schermer B, Obara T, O'Toole JF. Mutations in INVS encoding inversin cause nephronophthisis type 2, linking renal cystic disease to the function of primary cilia and left-right axis determination. *Nat Genet.* 2003;34:413–420

17. Olbrich H, Fliegauf M, Hoefele J, Kispert A. Mutations in a novel gene, NPHP3, cause adolescent nephronophthisis, tapeto-retinal degeneration and hepatic fibrosis. *Nat Genet.* 2003;34:455–459

18. Parfrey PS. Autosomal-recessive polycystic kidney disease. *Kidney Int.* 2005;67:1638–1648

19. Guay-Woodford LM, Desmond RA. Autosomal recessive polycystic kidney disease: the clinical experience in North America. *Pediatrics.* 2003;111:1072–1080

20. Alvarez F, Bernard O, Brunelle F. Congenital hepatic fibrosis in children. *J Pediatr.* 1981;99:370–375

21. Sedman A, Bell P, Manco-Johnson M, et al. Autosomal dominant polycystic kidney disease in childhood. A longitudinal study. *Kidney Int.* 1987;31:1000–1005

22. Peters DJ, Spruit L, Ravine D, et al. Chromosome 4 localization of a second gene for autosomal dominant polycystic kidney disease. *Nat Genet.* 1993;5:359–362

23. Abdollah Shamshirsaz A, Reza Bekheirnia M, Kamgar M, et al. Autosomal-dominant polycystic kidney disease in infancy and childhood: progression and outcome. *Kidney Int.* 2005;68:2218–2224

24. Watson ML. Complications of polycystic kidney disease. *Kidney Int.* 1997;51:353–365

25. Chertin B, Puri P. Familial vesicoureteral reflux. *J Urol.* 2003;169:1804–1808

Prenatal Diagnosis of Renal and Urinary Tract Abnormalities

Eliza M. F. Berkley and Alfred Z. Abuhamad

Abbreviations

ADPKD	Autosomal dominant polycystic kidney disease
PUV	Posterior urethral valve
UPJ	Ureteropelvic junction
UVJ	Ureterovesical junction
VUR	Vesicoureteral reflux

Introduction

Ultrasound is crucial to prenatal diagnosis and antenatal management of genitourinary abnormalities, which comprise approximately half of all fetal malformations. Accurate diagnosis and long-term outcome assessments over the past decade have greatly enhanced our ability to provide informative genetic counseling for families diagnosed with fetal renal and urinary tract anomalies.

Embryology

Prenatal ultrasonography is an invaluable tool in the diagnosis of fetal genitourinary abnormalities. Because sound waves readily penetrate fluid-filled structures, prenatal ultrasound is an excellent means to detect common fetal renal anomalies. Following the prenatal diagnosis of a genitourinary abnormality, thorough evaluation of the entire fetal anatomy is performed to provide accurate prenatal diagnosis and genetic counseling. The prenatal and postnatal risks, suspected course, and potential treatment options can then be discussed with the patient.

Knowledge of embryology is crucial in understanding normal and abnormal renal development. The proximity and complexity of the development of the urinary and genital systems results in a high incidence of fetal malformations.[1] Development of the urinary tract starts with embryonic folding of mesoderm during the fourth embryonic week, which gives rise to the urogenital ridge. From the urogenital ridge, a longitudinal mass known as the *nephrogenic cord* arises, and out of this the mesonephric duct develops. The mesonephric duct serves as a temporary excretory organ from the fourth through the eighth week after fertilization. The caudal segment of the duct opens into the cloaca, and the remainder differentiates into mesonephric vesicles, tubules, and glomeruli.[2]

In the fifth week, a diverticulum of the mesonephric duct anatomically close to the cloaca forms; it is called the *ureteric bud.* The stalk of this diverticulum will form the ureter when it is incorporated into the bladder wall. The tip of the diverticulum, or ampulla, expands and undergoes 15 subdivisions that eventually result in the renal collecting tubules. Dilation of these tubules during weeks 10 to 14 creates the renal pelvis and the major and minor calices.[1] Lack of this ureteric bud induction may result in renal agenesis. The relationship of the ureteric ampulla and the metanephric blastema derived from the nephrogenic cord is essential for creation of the urinary nephrons. Approximately 10 to 13 weeks after fertilization, urine production begins.[2]

Between weeks 5 and 8 after fertilization, the kidneys ascend to the level of the first through third lumbar spine. Arrest of this ascent may result in a horseshoe or pelvic kidney. In the seventh week after fertilization, as the metanephric ducts migrate they approach the aortic bifurcation, and if fusion occurs it results in a single horseshoe kidney blocked from further migration by the inferior mesenteric artery. Similarly, the umbilical artery may trap one kidney in the pelvis.[1]

> ❧ **Pearl**
>
> Urine production begins in weeks 10 to 13 of gestation.

Normal Anatomy

The fetal kidneys may be imaged as early as 9 weeks and should be visualized after 13 weeks on ultrasound examination. They appear as bilateral hyperechoic structures in a paraspinal location (Figure 17-1). The renal pelvis is often seen as an echolucent area within the kidney. The kidneys continue to grow throughout pregnancy, but the ratio of the kidney circumference to the abdominal circumference remains approximately the same at 0.3.

The bladder is visualized as a central sonolucent area within the fetal pelvis, and when using color Doppler the umbilical arteries are noted to bifurcate around it. It normally fills and empties approximately every 30 minutes. The ureters are not typically seen, and if noted raise concern for obstruction.

Until 16 weeks of gestation, amniotic fluid, which ranges from 500 mL to 2 L, is transudate from maternal plasma.[3] After 16 weeks, the amniotic fluid is largely urine produced by the fetal kidneys. The volume peaks at the end of the second trimester and gradually decreases late in the third trimester.[4] The amniotic fluid is hypotonic secondary to excessive renal tubule reabsorption of sodium and chloride over water.[5] In fact, prognosis of fetal renal function can be made by evaluating the amniotic fluid when treating fetuses with bilateral hydronephrosis and suspected bladder outlet obstruction. Glick et al[6] showed that those with normal hypotonic urine had good renal function. Furthermore Crombleholme et al[7] assessed fetal urine electrolyte levels and renal appearance and showed they were helpful in predicting neonatal outcome.

Between 18 and 20 weeks of gestation, a fetal anatomical survey is routinely performed, at which time the kidneys are seen as hyperechoic structures compared with the surrounding bowel. In a coronal plane, the adrenal gland appears as a hypoechoic crescent-shaped structure just superior to the kidney, and the psoas muscle borders the kidney medially. Within the kidney, the renal pyramids are noted as hypoechoic. In a transverse plane, the kidneys appear circular and the renal pelvis is easily visualized and can be measured. At less than 33 weeks of gestation, the measurement should be no greater than 4 mm. From 33 weeks until term, the normal pelvic measurement may increase to 7 mm.

> ### ﻬ Pearl
> Fetal kidneys should be visualized on ultrasound after 13 weeks.

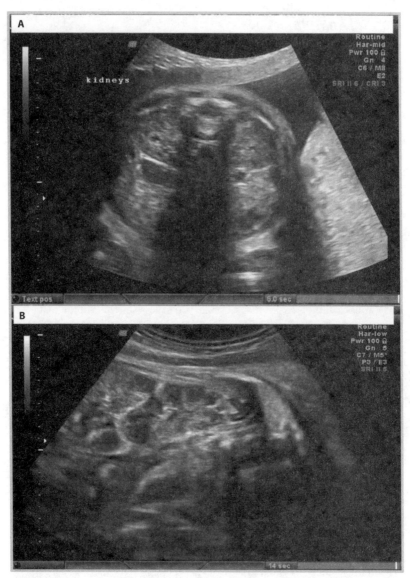

Figure 17-1.
Abdominal ultrasound showing normal fetal kidneys. **A.** Transverse plane of the fetal kidneys in a paraspinal location. **B.** Sagittal plane of a fetal kidney.

Hydronephrosis

Genitourinary tract anomalies may complicate 1% of pregnancies. The most common of these abnormalities is hydronephrosis, which may result from both obstructive and nonobstructive conditions. Hydronephrosis is usually diagnosed when the renal pelvis or calices are dilated. There is some debate over the degree of dilation that defines hydronephrosis, but anteroposterior renal pelvic diameters greater than 10 mm have been correlated with postnatal abnormalities[8,9] (Figure 17-2).

Many physicians use cutoff values of 4 and 7 mm for a gestational age less than and greater than 33 weeks, respectively. Using these cutoff criteria, Stocks et al[10] showed an increased incidence of UPJ obstruction. In addition, VUR has been observed in 12% of babies that had a fetal renal pelvic measurement between 4 and 10 mm.[11] Calyceal dilation also predicts more significant hydronephrosis.[12] Therefore, fetuses with pelvic diameters between 5 and 10 mm with associated calyceal dilation require follow-up ultrasound assessments in the third trimester and postnatally.

The goal of prenatal diagnosis is to determine the level of obstruction or cause of the hydronephrosis. Kaefer et al[13] showed that oligohydramnios

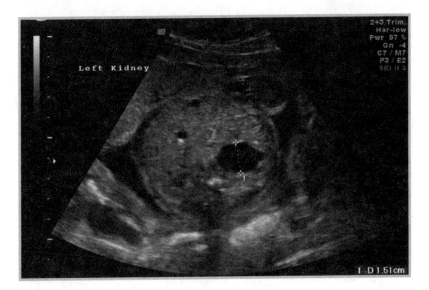

Figure 17-2.
Unilateral hydronephrosis. Abdominal ultrasound of the fetal kidneys in a transverse plane with the left renal pelvis measuring more than 10 mm in the anterior to posterior diameter.

and renal echogenicity predicted an obstructive etiology with a sensitivity of 100% and a specificity of 93%. Prenatal diagnosis also seeks to evaluate the fetal well-being, establish the gestational age and amniotic fluid level, and assess the need for any potential treatment or follow-up. If there is unilateral hydronephrosis, and the amniotic fluid volume is normal, there is no need for intervention. However, bilateral hydronephrosis with oligohydramnios and a dilated bladder, suggesting bladder outlet obstruction in a karyotypically normal fetus, may warrant prenatal intervention with a vesicoamniotic shunt. The Society of Fetal Urology grading system for anatomically detected hydronephrosis is presented in Figure 5-4, and the workup of prenatally detected hydronephrosis is presented in Figure 5-5.

ह Pearl

In the presence of unilateral hydronephrosis and normal amniotic fluid volume, there is no need for intervention.

Ureteropelvic Junction Obstruction

The obstruction of urine flow from the renal pelvis to the ureter, UPJ obstruction, is the most common cause of fetal hydronephrosis. The condition is unilateral in 90% of cases and more common in males.[14] The etiology of this congenital condition is unknown but may result from increased muscle thickness at the UPJ.

Diagnosis of UPJ obstruction is made when pelvicaliceal dilation is seen without evidence of ureteral enlargement, ectopic ureterocele, or bladder or posterior urethral dilation. The renal pelvis often appears "rounded" or "blunted" (Figure 17-3). In addition, oligohydramnios is rare and polyhydramnios may be seen. Progression of pelvic dilation occurs in less than half of the kidneys, but when noted increases the likelihood of postnatal surgery. Severe obstruction may result in rupture of the renal pelvis, development of a paranephric urinoma, and subsequent loss of renal function.

Twenty-five percent of contralateral kidneys have anomalies such as renal agenesis, VUR, or dysplasia.[15] Associated anomalies are seen in 12% of fetuses.[16] Prognosis of unilateral or bilateral UPJ obstruction without these additional findings is excellent, but postnatal follow-up is warranted.

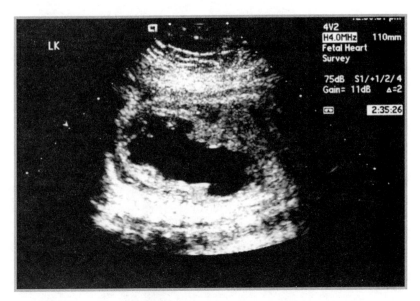

Figure 17-3.
Abdominal ultrasound in the sagittal plane of a fetal kidney with ureteropelvic junction obstruction. The renal pelvis is dilated and appears rounded, and the cortex is thin.

Ureterovesical Junction Obstruction

Ureterovesical junction obstruction is the least common cause of obstructive hydronephrosis. Stenosis, obstruction, or a lack of peristalsis of the distal ureter causes dilation of the renal pelvis and ureter. Like UPJ obstruction, UVJ obstruction is more common in males. Oligohydramnios is rare in unilateral obstruction but may be seen in bilateral obstruction. Again, renal anomalies may be seen in the contralateral kidney. The prognosis, even in bilateral UVJ obstruction, is good, and conservative management is the norm. However, ureteral enlargement greater than 10 mm usually requires surgical treatment.[17]

More commonly, ureterovesical pathology is the result of ureteral duplication with an ectopic ureter. Ultrasound findings include a dilated ureter with upper pole hydronephrosis and a cystic structure in the bladder. This ectopic ureterocele usually arises from the upper pole and is the result of stenosis at the level of the bladder. The duplex ureter may also be dilated secondary to ectopic insertion into the vagina, urethra, seminal vesicle, or vas deferens with increased pressure from the closed bladder neck. Resultant ureteral obstruction leads to hydronephrosis and cystic dysplasia.[18]

Sonographic detection of a hydroureter should suggest the possibility of a duplex ureter and a normal renal lower pole (Figure 17-4). When the lower pole is affected, this is usually secondary to VUR. Reflux is more common with a ureterocele than an ectopic ureter. If the ureterocele is large, the opposite kidney may become obstructed or urethral herniation may result in bladder outlet obstruction.[19] Unilateral involvement carries a good prognosis.

A third cause of ureteropelvic pathology is congenital megaloureter. This condition is more common in boys and more commonly seen on the left side. There has been documentation of spontaneous regression. However, a full postnatal evaluation of all of these UVJ pathologies is necessary.

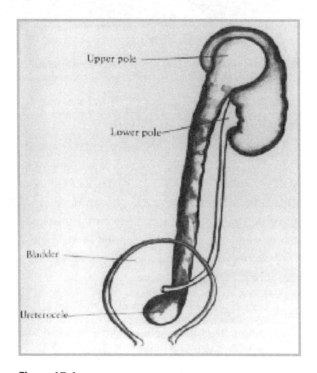

Figure 17-4.
The typical renal duplex anomaly diagnosed prenatally. A cystlike upper pole, a dilated ureter draining the upper pole, and a ureterocele in the bladder are common prenatal sonographic signs.

Bladder Outlet Obstruction and Posterior Urethral Valves

Bladder outlet obstruction almost always affects male fetuses secondary to PUVs. This condition affects approximately 1 in 5,000 to 8,000 newborns. Rarely, it may be seen in females as a result of a cloacal malformation.

A dilated bladder with a thickened bladder wall and dilated posterior urethra giving the appearance of a keyhole are characteristic signs of PUVs[20] (Figure 17-5). A massive bladder with bladder wall trabeculations may be identified on ultrasound examination. Ureteral dilation and bilateral hydronephrosis are also common. The obstruction may cause such high pressure that rupture of the bladder or kidney may occur and lead to urinary ascites. Oligohydramnios, cortical cysts, increased renal echogenicity, urinomas, urinary ascites, and early diagnosis confer a poor prognosis.[21-24]

Severe oligohydramnios and bilateral renal dysplasia lead to the development of Potter syndrome with pulmonary hypoplasia. In addition, it creates a Potter facies with low-set ears, micrognathia, and limb contractures. This has also been proposed as the cause of prune-belly syndrome, characterized by loose abdominal wall muscles and urinary tract defects.

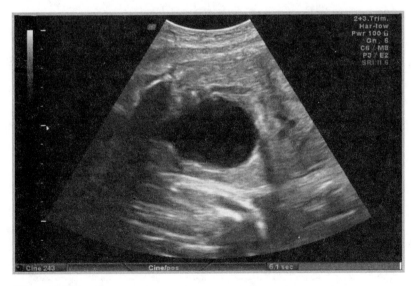

Figure 17-5.
Posterior urethral valves. A sagittal section through the fetal abdomen reveals a dilated bladder and posterior urethra, giving a keyhole appearance.

Pregnancy termination or conservative management with comfort care at delivery may be offered in cases with poor prognostic signs. In contrast, if the amniotic fluid volume remains normal and the hydronephrosis remains stable, repeat assessment with ultrasound until delivery at term is offered. The best predictor of renal function is provided through serial amniocentesis with bladder aspirations to assess urine electrolytes[25] (Table 17-1). In addition, after excluding other anomalies and verifying a normal karyotype, placement of a vesicoamniotic shunt can help decompress the bladder and kidneys if the gestation is less than 32 weeks. After 32 weeks, delivery with corrective surgery is recommended.[26]

♂ Pearl

Renal function can be predicted by bladder aspirations to assess urine electrolytes.

Similar to PUVs, urethral atresia and congenital megaloureter will result in bladder outlet obstructions. Marked bladder dilation, bilateral hydronephrosis, and oligohydramnios are usually seen on ultrasound. There is an increased risk of chromosomal defects, including trisomy 13, 18, and 21, in addition to a high risk of associated anomalies such as VATER.[27]

Megacystis-Microcolon-Intestinal Hypoperistalsis Syndrome

The rare megacystis-microcolon-intestinal hypoperistalsis syndrome has a female preponderance yet appears to have an autosomal recessive mode of inheritance. As the name implies, noted findings include a dilated bladder and a microcolon with a small bowel obstruction or malrotation. Although

Table 17-1. Fetal Urinary Biochemistry: Predictors of Good Renal Function[a]	
Chemical	**Measurement (mg/dL)**
Sodium	<100
Chloride	<90
Osmolality	<200
Calcium	<8 mg
β_2-Microglobulin	<4
Total protein	<20

[a]Reprinted with permission from Callen PW. *Ultrasonography in Obstetrics and Gynecology.* 4th ed. Philadelphia, PA: WB Saunders Co; 2000.

amniotic fluid volume may be normal, the prognosis is poor.[28] Vesicoamniotic shunting has not been found to improve outcomes in these pregnancies.

Vesicoureteral Reflux

Vesicoureteral reflux is the retrograde flow of urine from the bladder into the ureters and back to the renal pelvis. It affects 1% of all children and is believed to be responsible for up to 50% of childhood urinary tract infections.[29] In addition, VUR may account for 10% of fetal unilateral or bilateral hydronephrosis. Prenatal diagnosis has shown an increased incidence in males and a high recurrence rate in offspring.

Antenatal management includes repeat ultrasound assessment of the kidneys and amniotic fluid volume in the third trimester. Most cases have a normal amniotic fluid volume. Postnatal evaluation with ultrasound and/or a micturating cystoure-throgram is recommended. Although one-quarter to one-half of cases may resolve after birth, prophylactic antibiotics are probably beneficial.[5]

✐ Pearl

Vesicoureteral reflux accounts for 10% of fetal hydronephrosis.

Nonhydronephrotic Fetal Renal Abnormalities

Renal Agenesis

High-resolution real-time ultrasonography and color Doppler have increased the accuracy of diagnosing renal agenesis. Before making the diagnosis, it is important to rule out renal ectopia, severe hypoplasia, or the possibility of technical difficulties caused by fetal positioning and severe oligohydramnios. One may consider making the diagnosis of bilateral renal agenesis after excluding the preceding conditions and observing severe oligohydramnios, absence of the kidneys and bladder during a prolonged ultrasound examination of 60 to 90 minutes, and nonvisualization of the renal arteries with color Doppler[30] (Figure 17-6). In addition, an attempt to visualize the adrenal glands should be made. The lack of kidneys allows the adrenal glands to appear flat, with parallel hypoechoic and hyperechoic lines representing the adrenal cortex and medulla, respectively. The "lying down" adrenal sign also helps confirm renal agenesis.[31] Thorough ultrasound evaluation is crucial for prenatal counseling and management because bilateral

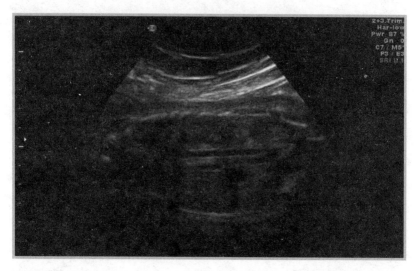

Figure 17-6.
Renal agenesis. Abdominal ultrasound in a coronal plane of the fetal pelvis with the aorta in the midline and absence of the kidneys. Severe oligohydramnios secondary to renal agenesis is noted.

renal agenesis is a lethal condition. Elective termination or expectant management may be offered.

> *Pearl*
>
> A thorough ultrasound evaluation is crucial for prenatal counseling of bilateral renal agenesis.

Unilateral renal agenesis, however, is usually a solitary finding with normal renal function and a normal life expectancy. An ultrasound is important to exclude other anomalies, because unilateral renal agenesis may be part of the VACTERL syndrome (vertebral defects, anal atresia, congenital cardiac disease, tracheoesophageal fistula, renal abnormalities, radial dysplasia, and other limb defects).

Renal Cystic Disease

Multicystic Dysplastic Kidneys

The most common cause for renal cysts in the fetus is a multicystic dysplastic kidney. Most cases are sporadic and unilateral, with an incidence of approximately 1 in 3,000 live births.[32] However, contralateral renal anomalies are observed in close to 40% of cases. The etiology of multicystic dysplasia is believed to be failed growth of the ureteric bud into the meta-nephros, creating early and severe renal obstruction.[33]

Ultrasound findings include multiple noncommunicating cysts of various sizes throughout the kidney (Figure 17-7). The ureter and bladder are not involved and thus appear normal. Unless there is bilateral involvement, the amniotic fluid level is normal. With bilateral multicystic renal dysplasia, the bladder is not visualized and oligohydramnios is present. This condition leads to lethal pulmonary hypoplasia.

Multicystic dysplasia is not to be confused with hydronephrosis, in which multiple cysts may be seen but careful evaluation reveals communication between them. Three-dimensional ultrasound with an inverse mode may help differentiate between these 2 potential etiologies.

Unilateral multicystic renal dyspla-sia has a good prognosis if the opposite kidney is normal. Typically, the normal kidney measures more than 90% of full size. Prenatal management includes repeat

⋙ *Pearl*

Neonatal renal evaluation of a multicystic dysplastic kidney is recommended.

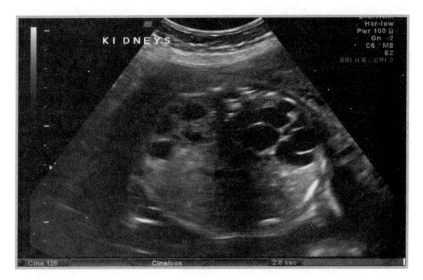

Figure 17-7.
Multicystic dysplastic kidneys. Abdominal ultrasound of the fetal pelvis in a transverse plane with the kidneys in a paraspinal location showing multiple dilated cysts of various shapes and sizes in no distinct pattern, most consistent with a multicystic dysplastic kidney.

ultrasound examination in the third trimester to assess both kidneys. Neo-natal renal evaluation is also recommended because there are rare reports of malignant transformation. Because most dysplastic kidneys involve in the first few years, most are managed conservatively.[34]

Autosomal Recessive Polycystic Kidney Disease

Autosomal recessive polycystic kidney disease has an incidence of about 1 in 45,000 live births (Chapter 16). The diagnosis is usually made after identifying bilaterally enlarged, echogenic kidneys with a small or absent bladder and oligohydramnios (Figure 16-1). At delivery, Potter facies and pulmonary hypoplasia result from severe oligohydramnios.[35,36] Autosomal recessive polycystic kidney disease cannot be excluded until late in the third trimester. Occasional first trimester cases have been detected based on endovaginal ultrasound measurements revealing enlarged kidneys and faster than normal growth. Prenatal diagnosis can be made with detection of the gene for infantile polycystic kidney disease on the short arm of chromosome 6.[37]

Autosomal Dominant Polycystic Kidney Disease

Autosomal dominant polycystic kidney disease is a genetic disorder with an incidence of 1 in 1,000 live births. It is characterized by cyst formation in the kidneys and liver, as well as other organs, and presents in adult life with renal failure and hypertension (Chapter 16). At diagnosis, enlarged echogenic kidneys with multiple cysts of varying size may be seen on ultrasound[38] (Figure 16-2). Rarely, this condition may be diagnosed during prenatal ultrasound examination. If associated anomalies are noted, an amniocentesis for karyotype should be offered. Even if ultrasound reveals otherwise normal fetal morphology, a prenatal diagnosis of adult polycystic kidney disease carries a poor prognosis. The outcome is more severe, with close to 50% mortality in infancy.[39]

Most cases are caused by a mutation on chromosome 16, but approximately 5% are connected with chromosome 4.[40,41] As such, prenatal diagnosis with chorionic villus sampling or amniocentesis can be provided. Again, if there is a family history of ADPKD, one must be careful not to exclude this diagnosis early in gestation because the kidneys may appear normal.

❧ Pearl

Prenatal diagnosis of ADPKD carries a poor prognosis.

Summary

Fetal genitourinary abnormalities range from incidental findings to lethal anomalies. Prenatal diagnosis of these findings using ultrasound has greatly enhanced our understanding of these conditions and at times has allowed us to intervene and improve the outcome. However, there is a dearth of high-quality evidence to guide clinical management in certain rare conditions like lower urinary tract obstructions. In select cases of genitourinary anomalies, fetal intervention has been shown to improve outcome. For instance, placing a vesicoamniotic shunt in fetuses with bladder outlet obstruction has resulted in a lower incidence of pulmonary hypoplasia.[42] Further research is needed, however, to fully explore the value of prenatal intervention. Therefore, continued research and randomized multicentered trials are ongoing to answer these questions.

References

1. DeUgarte CM, Bast JD. Embryology of the urogenital system and congenital anomalies of the female genital tract. In: DeCherney AH, Nathan L, Goodwin TM, Laufer N, eds. *Current Diagnosis and Treatment Obstetrics and Gynecology.* 10th ed. New York, NY: McGraw-Hill; 2007:64–94

2. O'Rahilly R, Müller F. *Human Embryology and Teratology.* New York, NY: Wiley-Liss; 1992:193–199

3. Behrman RE, Parer JT, De Lannoy CW Jr. Placental growth and the formation of amniotic fluid. *Nature.* 1967;214:678–680

4. Queenan JT, Thompson W, Whitfield C. Amniotic fluid volume in normal pregnancy. *Am J Obstet Gynecol.* 1972;114:34–38

5. Hubert KC. Current diagnosis and management of fetal genitourinary abnormalities. *Urol Clin North Am.* 2007;34:89–101

6. Glick PL, Harrison MR, Golbus MS, et al. Management of the fetus with congenital hydronephrosis, II: prognostic criteria and selection for treatment. *J Pediatr Surg.* 1985;20:376–387

7. Crombleholme TM, Harrison MR, Golbus MS, et al. Fetal intervention in obstructive uropathy: prognostic indicators and efficacy of intervention. *Am J Obstet Gynecol.* 1990;162:1239–1244

8. Tam JC, Hodson EM, Choong KK, et al. Postnatal diagnosis and outcome of urinary tract abnormalities detected by antenatal ultrasound. *Med J Aust.* 1994;160:633–637

9. Dillon E, Walton SM. The antenatal diagnosis of fetal abnormalities: a 10-year audit of influencing factors. *Br J Radiol.* 1997;70:341–346

10. Stocks A, Richards D, Frentzen B, Richard G. Correlation of renal pelvic anteroposterior diameter with outcome in infancy. *J Urol.* 1996;155:1050–1052

11. Marra G, Barbieri G, Dell'Angola CA, Caccamo ML, Castellani MR, Assael BM. Congenital renal damage associated with primary vesicoureteral reflux detected prenatally in male infants. *J Pediatr.* 1994;124:726–730

12. Grignon A, Filion R, Filiatrault D, et al. Urinary tract dilatation in utero: classification and clinical applications. *Radiology.* 1986;160:645–647

13. Kaefer M, Peters CA, Retik AB, Benacerraf BB. Increased renal echogenicity: a sonographic sign for differentiating between obstructive and nonobstructive etiologies of in utero bladder distension. *J Urol.* 1997;158:1026–1029

14. Kleiner B, Callen P, Filly R. Sonographic analysis of the fetus with ureteropelvic junction obstruction. *Am J Roentgenol.* 1987;148:359–363

15. Drake DP, Stevens PS, Eckstein HB. Hydronephrosis secondary to ureteropelvic obstruction in children: a review of 14 years of experience. *J Urol.* 1978;119:649–651

16. Bosman G, Reuss A, Nijman JM, Wladimiroff JW. Prenatal diagnosis, management and outcome of fetal ureteropelvic junction obstruction. *Ultrasound Med Biol.* 1991;17:117–120

17. Liu HY, Dhillon HK, Yeung CK, Diamond DA, Duffy PG, Ransley PG. Clinical outcome and management of prenatally diagnosed primary megaureters. *J Urol.* 1994;152:614–617

18. Abuhamad AZ, Horton CE, Evans AT. Renal duplication anomalies in the fetus: clues for prenatal diagnosis. *Ultrasound Obstet Gynecol.* 1996;7:174–177

19. Sherer DM, Menashe M, Lebensart P, Matoth I, Basel D. Sonographic diagnosis of unilateral fetal renal duplication with associated ectopic ureterocele. *J Clin Ultrasound.* 1989;17:371–373

20. Cendron M, Elder JS, Duckett JW. Perinatal urology. In: Gillenwater JY, Grayhack JT, Howard SS, Duckett JW, eds. *Adult and Pediatric Urology.* 3rd ed. St Louis, MO: Mosby Year-Book; 1996:2075

21. Jee LD, Rickwood AM, Turnock RR. Posterior urethral valves: does prenatal diagnosis influence prognosis? *Br J Urol.* 1993;72:830–833

22. Kaefer M, Keating M, Adams M, Rink R. Posterior urethral valves: pressure pop-offs and bladder function. *J Urol.* 1995;154:708–711

23. Hutton KAR, Thomas DFM, Davies B. Prenatally detected posterior urethral valves: qualitative assessment of second trimester scans and prediction of outcome. *J Urol.* 1997;158:1022–1025

24. Hutton KA, Thomas DF, Arthur RJ, Irving HC, Smith SE. Prenatally detected posterior urethral valves: is gestational age at detection a predictor of outcome? *J Urol.* 1994;152:698–701

25. Crombleholme TM, D'Alton M, Cendron M, et al. Prenatal diagnosis and the pediatric surgeon: the impact of prenatal consultation on perinatal management. *J Pediatr Surg.* 1996;31:156–163

26. Cendron M, D'Alton ME, Crombleholme T. Prenatal diagnosis and management of the fetus with hydronephrosis. *Semin Perinatol.* 1994;18:163–181

27. Hayden SA, Russ PD, Pretorius DH, Manco-Johnson ML, Clewell WH. Posterior urethral obstruction: prenatal sonographic findings and clinical outcome in fourteen cases. *J Ultrasound Med.* 1988:371–375

28. Stamm E, King G, Thickman D. Megacystis-microcolon-intestinal hypoperistalsis syndrome: prenatal identification in siblings and review of the literature. *J Ultrasound Med.* 1991;10:599–602

29. Ferrer FA, McKenna PH, Hochman HI, Herndon A. Results of a vesicoureteral reflux practice pattern survey among American Academy of Pediatrics, section on pediatric urology members. *Am Urol Assoc.* 1998;160:1031–1037

30. Romero R, Cullen M, Grannum P, et al. Antenatal diagnosis of renal anomalies with ultrasound, III: bilateral renal agenesis. *Am J Obstet Gynecol.* 1985;151:38–43

31. Hoffman CK, Filly RA, Callen PW. The "lying down" adrenal sign: a sonographic indicator of renal agenesis or ectopia in fetuses and neonates. *J Ultrasound Med.* 1992;11:533–536

32. Gough DC, Postlethwaite RJ, Lewis MA, Bruce J. Multicystic renal dysplasia diagnosed in the antenatal period: a note of caution. *Br J Urol.* 1995;76:244–248

33. Thomsen HS, Levine E, Meilstrup JW, et al. Renal cystic diseases. *Eur Radiol.* 1997;7: 1267–1275

34. Strife JL, Souza AS, Kirks DR, Strife CF, Gelfand ML, Wacksman J. Multicystic dysplastic kidney in children: US follow-up. *Radiology.* 1993;186:785–788

35. Osathanondh V, Potter EL. Pathogenesis of polycystic kidneys: type 1 due to hyperplasia of interstitial portions of collecting tubules. *Arch Pathol.* 1964;77:466–473

36. Blyth H, Ockenden BG. Polycystic disease of kidney and liver presenting in childhood. *J Med Genet.* 1971;8:257–284

37. Guay-Woodford LM, Muecher G, Hopkins SD, et al. The severe perinatal form of autosomal recessive polycystic kidney disease maps to chromosome 6p21.1-p12: implications for genetic counseling. *Am J Hum Genet.* 1995;56:1101–1107

38. Parfrey PS, Bear JC, Morgan J, et al. The diagnosis and prognosis of autosomal dominant polycystic kidney disease. *N Engl J Med.* 1990;323:1085–1090

39. MacDermot KD, Saggar-Malik AK, Economides DL, Jeffery S. Prenatal diagnosis of dominant polycystic kidney disease (PKD1) presenting in utero and prognosis for every early onset disease. *J Med Genet.* 1998;35:13–16

40. Reeders ST, Breuning MH, Davies KE, et al. A highly polymorphic DNA marker linked to adult polycystic kidney disease on chromosome 16. *Nature.* 1985;317:542–544

41. Kimberling WJ, Kumar S, Gabow PA, Kenyon JB, Connolly CJ, Somlo S. Autosomal dominant polycystic kidney disease: localization of the second gene to chromosome 4q13-q23. *Genomics.* 1993;18:467–472

42. Clark TJ, Martin WL, Divakaran TG, Whittle MJ, Kilby MD, Khan KS. Prenatal bladder drainage in the management of fetal lower urinary tract obstruction: a systematic review and meta-analysis. *Obstet Gynecol.* 2003;102:367–382

Chapter 18

Pediatric Urology and Congenital Anomalies of the Kidney and Urinary Tract

Andy Y. Chang and Douglas A. Canning

Abbreviations

ARPKD	Autosomal recessive polycystic kidney disease
CT	Computed tomography
DMSA	Dimercaptosuccinic acid
ESRD	End-stage renal disease
IVP	Intravenous pyelography
MAG3	Mercaptoacetyl triglycine
MCDK	Multicystic dysplastic kidney
MNE	Monosymptomatic enuresis
MRA	Magnetic resonance angiography
MRI	Magnetic resonance imaging
PUV	Posterior urethral valve
Tc-99m	Technetium 99
UPJ	Ureteropelvic junction
UTI	Urinary tract infection
UVJ	Ureterovesical junction
VCUG	Voiding cystourethrogram
VUR	Vesicoureteral reflux

Introduction

Pediatric urology encompasses myriad disorders, from complex bladder and genital reconstructions to more routine problems of UTIs. Many of these are congenital. In this chapter, congenital abnormalities of the kidney, ureter, and bladder are discussed. These organs are intimately involved in organogenesis. A solid understanding of embryology will facilitate better comprehension of congenital ailments and associated diseases of these organs.

Knowledge of embryology of the kidney and urinary tract is important to understand anomalies of the kidney and urinary tract and is presented briefly in Chapter 17 and another reference.[1] Development of the kidney starts at the fourth week of gestation, and nephrogenesis is complete before birth. However, kidney maturation continues postnatally. Renal tumors and genital abnormalities are presented in Chapter 5. This chapter and Chapter 5 cover most urologic problems encountered in pediatrics.

Anomalies of Number

Bilateral renal agenesis occurs in 1 in 4,800 to 10,000 births,[2,3] occurs mainly in males, and is incompatible with life. The mechanism of maldevelopment is unknown. Functional kidneys are not found, but rarely masses of poorly organized mesenchyme can exist that contain small arteries emanating from the aorta. The ureters and bladder are absent in 50% of patients, and when present the bladder is hypoplastic.

Infants with bilateral renal agenesis have oligohydramnios, low birth weight, typical Potter facies (flattened midportion of the face, wide-set eyes, beaked nose, and low-set ears; Figure 18-1), bowed and clubbed lower extremities with occasional sirenomelia, pulmonary hypoplasia, bell-shaped chest, cryptorchidism, and high prevalence of genitourinary abnormalities in females.

The diagnosis is easily made at birth when the infant has the characteristic Potter facies in the presence of oligohydramnios. These findings are pathognomonic but can be confirmed with ultrasound examination of the kidneys and bladder or nuclear renal scan. Prognosis is dismal. Nearly 40% of affected infants are stillborn, and most will die within 24 to 48 hours of birth.

Unilateral renal agenesis, or the absence of one kidney, is less obvious because there are no identifying signs, as with bilateral renal agenesis. Because of this the true incidence is not known, but it is reported to be 1 in 1,100 to 5,000 births.[4,5] Although Doroshow and Abeshouse[4] found a slight male predominance (M/F, 1.8:1); the large series of Sheih et al[5] found an equal sex distribution. The left kidney is absent slightly more often than the right one, and an autosomal dominant transmission exists with a 50% to 90% penetrance.[6] The exact mechanism is not known. Besides renal ectopia

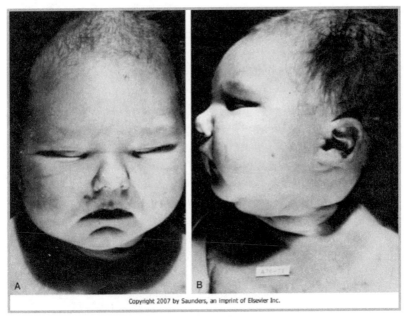

Figure 18-1.
An anephric infant who lived 2 days had a typical Potter facial appearance. **A.** Note the prominent fold and skin crease beneath each eye, blunted nose, and depression between lower lip and chin. **B.** The ears give an impression of being low set because the lobes are broad and drawn forward, but actually the ear canals are located normally. (Reprinted with permission from Wein AJ, Kavoussi LR, Novick AC, Partin AW, Peters CA, eds. *Campbell-Walsh Urology.* Philadelphia, PA: Saunders; 2006:3271.)

or malrotation, contralateral renal anomalies are uncommon. Contralateral collecting system abnormalities, however, do exist; the most prevalent being VUR in 28% to 30% of patients.[7] Contralateral UVJ and UPJ obstructions were found to be 11% and 7%, respectively. Genital abnormalities range from 20% to 40% of patients; girls have more malformations than do boys. The ipsilateral Wolffian and Müllerian duct structures are often maldeveloped, with 50% of boys having absent Wolffian duct-derived structures and roughly 33% of females having abnormalities of the internal genitalia.[8] Conversely, 79% of males with absent vas deferens and 43% of females with genital anomalies have ipsilateral missing kidneys.[8] Abnormalities of the cardiovascular (30%), gastrointestinal (25%), and musculoskeletal (14%) systems may also be present. The absence of a kidney is also associated with several syndromes, including Turner syndrome, Poland syndrome, DiGeorge syndrome, Kallmann syndrome, and VACTERL syndrome (vertebral defects, anal atresia, congenital cardiac disease, tracheoesophageal fistula, renal abnormalities, radial dysplasia, and other limb defects).[8]

Diagnosis is made by imaging: ultrasound, nuclear scans, IVP, CT scan, or MRI. Plain films may hint at left unilateral renal agenesis if the gas pattern of the large bowel fills the area of the renal fossa, where normally the gas pattern is medially displaced. The solitary kidney develops compensatory hypertrophy. Despite reports of hypertension and proteinuria, patients with isolated unilateral renal agenesis usually enjoy a normal life span.[9]

Supernumerary kidneys are accessory organs with their own blood supply and collecting system. They should not be confused with a duplex system. This kidney exists in addition to 2 normal kidneys. Incidence is not known. The supernumerary kidney is uniform in shape and smaller than the other 2 normal kidneys. The kidney is abnormal in one-third of cases, and the collecting system is dilated in half of cases.[8] The vasculature is anomalous. Besides ectopic ureter, no other clusters of genitourinary or other organ anomalies exist in association with the supernumerary kidney.

❧ Pearl

Patients with isolated unilateral renal agenesis usually enjoy a normal life span.

Supernumerary kidneys are usually not identified until adulthood following complaints of pain, fever, hypertension, and palpable abdominal mass. Urinary tract infection, obstruction, or both lead to the workup and eventual diagnosis through ultrasound examination, intravenous pyelogram, CT scan, or MRI. Prognosis is unknown because of the infrequency of diagnosis in asymptomatic patients.

Anomalies of Position

Renal ectopia describes a kidney that is not located in the renal fossa (lateral to the vertebral column from T11 to L3 and bounded by the diaphragm, quadratus lumborum, and psoas major muscles posteriorly). Ectopic kidneys can be pelvic, iliac, abdominal, thoracic, or crossed in location. The incidence of simple renal ectopia is 1 in 500 to 1,200, with an average incidence of 1 in 900.[8] There is no sex preponderance. Pelvic kidneys are found in 1 in 2,100 to 3,000 in autopsy series, with solitary pelvic kidneys being rare (occurring in 1 in 22,000).[8] Bilateral ectopia is extremely rare and accounts for only 10% of all ectopic kidneys.[10]

An ectopic kidney is smaller than a normal kidney. Hydronephrosis is found in 56% of ectopic kidneys secondary to UPJ or UVJ obstruction. Grade III, IV, or V VUR contributes to the hydronephrosis in 26% of cases. There may be anomalies of the contralateral kidney, including agenesis. Hydronephrosis due to obstruction or reflux is found in 25% of normally positioned contralateral kidneys. Genital anomalies are found in 15% to 45% of affected patients, more often in females. Associated anomalies in other organ systems, namely cardiac and skeletal, occur in 20% of patients.[11]

> **Pearl**
>
> Most ectopic kidneys are asymptomatic and are discovered on incidental radiologic examination.

Most ectopic kidneys are asymptomatic and are discovered on incidental radiologic examination. They can initially present with UTI or a palpable abdominal mass. Because of the ectopic position, renal colic may be mistaken for other abdominal or pelvic processes, such as appendicitis or pelvic inflammatory disease. Diagnosis can be made by ultrasound, IVP, CT scan, renal scan, or MRI. Patients with simple renal ectopia have higher incidences of hydronephrosis and nephrolithiasis. Otherwise, the ectopic kidney is at no greater risk to any other disease process than a normally positioned kidney.

When the kidney lies partially or completely above the diaphragm in the posterior mediastinum without any abdominal organs, it is a thoracic ectopic kidney. This position accounts for 5% of renal ectopia. Most patients with thoracic kidneys are asymptomatic and are discovered by chance on a chest x-ray. Besides an ectopic location and rare lower lung lobe hypoplasia, the thoracic kidney is not known to have any effect on the health of the patient.

Anomalies of Form and Fusion

A kidney is defined as crossed if it is located opposite the side in which its ureter inserts into the bladder. Ninety percent of crossed ectopia are fused to the other kidney (Figure 18-2). The incidence of cross-fused ectopia is 1 in 1,000 live births.[12] Male predominance exists, as well as left-to-right ectopia. The etiology of crossed ectopia is idiopathic.

Most ectopic kidneys have the superior poles fused to the lower poles of the "normal" kidneys. Anomalous vasculature is normal. The ureters of ectopic kidneys are orthotopic, although VUR is quite common at 15%.[8] Simi-

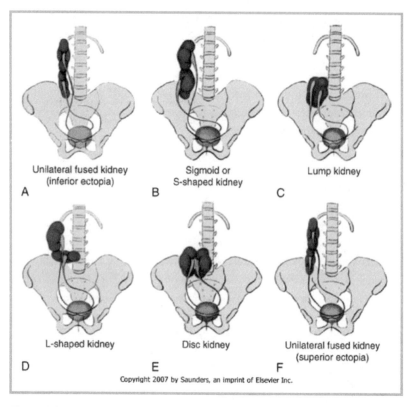

Figure 18-2.

Six forms of crossed renal ectopia with fusion. (Reprinted with permission from Wein AJ, Kavoussi LR, Novick AC, Partin AW, Peters CA, eds. *Campbell-Walsh Urology.* Philadelphia, PA: Saunders; 2006:3284.)

larly, UPJ obstruction of the ectopic kidney is found in 29% of patients.[8] The orthotopic kidneys generally do not have any associated anomalies. Skeletal (50%) and genital (40%) anomalies may be found in patients with solitary crossed ectopia.[8] Most crossed ectopic kidneys are asymptomatic.

Diagnosis can be made with any type of imaging. Cystoscopy and retrograde pyelography can be useful in delineating the collecting system if surgery is planned. Because of anomalous vasculature, angiogram, CT angiography, or MRA is recommended before surgical intervention. Patients with crossed renal ectopia generally have normal life spans, although UTIs and nephrolithiasis may develop in those with obstructed collecting systems.

Horseshoe kidney is the most common of the fused renal anomalies. It occurs in 1 in 400 individuals and is more common in males, with a male/female ratio of 2:1.[8] The kidneys are located on either side of the midline, with fusion occurring at the lower poles (95%) with an isthmus. The etiology is

₰ Pearl

The horseshoe kidney is asymptomatic but may be associated with congenital anomalies of the skeletal, cardiovascular, and central nervous systems.

unknown; however, the anomaly occurs early in gestation. The number of calyces is normal. The vasculature to the horseshoe kidney is anomalous.

The horseshoe kidney by itself is asymptomatic; however, it is often associated with congenital anomalies of the skeletal, cardiovascular, and central nervous systems. Horseshoe kidneys are found in 20% of patients with trisomy 18, 7% to 15% of females with Turner syndrome, and 3% of patients with neural tube defects. Hypospadias (4%); cryptorchidism (4%); and bicornuate uterus, septate vagina, or both were observed in patients with horseshoe kidney.[13] Duplicated ureters (10%), ectopic ureteroceles, VUR (50%), and MCDKs are also seen.[8]

Although many patients with horseshoe kidney go through life without symptoms, many present with hydronephrosis secondary to UPJ obstruction (33%), UTI (30%), or nephrolithiasis (20%–80%).[8] Sixty percent of patients are symptom-free for an average of 10 years.

Diagnosis can be made by ultrasound or IVP. Confirmatory studies include cystoscopy with retrograde pyelogram, CT scan, or magnetic resonance urogram. Life span is normal if those patients with severe congenital anomalies are excluded. Although only 13 of the 2,961 patients in the National Wilms Tumor Study have horseshoe kidneys, the incidence is double that of the general population.[14] The low retroperitoneal or pelvic location of the kidneys should not interfere with pregnancy or delivery.

Anomalies of Rotation

Normally, the kidney rests in the renal fossa with the calyces oriented laterally and the pelvis facing medially. Malrotation exists if the kidney is not in this position and orientation. Rotation occurs between the fourth and the ninth weeks of gestation, with an incidence of 1 in 390 patients and 1 in

939 autopsies.[8] The malrotated kidney can be described by the location of its pelvis; the most common position is ventral. Symptoms from a malrotated kidney are due to obstruction from the fibrous tissue or vasculature compressing the pelvis, UPJ, and proximal ureter. Infection, hematuria, and nephrolithiasis may also be seen.

Diagnosis is made by ultrasound, IVP, retrograde pyelogram, CT urogram, or magnetic resonance urogram. Bilateral malrotation, which occurs more often than expected, can lead to the misdiagnosis of horseshoe kidney. The presence of an isthmus can easily distinguish the 2 anomalies. Patients with renal malrotation have normal life spans.

Anomalies of Renal Vasculature

Vascular anatomy is of paramount importance to urologic surgeons because each renal segment is supplied by an end artery without collateralization. The term *multiple renal arteries* should be used to describe any kidney that is supplied by more than one artery. *Anomalous* or *aberrant* is reserved for describing vessels that do not originate from the aorta or main renal artery. When 2 or more arteries supply a renal segment, they are described as *accessory arteries.*[8] Only one renal artery is found in 70% to 85% of kidneys.

Symptoms result from obstruction of the collecting system by multiple, aberrant, or accessory arteries. Hydronephrosis secondary to UPJ or infundibular obstruction, infection, or nephrolithiasis can occur. Aberrant, accessory, or multiple renal vessels can be suspected on IVP, but definitive diagnosis is made with angiography, CT angiogram, or MRA. Deviations from the norm of one renal artery per kidney do not increase renal disease, and patients with renal vascular deviations have normal longevity and health.

Renal artery aneurysm occurs in 0.1% to 0.3% of people.[8] Aneurysms are classified as saccular, fusiform, dissecting, and arteriovenous. Saccular aneurysms are the most common (93%) and are outpouchings that communicate with the arterial lumens through narrow or wide necks. Most renal artery aneurysms, which can range from 1 to 10 cm, are less than 2 cm (90%) and are usually asymptomatic, especially in children. When present, symptoms consist of renin-mediated hypertension (55%), microscopic or gross hematuria (30%), and pain (15%).[8]

Renal aneurysms are suspected if bruits are heard during abdominal auscultation, pulsatile masses are appreciated over the renal hila, or ringlike calcifications are visualized in the areas of renal arteries or branches.[8] Although IVP may suggest the presence of an aneurysm, definitive diagnosis is made by angiography, color Doppler ultrasound, CT angiography, or MRA. Treatment is recommended if hypertension cannot be controlled, if the aneurysm is greater than 2.5 cm, in females of childbearing age fearing rupture during pregnancy, or if the aneurysm is progressively enlarging.[8] Methods of treatment can be endovascular stenting or surgical excision, either open or laparoscopic.

Renal arteriovenous fistula may be congenital (25%), idiopathic, or acquired (70%).[8] Acquired fistulae are due to trauma, inflammation, surgery, or percutaneous needle biopsy. All 3 types of fistulae have the same types of symptoms depending on the size and age; these symptoms include loud abdominal bruit (75%), hematuria (33%), diastolic hypertension (40%–50%), tachycardia, palpable flank mass, cardiomegaly, and congestive heart failure (50%).[8,15] Diagnosis is made by 3-dimensional Doppler ultrasound or angiography. Treatment options include total or partial nephrectomy, vascular ligation, or endovascular balloon or coil occlusion.

Abnormalities of the Collecting System

A calyceal diverticulum is a transitional epithelium-lined cystic cavity within the renal parenchyma and connected to a minor calyx by a narrow channel.[8] Incidence is 4.5 per 1,000 intravenous pyelograms.[16] The etiology is unknown. Nephrolithiasis with symptoms of infection or pain occurs in 39% of patients.[16] Diagnosis is made by IVP. Retrograde pyelogram, CT scan, MRI, and ultrasound may also be useful in making the diagnosis. Vesicoureteral reflux may be associated with calyceal diverticulum. Treatment is only recommended for symptomatic children and those with stone disease.

When the major calyces and renal pelvis are located outside the renal parenchyma, they are known as extrarenal calyces. Extrarenal pelvis is a normal anatomical variant in which the pelvis is found outside the renal sinus. Symptoms are associated with the numerous anomalies that occur with extrarenal pelvis and cause urinary stasis or obstruction. A bifid pelvis is a normal anatomical variant in which the pelvis divides into 2 major calyces at or just distal from the renal parenchyma.

Cystic Abnormalities of the Kidney

Autosomal Recessive Polycystic Kidney Disease

Infants with ARPKD have extremely enlarged kidneys and renal failure. Incidence is 1 in 5,000 to 40,000 children.[17,18] More than 75% of children with ARPKD present in the newborn period. Oligohydramnios is common with resultant Potter facies, limb deformities, and respiratory distress secondary to pulmonary hypoplasia. Besides renal and hepatic failure, these patients can suffer from hypertension, UTI, portal hypertension, esophageal varices, and hepatosplenomegaly. Diagnosis is made if the ultrasound reveals small renal cysts (Figure 16-1), liver biopsy shows congenital hepatic fibrosis, and family history is significant for recessive inheritance of cystic renal disease. Nephrectomies can be performed for a mass effect that impedes respiration. Dialysis and renal transplant may be necessary. Sclerotic therapy has also been employed for bleeding varices. The prognosis is poor for neonates; 50% die within the first few days of life.[17] If they live beyond the first year, patients with ARPKD have better prognosis, with 50% of the patients alive at 10 years of age.[19] Eventually, most children will require dialysis or renal transplantation. Chapter 16 covers this condition in more detail.

Autosomal Dominant Polycystic Kidney Disease

Autosomal dominant polycystic kidney disease is the most common of all cystic diseases. Most patients are diagnosed between 30 and 50 years of age with symptoms of pain (59%), UTI (53%), hypertension, hematuria (64%), and flank mass (60%).[16] Renal ultrasound may show cysts in the kidney and other organs (Figure 16-2). Genetic counseling and ultrasound examination of all children of the affected individual is necessary because of the autosomal dominant nature of the disease. Treatment consists of medical management of the renal failure, hypertension, pain, and recurrent UTI. Dialysis and a renal transplant may eventually be needed. Invasive procedures for pain consist of percutaneous cyst aspiration and sclerosis, open or laparoscopic cyst decompression, and laparoscopic denervation.[20] Nephrectomies may be indicated in patients in ESRD who have uncontrolled pain, recurrent UTI, or extremely large kidneys that interfere with respiration or placement of future transplant kidneys. Refer to Chapter 16 for more details.

Medullary Sponge Kidney

Medullary sponge kidney is a collection of dilated distal collecting ducts with small medullary cysts (1–8 mm) and diverticula. Bilateral disease is seen in 75% of patients.[21] The estimated incidence in the general population is 1 in 5,000 to 20,000.[18] The average age of presentation is 20, although symptoms of renal colic (50%–60%), UTI (20%–30%), and gross hematuria (10%–18%) can present between 3 weeks and 71 years of age.[18] Patients

> ## ❧ Pearl
>
> Patients with nephrolithiasis have a 3% to 21% chance of having medullary sponge kidney.

with nephrolithiasis have a 3% to 21% chance of having medullary sponge kidney, and one-third to one-half of patients have hypercalcemia and increased parathyroid hormone levels.[18] Associated anomalies include hemihypertrophy, Beckwith-Wiedemann syndrome, and Ehlers-Danlos syndrome.[18]

Diagnosis is usually made on ultrasound or IVP. The findings are of enlarged kidneys with or without calcification, contrast-filled elongated papillary tubules or cavities, and persistently opacified medulla and papillary contrast blush.[18] Treatment is for the sequelae, namely, kidney stones and UTI. Long-term prognosis is poor for 10% of these patients secondary to septicemia, stone disease, and renal failure.

Juvenile Nephronophthisis and Medullary Cystic Disease

Juvenile nephronophthisis and medullary cystic disease appear similar clinically and histologically. The first is characterized by early onset, longer duration, and recessive inheritance, and the second by late onset, rapid progression, and autosomal dominant inheritance.[18] Incidence is 1 in 50,000 for juvenile nephronophthisis and 1 in 100,000 for medullary cystic disease.[22,23]

Patients with either disease have polydipsia and polyuria (80%). Hypertension is seen with medullary cystic disease but not juvenile nephronophthisis. Association of juvenile nephronophthisis and autosomal recessive retinitis pigmentosa (16%) is termed *renal-retinal syndrome* or *Senior-Loken syndrome*.[24] Computed tomography scan

> ## ❧ Pearl
>
> Juvenile nephronophthisis is responsible for 10% to 20% of pediatric ESRD.

may be a better modality for diagnosis and visualization of cysts than ultrasound or IVP.[18]

Juvenile nephronophthisis is responsible for 10% to 20% of pediatric ESRD, with renal failure developing, on average, at 13 years and always before age 25.[18] Renal failure occurs in patients with medullary cystic disease by age 32.[25] Dialysis and renal transplantation will be needed later in life. Because hepatic disease has occasionally been associated with juvenile nephronophthisis, which can result in portal hypertension, liver biopsy should be considered before renal transplant.

Multicystic Dysplastic Kidney

Multicystic dysplastic kidney is the most common finding in a newborn with an abdominal mass. The kidney is severely dysplastic and composed of multiple cysts of varying sizes without a central cyst, giving the typical appearance of "a bunch of grapes" (Figure 18-3). Generally, little renal

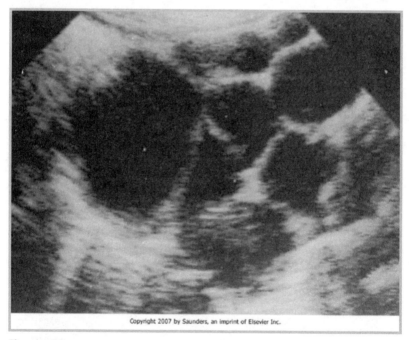

Copyright 2007 by Saunders, an imprint of Elsevier Inc.

Figure 18-3.
Female neonate with left multicystic kidney. Note large cysts arranged haphazardly without evidence of connections to or the presence of a large central or medial cyst. (Reprinted with permission from Wein AJ, Kavoussi LR, Novick AC, Partin AW, Peters CA, eds. *Campbell-Walsh Urology.* Philadelphia, PA: Saunders; 2006:3338.)

parenchyma is present. Males are more likely to have a unilateral MCDK; bilateral disease is more often found in females.

The etiology is unknown. Symptoms result from the initial large size of the kidneys. Unilateral disease is asymptomatic except for a palpable abdominal mass. Bilateral disease is incompatible with life. Many genitourinary abnormalities are seen with MCDK. Contralateral UPJ obstruction is seen in 3% to 12% of patients, and VUR in 18% to 43%.[18] Beckwith[26] estimated that MCDKs have a 4-fold increase in developing Wilms tumor compared with normal kidneys but concluded

✒ Pearl

Diagnosis of MCDK is made by ultrasound on prenatal evaluation or after an abdominal mass is discovered in infancy.

that prophylactic nephrectomies are not warranted. Noe et al[27] estimated that 2,000 prophylactic nephrectomies would need to be performed to prevent one case of Wilms tumor developing in MCDK. Hypertension occurs in 0.7% of patients, and prophylactic nephrectomy to prevent hypertension is generally not warranted.[18]

Diagnosis is typically made by ultrasound either on routine prenatal evaluation or after an abdominal mass is discovered in infancy. Sometimes it is difficult to distinguish a profoundly hydronephrotic kidney from an MCDK by ultrasound (Chapter 5). A Tc-99m-MAG3 scan shows no uptake in an MCDK but some function in hydronephrosis. Most MCDKs involute over time and do not need to be removed. Periodic blood pressure monitoring is recommended. With laparoscopic surgery being more common, removal of MCDKs may gain favor in some circles. The persistence or enlargement of an MCDK may prompt some to remove the kidney.

Ureteropelvic Junction Obstruction

Ureteropelvic junction obstruction occurs because of a kink or intrinsic narrowing at the junction between the renal pelvis and the ureter, resulting in hydronephrosis. Ureteropelvic junction obstruction occurs in 1 in 500 patients, more often on the left side (67%), and more often in males (M/F, 2:1).[28,29] It is bilateral in 10% to 40% of cases. On rare occasions when UPJ obstruction occurs in a duplicated system, the lower pole moiety is nearly always the one affected.

Ureteropelvic junction obstruction may be intrinsic, extrinsic, or secondary to high-grade VUR (10%).[30] Common associated anomalies include MCDK, renal dysplasia, unilateral renal agenesis, VUR (40%), and VATER syndrome (vertebral defects, anal atresia, tracheoesophageal fistula, esophageal atresia, and radial dysplasia). Twenty percent of patients with VATER syndrome have UPJ obstruction.[28]

Most children diagnosed during infancy are asymptomatic and discovered to have hydronephrosis on antenatal ultrasound (Chapter 17). If diagnosed after birth, UPJ obstruction may present as a palpable abdominal mass. Older children may have episodic flank or upper abdominal pain, nausea, emesis, hematuria and, rarely, hypertension. Diagnosis is made by history and radiographic imaging. When hydronephrosis is found prenatally, postnatal ultrasound examination is recommended after the third day of life to allow recovery from relative oliguria and minimize the potential for false-negative results. If hydronephrosis is present, a repeat renal ultrasound with a VCUG is obtained between 6 and 8 weeks of life to rule out VUR. A Tc-99m-MAG3 renal scan with furosemide (Lasix, Sanofi-Aventis, Bridgewater, NJ) allows assessment of renal vascular flow, differential function, and imaging of the collecting system. Magnetic resonance urography for assessment of UPJ obstruction is being developed and shows promise in providing both functional and anatomical data.

≥≈ Pearl

Prognosis of UPJ obstruction is good if repaired early in childhood.

Prognosis is good if the obstructed UPJ is repaired early in childhood. Most children will undergo dismembered pyeloplasty, using an open, laparoscopic, or robotic-assisted laparoscopic approach, with success rates greater than 90%.[28]

Ureteral Anomalies

A duplex kidney has 2 separate pelvicaliceal systems with an upper and a lower pole.[31] The vascular supply and collecting systems, including the ureters, are separate. Partial duplications can also exist. Partially duplicated systems are further described by the level at which the ureters converge. If the 2 systems join at the UPJ, it is called a *bifid system*. If the ureters join distal from the UPJ but proximal to the bladder, then bifid ureters exist. Duplicated ureters separately drain into the bladder.

Ureteral duplication is the most common anomaly of the ureters, with autopsy incidence of 1 in 125 (40% bilateral).[32] An autosomal dominant transmission exists with incomplete dominance. Incidence of sibling ureteral duplication is 1 in 8 to 25.[32] The upper pole ureter inserts in the bladder medially and caudally, and the lower pole ureter inserts into the bladder laterally and cranially. Associated anomalies include VUR (42%), renal dysplasia (29%), hydronephrosis, ureteroceles, and increased incidence of UTI.[33] Diagnosis can be made by IVP, renal scan, CT urogram, or magnetic resonance urogram. Ultrasound may also be useful. Treatment is individualized and driven by associated obstruction, which is common in the upper pole moiety, or VUR, which is more common in the lower pole ureter.

Ureterocele is a cystic dilation of the terminal, intravesical submucosal end of the ureter. Ureteroceles are categorized as intravesical (contained entirely within the bladder) or ectopic (have portions at the bladder neck or within the urethra). Incidence is 1 in 4,000 autopsies and 1 in 5,000 to 12,000 pediatric admissions.[34,35] Ureteroceles are bilateral in 10% of cases. Most ureteroceles are associated with duplicated ureters. Single-system ureteroceles are usually rare and generally found in boys.

Ureteroceles are often diagnosed prenatally on ultrasound (Chapter 17). If not identified in utero, most girls present with a UTI. If the ureterocele results in bladder outlet obstruction, the distended bladder can be palpated as a lower abdominal mass. In girls, the ureterocele may prolapse into the urethra and exit the urethral meatus. Vesicoureteral reflux is often seen with ureteroceles. In duplex systems, VUR to the ipsilateral lower pole ureter is roughly 50%. Contralateral reflux occurs in 25% of cases. Vesicoureteral reflux occurs in the ureter with the ureterocele 10% of the time.

Ureteroceles are usually identified with ultrasound, showing a well-defined cyst along the posterior wall of the bladder (Figure 18-4). Intravenous pyelography can also be used, where a "cobra head" is seen in the bladder at the distal, terminal end of the ureter. Voiding cystourethrography is important to identify associated VUR. Care must be taken when performing VCUG because overfilling the bladder may efface the ureterocele, which makes it harder to appreciate and more likely to be mistakenly diagnosed as a bladder diverticulum.

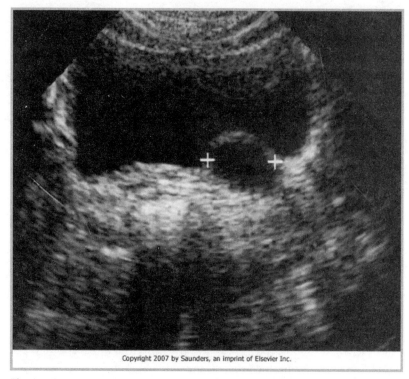

Figure 18-4.
An intravesical ureterocele in a 2-month-old girl is outlined by the cursors on an ultrasound image. (Reprinted with permission from Wein AJ, Kavoussi LR, Novick AC, Partin AW, Peters CA, eds. *Campbell-Walsh Urology*. Philadelphia, PA: Saunders; 2006:3399.)

Treatment of the ureterocele is variable, with the goals of infection control, protection of the normal renal units, preservation of renal function, and maintenance of continence. Endoscopic decompression of ureteroceles is a widely accepted form of initial treatment. This effectively decompresses an obstructed system and reduces risk of further renal deterioration. Success rates vary depending on whether the ureterocele is intravesical or ectopic.

Ectopic ureter is defined as a ureter that opens at or distal from the bladder neck. Incidence is 1 in 1,900 autopsies.[32] In more than 80% of cases, the ectopic ureters are the upper pole ureters of duplicated systems. They occur more often in females than in males (M/F, 1:3). Bilateral ectopia is found in 10% of patients.[32] The ectopic ureter can terminate anywhere along the urinary tract or genital structures derived from the Wolffian duct.

Symptoms in males are UTI, urinary urgency and frequency, epididymitis, constipation, abdominal and pelvic pain, discomfort with ejaculation, and infertility. In females, ectopic ureters can present as urinary incontinence, persistent vaginal discharge, UTI, abdominal pain, failure to thrive, reflux, hydronephrosis, hydroureter, or abdominal mass. Associated findings are VUR into the lower pole ureter of duplicated systems (50%), as well as into the ectopic ureter, which is usually the upper pole system. The severity of the renal dysplasia in the segment drained by the ectopic ureter usually correlates with the degree of ectopia—the more abnormally placed the ureteral orifice, the more renal dysplasia.

Ectopic ureters are best identified with ultrasound, with which a dilated upper pole ureter is identified. Intravenous pyelography and, more recently, magnetic resonance urography are the definitive examinations that delineate the course of the ectopic ureter. A DMSA scan can assess function of the associated moiety. A VCUG is obtained to diagnose associated VUR. Computed tomography or magnetic resonance urography can be helpful in identifying small, poorly functioning upper pole moieties. Cystoscopy and vaginoscopy with retrograde pyelogram are other tools useful in identifying ectopic ureters. Treatment usually involves complete or partial nephroureterectomy of the corresponding renal moiety to the ectopic ureter. Most children have poorly functioning parenchyma associated with the ectopic ureter.

Megaureter is a loose term that defines a dilated ureter diameter of greater than 7 mm (Chapter 5). It can be grouped into 3 categories: refluxing, obstructed, and nonrefluxing and nonobstructed.[35] The refluxing megaureter can be further subcategorized into primary and secondary. A small number of these (2%) are also obstructed. Patients tend to have bilateral disease and present with signs and symptoms of UTI. Boys are more affected than girls. Older children may have hypertension. Secondary UPJ obstruction may result. Secondary refluxing megaureters are due to functional or anatomical bladder outlet obstruction. These can occur in children who fail to empty their bladders because of a neurologic problem or from behavioral inability to relax the external sphincter. Anatomical causes of outlet obstruction include PUVs, ball valving ureteroceles, or urethral stricture.

The primary obstructive megaureter is typically caused by a 3- to 4-cm aperistaltic segment of the ureter at the area of the vesicoureteral junction. This portion of ureter inhibits the proper flow of urine into the bladder. Less common etiologies are congenital ureteral strictures and ureteral valves. The 2 most common causes of secondary obstructive megaureter are dysfunctional voiding or PUVs. Other causes of secondary obstructive megaureter are ureteroceles, ureteral ectopia, bladder diverticula, periureteral post-reimplantation fibrosis, neurogenic bladder, and external compression because of tumors, masses, or anomalous vessels.

The etiology of primary nonrefluxing, nonobstructive megaureter is unknown and is a diagnosis of exclusion. Secondary nonrefluxing, nonobstructive megaureter can be due to high volume and flow seen in diabetes insipidus or compulsive water intake. Residual ureteral dilation after PUV ablation or ureteral reimplantation can also account for this type of secondary megaureter. Urinary tract infection may also be a cause. Ultrasound can distinguish a UPJ obstruction from a megaureter. After a diagnosis of megaureter has been established, a VCUG will identify VUR or bladder outlet obstruction if present. A renal scan is helpful to determine whether ureteral obstruction is present.

Management varies. For children with a nonobstructive megaureter and good renal function, no therapy is indicated. However, some may opt for surgical intervention for children with higher-volume VUR. Controversy exists over the management of primary obstructive megaureters. Some recommend long-term observation, and others advocate surgical correction. If surgical intervention is indicated or chosen, urinary diversion through cutaneous ureterostomy is recommended in infants. Children older than 1 year may undergo primary ureteral reimplantation if indicated. Although surgery does little to improve renal function in older children, it does improve pain and help control recurrent infections. Nephrectomy is an option if renal function is less than 10% and the function of the contralateral kidney is normal.

> ### ?» Pearl
>
> The term *megaureter* defines a dilated ureter with a diameter greater than 7 mm.

Vesicoureteral Reflux

Vesicoureteral reflux is defined as the retrograde flow of urine from the bladder into the ureter and kidney. The incidence of VUR is less than 1% of the general population.[36] However, in infants who present with UTI, the incidence is as high as 70%.[37] When intrarenal reflux coexists with UTI, the kidney is at risk for scarring and ultimately ESRD. Progressive scarring from pyelonephritis clearly occurs. Yet some infants with severe VUR are born with renal dysplasia and have no history of UTI.

Although the need for treatment of VUR is debated, we present the more accepted algorithm (Figure 18-5). Workup should be initiated if hydronephrosis is discovered antenatally or UTI occurs (29%–50% of

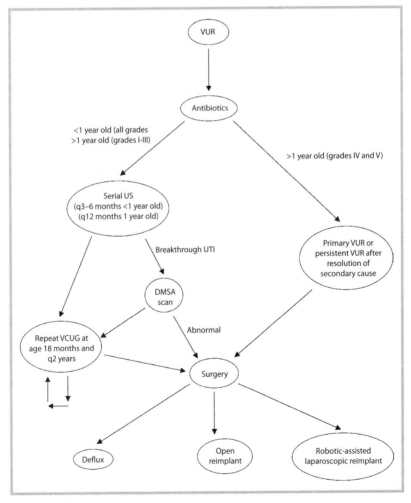

Figure 18-5.
Algorithm outlining the management of VUR. VUR indicates vesicoureteral reflux; US, ultrasound; q, every; UTI, urinary tract infection; DMSA, dimercaptosuccinic acid.

patients will have VUR).[38] Evaluation of siblings of refluxing children is also recommended. Associated anomalies are UPJ obstruction (5%–25%), ureteral duplication, bladder diverticula, renal agenesis, MCDK, mega-cystis-megaureter syndrome, VACTERL syndrome, imperforate anus, and CHARGE syndrome (coloboma, heart defects, atresia choanae, retarded growth and development, genitourinary abnormalities, and ear anomalies or deafness).[36]

Diagnosis is made by VCUG. Cyclic VCUG with 2 or more voiding cycles is recommended to diagnose the 12% of patients that can be missed with just one voiding cycle.[37] Vesicoureteral reflux is graded from I to V according to the classification developed by the International Reflux Study in Children (Figure 5-13). Nuclear VCUG can also be employed, with the benefit of lower radiation exposure for the children. However, less anatomi-cal detail can be obtained from a nuclear VCUG. Renal ultrasound is help-ful in identifying those with dilated upper tracts, but it is not an adequate substitute for VCUG and cannot be used for the diagnosis of VUR. A DMSA scan can delineate the presence of acute pyelonephritis, renal scar, or renal dysplasia and aid in the management of VUR.

Management of reflux is divided into medical and surgical treatment. Medical management is based on the observation that low-grade reflux will resolve spontaneously in approximately 80% of patients, with the resolu-tion rate for high-grade reflux at 20%.[39] Medical management entails daily prophylactic antibiotics with serial radiographic follow-up. Surgical man-agement is considered when breakthrough UTI occurs despite appropriate antibiotic prophylaxis.[39] Surgical intervention includes open reimplant, robotic-assisted laparoscopic reimplant, or endoscopic subureteric injection of a bulking agent (DeFlux, Q-Med Scandinavia, Uppsala, Sweden).

Management of secondary reflux is directed at the primary etiology. Reflux often improves when intravesical pressure returns to normal. Anti-

ஐ *Pearl*

Of patients with VUR, 30% develop ESRD.

reflux surgery should be done only after careful consideration in patients with history of PUVs, neuropathic bladder, or dysfunctional voiding sec-ondary to the high failure rate if these diseases are not adequately treated. If recurrent pyelonephritis exists despite prophylactic antibiotic treatment in these patients, vesicostomy is a better option.

Children with VUR are followed for at least 1 year regardless of the grade of reflux. Infants void with high pressures that decrease with age. Thus vast improvements in VUR can be seen in the first year of life.[39] The sequelae of VUR can be serious, with up to 30% of patients developing ESRD.[40] In a long-term study, hypertension occurred in 12.8% of patients with successfully reimplanted ureters.[41]

Bladder and Urethral Anomalies

Classic bladder exstrophy and epispadias can be viewed as the continuum of a spectrum of disease. In bladder exstrophy, the patient presents with a bladder plate that is contiguous with the abdominal wall and the urethra is open dorsally. With epispadias, the bladder is intact and located within the pelvis but the urethra is open dorsally, usually beginning at the penopubic junction. In some cases, the urethral meatus may be more distal, even placed within the glans. When either epispadias or bladder exstrophy is present, the pubic symphysis is variably separated and the penis is broad and shortened. In females, the clitoris is bifid. The incidence of classic bladder exstrophy is 1 in 10,000 to 50,000 births with a 3:1 male/female predominance.[42,43] The incidence of male epispadias is 1 in 117,000.[43] Female epispadias occurs at a rate of 1 in 484,000.[44]

Associated findings in classic bladder exstrophy are undescended testicles, inguinal hernias (56% for males and 15% for females),[45] VUR (100%), failure of infraumbilical rectus muscle development, vaginal stenosis, bifid uterus, and duplicated collecting systems. Of males with epispadias, 70% are incontinent and 30% to 40% have VUR.[44] Vesicoureteral reflux occurs in 20% to 75% of females with epispadias.[44]

Treatment of classic bladder exstrophy may be in stages or as a primary single repair. The staged (Jeffs) repair begins with bladder closure during the newborn period, with simultaneous release of the penile corpora from the attachments to the pubic bone to gain length. The second stage consists of epispadias repair that occurs when the patient is 1 to 2 years of age. The third stage is the tubularization of the bladder neck, performed only when the bladder volume is deemed sufficiently large (>85 mL). A 60% continence rate is achieved with the staged approach. Patients that fail the initial staged closure can have bladder augmentation, which will require them to perform clean intermittent catheterization thereafter. The second option is bladder closure, bladder neck repair, penile disassembly, and epispadias repair performed together (Mitchell repair). Of the small numbers of patients who have undergone a single-stage repair and are toilet trained, up to 80% have potential for urinary continence.[42,44] Surgical repair of epispadias is the same as that for exstrophy. The goal is to achieve urinary continence with a cosmetically acceptable penis. Continence is achieved in 84%, and 56% of the patients had erections that allowed satisfactory sexual intercourse.[46]

Patients with untreated bladder exstrophy have a 235-fold increased likelihood of developing bladder cancer compared with a person with a normal bladder.[45] All patients are carefully followed throughout life with radiographs of the upper tracts (IVP or ultrasound), monitoring of acid-base balance, renal function assays, and supportive counseling.

Cloacal exstrophy is the occurrence of omphalocele, prolapsed terminal ileum, exstrophied ileocecal intestine, and exstrophied hemibladders. The incidence is 1 in 200,000 to 400,000 births. Patients with cloacal exstrophy are some of the most challenging patients to care for. Numerous anomalies exist with cloacal exstrophy. Sixty-seven percent of the patients have renal anomalies: pelvic kidney, cross-fused ectopia, ureteral duplication, renal agenesis, horseshoe kidney, single-system ureteral ectopia, and UPJ obstruction. Bifid genitalia exist. In females, uterus didelphys (94%), vaginal duplication (54%), vaginal agenesis (20%), and clitoral agenesis (17%) occur. Besides the obvious and previously listed bowel anomalies, bowel duplication, malrotation, intestinal atresia, inguinal hernias, and Meckel diverticulum can be present. Neurologic abnormalities of the lower spinal cord are seen in 50% to 100% of patients.[45] Treatment can be performed in one or multiple stages.

The patent urachus (15%) exists as a persistently open urachus with partial distention of the bladder or a fistula between the bladder and the umbilicus. A urachal cyst (36%) can form anywhere along the urachal canal and is often connected to the bladder through a persistent tract. Such cysts often become infected. A urachal sinus (49%) is the persistence of the urachal apex that drains into the umbilicus. An infected urachal cyst can become a urachal sinus if the cyst starts to drain into the bladder or umbilicus. Finally, urachal diverticulum is a blind sinus that drains into the apex of the bladder and is usually an incidental finding on radiograph.

Symptoms are periumbilical discharge (42%), umbilical cyst or mass (33%), abdominal or periumbilical pain (22%), and dysuria (2%).[47] Diagnosis can be made using VCUG for a patent urachus or a sonogram for a urachal cyst or sinus. In addition, analysis of the periumbilical fluid for urea and creatinine can be helpful. Treatment involves surgical excision of the urachus. Late occurrence of bladder adenocarcinoma has been reported in patients with urachal anomalies. The umbilicus can be left intact in most pediatric patients. If infection is present, treatment with antibiotics for several weeks before excision is recommended.

Dysfunctional Voiding

Dysfunctional voiding is a nonspecific term encompassing any child who presents with voiding symptoms or incontinence without anatomical or neurogenic etiologies. Proper diagnosis of dysfunctional voiding relies heavily on a good history and physical examination. The detailed history should include onset of symptoms, age of toilet training, time of day or night enuresis, past UTI, associated family history, fluid intake, and bowel habits—constipation, encopresis, and diarrhea.

Physical examination begins as the child walks into the room, observing for abnormal gait. Careful examination of the sacral spine (dimples, boney abnormalities, and hair tufts) and buttocks (asymmetry) can raise the suspicion of neurogenic etiology. A thorough neurologic examination is also needed. Urinalysis and urine culture should be obtained. Radiologic studies are not always necessary but, if needed, may start with an ultrasound followed by VCUG and fluorourodynamics.

Unstable bladder is the most common of the voiding dysfunctions and has been termed *overactive bladder.* Up to 57% of symptomatic patients between 3 and 14 years of age have unstable bladders.[48] Uncontrolled contractions are normal for infant voiding and represent a delay in developmental maturation if present in childhood. One subcategory, urgency-incontinence syndrome (60%–70%), occurs when urgency and frequency (signs of bladder instability) elicit a weak or absent sphincter response. Another subcategory often associated with UTI is small-capacity, hypertonic bladder with detrusor-sphincter dyssynergia, which has decreased functional capacity. Treatment is with anticholinergics, fluid restriction, frequent voids, and restricting caffeine intake. A high index of suspicion for tethered spinal cord should exist if the preceding symptoms, especially significant urgency and urge incontinence, develop in an older child who was previously normal.

Infrequent voiding occurs more often in girls than in boys and includes a spectrum of disorders from infrequent micturition to the rare psychogenic urinary retention, which is diagnosed by exclusion. Infrequent voiders can have incontinence, UTI, and idiopathic retention. Radiographs and urodynamics are obtained if symptoms are significant. Usually, these tests are negative except for a larger than expected bladder capacity.[48] Treatment involves timed voiding every 3 hours to retrain the bladder, which gives good results. In addition, voiding diaries, treatments of constipation and fecal retention and, in extreme cases, clean intermittent catheterizations are employed in the treatment of these problems.

Constipation, as defined as fewer than 3 hard bowel movements in a week, is closely related to dysfunctional voiding. A rectum filled with stool can distort the shape of the bladder neck and urethra, which can cause staccato patterns of voiding and even urinary retention. Diagnosis is made with emphasis on bowel habits, palpable stool during abdominal and rectal examination, and abdominal plain film looking for stool. Treatment starts with enemas and laxatives, followed by a bowel regimen that includes stool softeners or laxatives and dietary changes (increased fiber, fruits, and vegetables). Increased water intake is also recommended because dehydration can lead to constipation. The goal is to have soft bowel movements daily. Numerous studies link constipation, dysfunctional voiding, UTI, and VUR.[48] Successful treatment of constipation may reduce or eliminate UTI and VUR.

Giggle incontinence is the occurrence of incontinence during laughter. It is surprisingly common in girls, with a report citing 25% of nursing students having giggle incontinence at some time in their lives.[49] The pathology is unknown, and diagnosis is made by history only. Patients have otherwise normal voiding patterns. Treatment consists of frequent voiding, especially before incontinence-provoking events. Central nervous system stimulants used to treat narcolepsy can also be used.[48]

Postvoid dribbling occurs in girls who have completed toilet training. The cause is vaginal reflux. The urine drips out shortly after micturition. History is used to make the diagnosis. Prevention of urine from refluxing into the vagina will treat the problem, although improvement does occur with age and growth. Opening the introitus (spreading the legs or facing the toilet while voiding) or tilting the vaginal canal (touching the toes while sitting on the toilet after voiding) effectively cures the problem. Postvoid dribbling is not associated with any other problem.

Daytime urinary frequency syndrome is the sudden occurrence of severe diurnal urinary frequency without incontinence in otherwise healthy children. The average age of onset is 4.5 years. Voiding can happen as often as every 15 to 20 minutes and generally dissipates once the child is asleep. Etiology is idiopathic. Thirty percent of these children have hypercalciuria.[48] Diagnosis is by exclusion, and workup includes history with physical examination to rule out occult neuropathy. Renal ultrasound is obtained to exclude anatomical abnormalities that can be the root cause. No known effective treatment exists; however, daytime urinary frequency resolves spontaneously after a few months.

Enuresis (previously referred to as nocturnal enuresis; see Chapter 2) is defined as intermittent voiding. Roughly 15% of 5-year-old children are enuretic at night.[48] Enuresis is not a problem until parents or children deem it socially unacceptable. Enuresis has a spontaneous resolution rate of 15% per year. Only 1% of 15-year-olds have enuresis. This voiding is hereditary, with variable autosomal dominant penetrance. Children of both parents, one parent, and no parents who were enuretic have a 77%, 43%, and 15% chance of having enuresis, respectively.[48] It happens more often in boys than in girls.

Patients with primary enuresis have never been dry. Patients with secondary enuresis have histories of being dry for at least 6 months. If enuresis is an isolated event, without any of the preceding disorders, the disorder is termed *ME*. Patients with ME have reduced functional bladder capacity.[48] Incontinence is not due to bladder instability or sleep disturbances (deep sleepers) but is possibly a symptom of delayed development. A decrease in serum vasopressin has been observed in children with ME. However, the circadian rhythm of lower nocturnal vasopressin can be the cause or result of enuresis. Diagnosis is again one of exclusion, with careful history and physical examination. Ultrasound is a reasonable, noninvasive test to perform if obstruction is suspected.

Treatment should not be initiated until the child is motivated to remain dry and is at least 7 years of age. Behavior modification, consisting of bladder training (progressive increase in voiding intervals to increase bladder capacity), responsibility to change wet sheets and rewards for dry nights, and conditional therapy (urinary alarm), is more successful than pharmacologic agents. Urinary alarms are extremely effective, with success rates of 60% to 100%, but 25% relapse. Most patients respond to retreatment. Parents and children need to be committed to urinary alarms for up to 4 months. Pharmacotherapy is less effective. The most commonly used medication is desmopressin (DDAVP, Sanofi-Aventis, Bridgewater, NJ, US) in nasal (20–40 μg) or oral (0.2–0.6 μg) forms. After DDAVP is discontinued, 50% to 90% of patients relapse. Water intake should be limited to 8 ounces a night when used to decrease the likelihood of water intoxication and hyponatremic seizure. One effective use of DDAVP is the temporary relief for children with ME during a sleepover. Combination therapy of urinary alarms with medications or behavior modification produces response rates of 80%.[48] Patients with enuresis and diurnal symptoms or neurogenic etiology should have the other problems addressed first. The successful treatment of diurnal symptoms or neurogenic bladder can often result in resolution of enuresis.

References

1. Park JM. Normal and anomalous development of the urogenital system. In: Walsh PC, Retik AB, Darracott E, Vaughan J, Wein AJ, eds. *Campbell's Urology*. 8th ed. Philadelphia, PA: Saunders; 2002:1737–1764

2. Potter E. Bilateral renal agenesis. *J Pediatr*. 1946;29:68

3. Wilson RD, Baird PA. Renal agenesis in British Columbia. *Am J Med Genet*. 1985; 21:153–169

4. Doroshow LW, Abeshouse BS. Congenital unilateral solitary kidney: report of 37 cases and a review of the literature. *Urol Surv*. 1961;11:219–229

5. Sheih CP, Hung CS, Wei CF, Lin CY. Cystic dilatations within the pelvis in patients with ipsilateral renal agenesis or dysplasia. *J Urol*. 1990;144:324–327

6. McPherson E, Carey J, Kramer A, et al. Dominantly inherited renal adysplasia. *Am J Med Genet*. 1987;26:863–872

7. Cascio S, Paran S, Puri P. Associated urological anomalies in children with unilateral renal agenesis. *J Urol*. 1999;162:1081–1083

8. Bauer SB. Anomalies of the upper urinary tract. In: Walsh PC, Retik AB, Darracott E, Vaughan J, Wein AJ, eds. *Campbell's Urology*. Philadelphia, PA: Saunders; 2002:1885–1924

9. Emanuel B, Nachman R, Aronson N, Weiss H. Congenital solitary kidney: a review of 74 cases. *Am J Dis Child*. 1974;127:17–19

10. Malek RS, Kelalis PP, Burke EC. Ectopic kidney in children and frequency of association with other malformations. *Mayo Clin Proc.* 1971;46:461–467

11. Downs RA, Lane JW, Burns E. Solitary pelvic kidney: its clinical implications. *Urology.* 1973;1:51–56

12. Abeshouse BS, Bhisitkul I. Crossed renal ectopia with and without fusion. *Urol Int.* 1959;9:63–91

13. Boatman DL, Cornell SH, Kolln CP. The arterial supply of horseshoe kidneys. *Am J Roentgenol Radium Ther Nucl Med.* 1971;113:447–451

14. Mesrobian HG, Kelalis PP, Hrabovsky E, Othersen HB Jr, deLorimier A, Nesmith B. Wilms tumor in horseshoe kidneys: a report from the National Wilms Tumor Study. *J Urol.* 1985;133:1002–1003

15. Novick AC, Fergany A. Renovascular hypertension and ischemic nephropathy. In: Walsh PC, Retik AB, Darracott E, Vaughan J, Wein AJ, eds. *Campbell's Urology.* Philadelphia, PA: Saunders; 2002:229–271

16. Timmons JW Jr, Malek RS, Hattery RR, Deweerd JH. Caliceal diverticulum. *J Urol.* 1975;114:6–9

17. Lippert MC. Renal cystic disease. In: Gillenwater JY, Grayhack JT, Howards SS, Mitchell ME, eds. *Adult and Pediatric Urology.* Philadelphia, PA: Lippincott, Williams & Wilkins; 2002

18. Glassberg KI. Renal dysgenesis and cystic disease of the kidney. In: Walsh PC, Retik AB, Darracott E, Vaughan J, Wein AJ, eds. *Campbell's Urology.* Philadelphia, PA: Saunders; 2002:1925–1994

19. Kaplan BS, Kaplan P, Rosenberg HK, Lamothe E, Rosenblatt DS. Polycystic kidney diseases in childhood. *J Pediatr.* 1989;115:867–880

20. Resnick M, Chang AY, Casale P. Laparoscopic renal denervation and nephropexy for autosomal dominant polycystic kidney disease related pain in adolescents. *J Urol.* 2006;175:2274–2276; discussion 6

21. Kuiper JJ. Medullary sponge kidney. *Perspect Nephrol Hypertens.* 1976;4:151–171

22. Lirenman DS, Brianlowry R, Chase WH. Familial juvenile nephronophthisis: experience with eleven cases. *Birth Defects Orig Artic Ser.* 1974;10:32–34

23. Reeders ST. The genetics of renal cystic disease. In: Gardner KD Jr, Bernstein J, eds. *The Cystic Kidney.* The Netherlands: Kluwer Academic Publishers; 1990:117–146

24. Hildebrandt F, Singh-Sawhney I, Schnieders B, Centofante I, et al. Mapping of a gene for familial juvenile nephronophthisis: refining the map and defining flanking markers on chromosome 2. APN Study Group. *Am J Hum Genet.* 1993;53:1256–1261

25. Gardner KD Jr. Juvenile nephronophthisis and renal medullary cystic disease. In: Gardner KD Jr, ed. *Cystic Diseases of the Kidney.* New York, NY: John Wiley & Sons; 1976:173

26. Beckwith JB. Wilms tumor and multicystic dysplastic kidney disease: editorial comment. *J Urol.* 1997;158:2259–2260

27. Noe HN, Marshall JH, Edwards OP. Nodular renal blastema in the multicystic kidney. *J Urol.* 1989;142:486–488; discussion 9

28. Carr MC. Anomalies and surgery of the ureteropelvic junction in children. In: Walsh PC, Retik AB, Darracott E, Vaughan J, Wein AJ, eds. *Campbell's Urology*. Philadelphia, PA: Saunders; 2002:1995–2006

29. Arger PH, Coleman BG, Mintz MC, et al. Routine fetal genitourinary tract screening. *Radiology*. 1985;156:485–489

30. Lebowitz RL, Blickman JG. The coexistence of ureteropelvic junction obstruction and reflux. *Am J Roentgenol*. 1983;140:231–238

31. Timothy RP, Decter A, Perlmutter AD. Ureteral duplication: clinical findings and therapy in 46 children. *J Urol*. 1971;105:445–451

32. Cooper CS, Snyder HM III. Ureteral anomalies. In: Gillenwater JY, Grayhack JT, Howards SS, Mitchell ME, eds. *Adult and Pediatric Urology*. Philadelphia, PA: Lippincott, Williams & Wilkins; 2002:2155–2187

33. Schlussel RN, Retik AB. Ectopic ureter, ureterocele, and other anomalies of the ureter. In: Walsh PC, Retik AB, Darracott E, Vaughan J, Wein AJ, eds. *Campbell's Urology*. Philadelphia, PA: Saunders; 2002:2007–2052

34. Campbell M. Ureterocele: a study of 94 instances in 80 infants and children. *Surg Gynecol Obstet*. 1951;93:705

35. Malek RS, Kelalis PP, Stickler GB, Burke EC. Observations on ureteral ectopy in children. *J Urol*. 1972;107:308–313

36. American Academy of Pediatrics Committee on Quality Improvement, Subcommittee on Urinary Tract Infection. Practice parameter: the diagnosis, treatment, and evaluation of the initial urinary tract infection in febrile infants and young children. *Pediatrics*. 1999;103:843–852

37. Atala A, Keating MA. Vesicoureteral reflux and megaureter. In: Walsh PC, Retik AB, Darracott E, Vaughan J, Wein AJ, eds. *Campbell's Urology*. Philadelphia, PA: Saunders; 2002:2053–2116

38. International Reflux Study Committee. Medical versus surgical treatment of primary vesicoureteral reflux: report of the International Reflux Study Committee. *Pediatrics*. 1981;67:392–400

39. Canning DA, Kolu J, Meyers KEC. Vesicoureteral reflux. In: Kaplan BS, Meyers KEC, eds. *Pediatric Nephrology and Urology: The Requisites in Pediatrics*. Philadelphia, PA: Elsevier Mosby; 2004:340–345

40. Bailey RR. Sterile reflux: is it harmless? In: Hudson J, Kincaid-Smith P, eds. *Reflux Nephropathy*. New York, NY: Masson Publishing; 1979:334

41. Wallace DM, Rothwell DL, Williams DI. The long-term follow-up of surgically treated vesicoureteric reflux. *Br J Urol*. 1978;50:479–484

42. Casale P, Canning DA. Congenital anomalies. In: Hanno PM, Malkowicz SB, Wein AJ, eds. *Penn Clinical Manual of Urology*. Philadelphia, PA: Saunders Elsevier; 2007:893–918

43. Lattimer JK, Smith MJ. Exstrophy closure: a follow-up on 70 cases. *J Urol*. 1966;95:356–359

44. Gearhart JP. Exstrophy, epispadias, and other bladder anomalies. In: Walsh PC, Retik AB, Darracott E, Vaughan J, Wein AJ, eds. *Campbell's Urology*. Philadelphia, PA: Saunders; 2002:2136–2196

45. Grady RW, Mitchell ME. Exstrophy and epispadias anomalies. In: Gillenwater JY, Grayhack JT, Howards SS, Mitchell ME, eds. *Adult and Pediatric Urology.* Philadelphia, PA: Lippincott, Williams & Wilkins; 2002:2269–2310

46. Mollard P, Basset T, Mure PY. Male epispadias: experience with 45 cases. *J Urol.* 1998; 160:55–59

47. Cilento BG Jr, Bauer SB, Retik AB, Peters CA, Atala A. Urachal anomalies: defining the best diagnostic modality. *Urology.* 1998;52:120–122

48. Bauer SB, Koff SA, Jayanthi VR. Voiding dysfunction in children: neurogenic and non-neurogenic. In: Walsh PC, Retik AB, Darracott E, Vaughan J, Wein AJ, eds. *Campbell's Urology.* Philadelphia, PA: Saunders; 2002:2231–2283

49. Christmas TJ, Noble JG, Watson GM, Turner-Warwick RT. Use of biofeedback in treatment of psychogenic voiding dysfunction. *Urology.* 1991;37:43–45

Chapter 19

Renal Calculi

Mark A. Williams and H. Norman Noe

Introduction

Pediatric urolithiasis is relatively uncommon. Nonetheless, urinary calculi in children are not rare, and failure to consider this diagnosis may lead to unnecessary or inappropriate treatment. There are wide variations in the etiology and presentation of pediatric urolithiasis. This overview attempts to provide a framework for the diagnosis and treatment of the most common clinical presentations of pediatric urolithiasis.

Epidemiology and Etiology

Historically, most occurrences of urinary calculi in children were thought to be related to some preexisting condition, including urologic factors (chronic UTI, obstruction, or neurogenic bladder), genetic disorders, nutritional deficiencies, and immobilization. However, in the industrialized world and especially in North America, in many cases the etiology of stones is similar to that seen in adults, including metabolic disorders (most commonly hypercalciuria). Environmental factors, diet, and family history are also important influences in pediatric kidney stone disease.[1,2]

Overall, about 7% of all urolithiasis cases occur in children younger than 16 years. A specific cause for the stone, either metabolic or urologic, can be determined in most cases.[3] Considerable geographic variation in the incidence and etiology of pediatric stone formation is possible. In the United States, metabolic causes such as hypercalciuria are the most common. In many European series, however, infection-related stones are still often seen.[2,4] White children, particularly those with a family history of stones, seem to be the most affected group; black and Hispanic children are significantly less affected.

Pediatric urolithiasis may develop at any age. Many adults with recurrent stones report their first episode during their teen years, but the average age at presentation is between 8 and 10 years. Stones may occur as early as the neonatal period, however, especially in low-birth-weight infants. Unlike adult cases, the male/female ratio is nearly equal in pediatric cases, although there is a slight male preponderance.

Stone composition can be quite variable and is influenced by the etiology of the stone (Table 19-1). Most stones in patients with hypercalciuria are composed of calcium oxalate. Patients with an intrinsic renal disorder such as distal renal tubular acidosis may be more likely to develop stones composed of calcium phosphate. Although hypercalciuria is the most common metabolic cause for stones, other less common conditions may be encountered. Hypocitraturia, or low urinary citrate concentrations, is associated with calcium stone formation in many patients. Less common are patients with cystinuria, an autosomal recessive disorder affecting cystine metabolism, which leads to the formation of cystine stones. Abnormal purine metabolism or hyperexcretion of uric acid may allow for the formation of uric acid stones. Patients with underlying urologic problems such as chronic UTI may secondarily develop stones composed of struvite (magnesium-ammonium-phosphate). These stones, commonly referred to as *infection stones,* develop when the urine is infected with urease-producing bacteria such as *Proteus, Pseudomonas, Klebsiella, Staphylococcus, Providencia, Serratia,* and *Ureaplasma.*

Table 19-1. Frequency of Various Types of Stones	
Calcium oxalate/calcium phosphate	70%–80%
Struvite	20%–25%
Uric acid	5%–10%
Cystine	2%–5%

Infection stones are usually large calculi within the renal collecting system that develop as a result of chronic or recurrent UTIs. They may fill the entire collecting system of the kidney, branching out into the calyces and forming a staghorn appearance. Once formed, these staghorn calculi harbor bacteria, making it impossible to eradicate infection. Chronic infection and chronic obstruction caused by the ever-growing stones eventually destroy the kidney. This is different from the situation in which a patient with a primary renal or ureteral stone develops a UTI. In this situation, a patient develops a UTI when the stone drops into the ureter and causes obstruction and stasis of urine. The combination of an obstructed hydronephrotic kidney and infection can quickly lead to bacteremia and sepsis, especially in young patients, and requires immediate surgical attention. Box 19-1 presents some clinical disorders associated with various types of urolithiasis.

> ව *Pearl*
>
> About 7% of all stone cases occur in patients younger than 16 years.

Box 19-1. Some Clinical Disorders Associated With Urolithiasis

Calcium stones
  Normocalcemic hypercalciuria
    Idiopathic hypercalciuria (calcium oxalate stones most common)
    Distal renal tubular acidosis (calcium phosphate)
    Furosemide (low-birth-weight infants)
  Hypercalcemic hypercalciuria
    Immobilization/fractures
    Primary hyperparathyroidism
  Hyperoxaluria
    Enteric hyperoxaluria (short gut, ileostomy, malabsorption)
    Hereditary hyperoxaluria (types I and II)
  Other causes
    Idiopathic calcium urolithiasis
    Hyperuricosuria (uric acid nidus for calcium oxalate crystallization)
Uric acid stones
  Hyperuricosuria (inflammatory bowel, ileostomy)
  Leukemia, lymphoma (secondary to massive cell death after chemotherapy)
  Lesch-Nyhan syndrome
Cystine stones (homozygous for cystinuria)
Struvite stones (chronic urinary tract infection with urease-producing bacteria)

Presenting Symptoms

Presenting symptoms in children with urinary stones are variable and depend on the age of the patient and the size and location of the stone. Other factors that may affect the presentation include whether the stone is of metabolic origin or it is the result of some underlying urologic problem such as obstruction or infection. Signs and symptoms range from asymptomatic microscopic hematuria discovered incidentally to the classic triad of severe colicky flank pain, nausea, and gross hematuria to sepsis in the patient with an obstructed ureter and secondary UTI. In general, younger patients have more atypical presenting symptoms, and the stone may be an unexpected finding. In very young patients the passage of small stone fragments into the diaper may be the first indication of a problem. Urolithiasis should be considered in any patient with painless microscopic or macroscopic hematuria and in any child being evaluated for UTI.

Pain, however, is frequently the initial manifestation of a stone in children and usually indicates an attempt to pass the stone into the ureter. The pain results from the obstructed flow of urine and concomitant distention of the urinary tract proximal to the stone. As the stone progresses toward the bladder, the ureter occasionally may become unobstructed and the pain may cease temporarily. This results in intermittent waves of pain. Younger children may have vague, generalized abdominal or genital pain. Older children are more likely to lateralize the pain to the affected kidney. When the stone is in the renal pelvis or proximal ureter, the pain is usually reported in the flank or costovertebral angle area. As the stone moves along the ureter, the location of the pain will migrate to the side and finally into the anterior lower quadrant. As the stone nears the bladder, many patients will report irritative bladder symptoms such as

ᣠ Pearl

The most common symptoms of a kidney stone are abdominal pain, nausea, and gross hematuria.

frequency and dysuria. The degree of hematuria often worsens as the stone moves nearer the bladder. Nausea and vomiting frequently accompany ureteral obstruction and renal colic. This is because of the shared autonomic nerve supply of the kidney and the stomach within the celiac ganglion. Gastrointestinal symptoms, including ileus, may predominate the clinical picture and lead to an incorrect diagnosis of gastroenteritis, appendicitis, or bowel obstruction.

Patients may have multiple stones in both kidneys at the time of the initial presentation. Although rare, a patient can present with anuria as a result of simultaneous bilateral obstructing ureteral stones. Rarely, a large stone may be impacted in the male urethra, producing acute urinary obstruction.

Physical Examination

Physical examination findings depend on the etiology and presentation of the stone. For children with asymptomatic microscopic hematuria, there may be no physical signs. Even gross hematuria may be seen in a child with a normal physical examination. When the stone causes acute ureteral obstruction, the patient has a general appearance of significant discomfort. The pain can be quite severe and the patient might writhe about in extreme discomfort, unable to find a comfortable position. A child also may be pale and diaphoretic. Severe vomiting and poor oral intake may lead to dehydration. Abdominal distention

ə Pearl

Younger patients frequently have atypical presenting signs and symptoms

secondary to intestinal ileus also may be seen, especially in younger patients. Children with a UTI associated with an obstructing calculus may appear quite ill, obtunded or hypotensive from sepsis. If a patient has a stone secondary to chronic urinary infection or other primary urologic or metabolic disorder, the physical examination findings may be dominated by the characteristics of the primary condition.

Laboratory Tests

Laboratory evaluation during an acute episode is usually limited, but it should always include a urinalysis. Occasionally, patients with stones will have a normal urinalysis, but usually there will be some degree of microscopic or macroscopic hematuria. Depending on the amount of blood in the urine and whether there is infection involved, examination of a centrifuged specimen may also reveal pyu-

ə Pearl

Pediatric patients with stones should undergo metabolic evaluation following the acute management.

ria. Proteinuria, red blood cell casts, and dysmorphic red cells generally are not encountered. Most stone types have characteristic crystals that may be seen on high-power magnification of centrifuged urine sediment; however, the absence of crystalluria does not rule out the presence of a stone (see Chapter 3). Other useful laboratory tests are presented in Box 19-2. Once the acute stone process is treated, a more extensive laboratory assessment is required to determine a possible metabolic cause of the stone.

Differential Diagnosis

Asymptomatic hematuria may occur in any nephrologic or urologic disorder ranging from cystitis to glomerulonephritis (see Chapter 7). Often a thorough urinalysis with microscopic examination of the sediment can help distinguish the cause. If hematuria is heavy, clots may form, and the painful passage of these clots along the ureter may mimic the passage of a stone. Any form of urinary tract obstruction or hydronephrosis, congenital or acquired, may produce a similar pain pattern. A common differential diagnosis would be congenital ureteropelvic junction obstruction with hydronephrosis and intermittent pain and nausea. When gastrointestinal symptoms are prominent, gastroenteritis, appendicitis, and small bowel obstruction should be considered. These can usually be sorted out with a careful physical examination, noting the absence of peritoneal irritation in cases of urinary stones.

Box 19-2. Baseline Metabolic Evaluation of Patients With Urolithiasis

Stone analysis
    Crystallographic evaluation: may be diagnostic with cystine, uric acid, and struvite stones
Urine
    Urinalysis: evaluate for RBCs, WBCs, crystals, pyuria
    Urine culture: note especially urease-producing bacteria
    Urine cystine screen: sodium nitroprusside test
    24-hour urine collection: volume, pH, creatinine, calcium oxalate, uric acid, citrate
Serum: electrolytes, calcium, phosphorus, uric acid, creatinine

---

Abbreviations: RBC, red blood cell; WBC, white blood cell.

Diagnostic Imaging

Imaging studies are required to confirm the diagnosis of a urinary stone. Previously, IVP was the gold standard for this diagnosis. More recently, however, less invasive and more accurate modalities, including ultrasound and noncontrasted CT, have largely replaced IVP as the first line of diagnostic imaging.[5] Although IVP is accurate in identifying the stone in most cases, it requires placement of an intravenous catheter and administration of contrast material. The discomfort and the potential for an allergic reaction to the iodinated contrast, as well as the excessive radiation exposure associated with IVP, make it a less attractive choice, especially in the acute care setting. Plain film radiography of the abdomen or a KUB film can sometimes suggest the presence of a stone (Figure 19-1); however, some stones, such as those composed of uric acid, are radiolucent, and others may be so faintly calcified as to be undetectable on plain film. In addition, overlying bowel gas may be

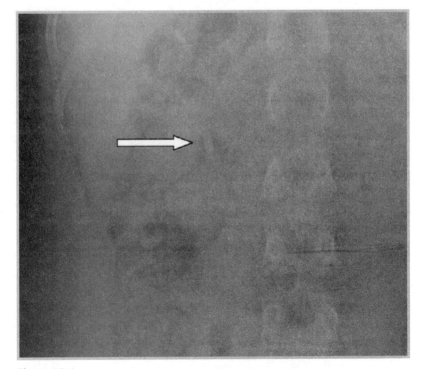

Figure 19-1.
Kidney, ureter, bladder plain film with calcification overlying right renal fossa (arrow).

excessive and may obscure visualization of the stone. When a calcification is seen, its location within the kidney or ureter may be suspected but can only be confirmed by proceeding to ultrasound or CT scan.

Ultrasound of the urinary tract is an attractive technique in evaluating a patient for a stone (Figure 19-2). Ultrasound is readily available, inexpensive, and noninvasive, and does not expose the child to ionizing radiation. It is particularly useful when repeated imaging is necessary, when following a stone for spontaneous passage, or when evaluating a child with recurrent stones. It is an excellent means of evaluating a patient with asymptomatic hematuria as a result of a stone located within the kidney. Ultrasound, however, lacks sensitivity in some cases, especially in the symptomatic child with a ureteral stone.[5] This lack of sensitivity must be considered when using ultrasound to evaluate a child with abdominal pain. Failure to identify a calculus with ultrasound in this situation does not rule out its presence. Although a ureteral stone may not be seen on ultrasound, the presence of the stone may be suspected in a symptomatic child if the ureter or renal pelvis is noted to be dilated. Here, the addition of a KUB film may

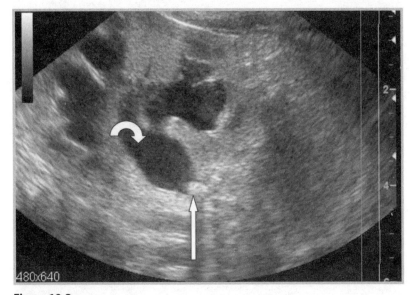

Figure 19-2.
Renal ultrasound with stone impacted at ureteropelvic junction (straight arrow). Note hydronephrosis proximal to stone (curved arrow).

allow visualization of a calcification, with the ultrasound confirming the obstructed ureter. The combination of these 2 studies is an excellent noninvasive way to diagnose and follow a ureteral stone.

A noncontrasted CT scan of the abdomen and pelvis using the helical or spiral technique is now the gold standard for evaluating patients suspected of harboring a urinary stone. The advantages of this technique are speed, availability, noninvasiveness, and especially accuracy and sensitivity.[5,6] This technique will identify and precisely locate virtually all stones, including very small calcifications, anywhere within the kidney (Figure 5-14) or ureter (Figure 19-3). In addition, the degree of obstruction can be determined by noting whether there is any dilation of the ureter or renal collecting system proximal to the stone. Finally, all stone types, even poorly calcified and fully radiolucent uric stones, can be seen with this technique. As a caveat, the ordering physician must suspect a stone and specify the CT scan be done using stone protocol and involving no contrast. The ability to identify the

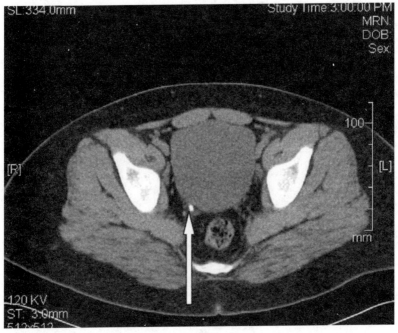

Figure 19-3.
Noncontrast computed tomography scan showing right distal ureteral stone (arrow).

✐ Pearl

A noncontrast helical or spiral CT of the abdomen and pelvis is the gold standard for diagnosing urolithiasis. An ultrasound with or without a KUB is adequate for follow-up.

stone may be lost once contrast fills the collecting system of the kidney. The principle drawback of noncontrasted CT scanning in children is the significant radiation exposure.[7] This is particularly true if repeated scanning is used to follow the patient with an active stone or recurrent stones. Newer CT protocols have been described that decrease the radiation exposure to children.[8] Nonetheless, judicious use of CT scanning in children is recommended. A preferred strategy might include use of noncontrast helical CT to confirm the initial diagnosis at the time of presentation, with follow-up using ultrasound with or without a KUB.

Treatment

Clinical evaluation of the child with urolithiasis is summarized in Figure 19-4. The proper treatment will be affected by several factors, including the presentation of the disease and the size, location, and type of stone. Children presenting with severe pain, high-grade ureteral obstruction, intractable nausea and vomiting, or evidence of a concomitant urinary infection will likely require admission to the hospital and urgent consultation with a pediatric urologist. These patients may need parenteral antibiotics and hydration and temporary ureteral stenting to relieve the obstruction and allow the condition to stabilize. Once this is accomplished, determination of how best to eliminate the stone can be done on a nonurgent basis.

Most children with an acute stone episode, however, can be managed initially on an outpatient basis with referral to a pediatric urologist within 24 to 72 hours. Outpatient management should consist of adequate pain and nausea control, usually with hydrocodone and antiemetics. Patients should remain well hydrated. If a patient is toilet trained, an attempt should be made to strain all urine for the purpose of capturing a spontaneously passed stone. Once the patient has been evaluated by the urologist, medical management may continue or surgical intervention may be prescribed based on the likelihood of stone passage. Spontaneous passage of the stone is the desirable outcome; however, this is not always possible. Most stones that pass do so within a few hours to days of the onset of symptoms. As long

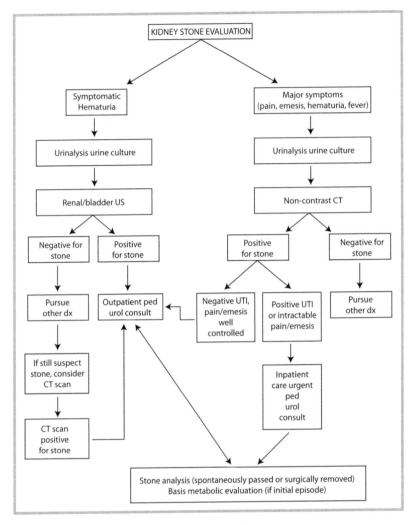

Figure 19-4.
Clinical evaluation of the child with urolithiasis. US indicates ultrasound; CT, computed tomography; dx, diagnosis; ped urol, pediatric urology; UTI, urinary tract infection.

as the pain and emesis are well controlled, a stone may be followed for 2 to 3 weeks, provided there is radiographic evidence that the stone is progressing along the ureter toward the bladder. If there is a lack of progress or if the patient's symptoms are difficult or impossible to control, surgical intervention is required.

Stones of any size can spontaneously pass; however, children with a stone larger than 4 mm are more likely to require surgical intervention.[9] Rarely, open surgical procedures are needed to treat a stone. Pediatric urologists are now able to manage most stones using less invasive procedures such as extracorporeal shockwave lithotripsy and ureteroscopy.[10,11] When the stone is found unexpectedly during evaluation of a nonacute patient, referral to a pediatric urologist or nephrologist may be done on an outpatient basis. Depending on the size and suspected composition of the stone, medical or surgical management may be prescribed.

Medical therapy, usually under the supervision of a pediatric nephrologist, is necessary for patients with certain metabolic conditions. This therapy is useful for treating an active stone or for the prevention of recurrent stones and usually involves altering the composition of the urine pharmacologically or by dietary manipulation. Hypercalciuria predisposes a child to recurrent stone formation. Therefore, an attempt to reduce the amount of calcium in the urine should be undertaken to reduce the number of stones that may occur during a child's lifetime. A detailed discussion of the pathophysiology of hypercalciuria is beyond the scope of this review. However, it should be pointed out that simply reducing the oral intake of calcium below the recommended daily allowance generally is not helpful in reducing the urine calcium level and is therefore not advised. The urine calcium level is more likely to be decreased by moderately reducing oral sodium consumption, limiting animal protein, and hydrating appropriately. Unfortunately, the fluid intake needed for adequate hydration (enough to maintain a urine output of about 35 mL/kg/d) is beyond the thirst level of most children and compliance is therefore difficult to maintain. These general dietary measures are useful for patients with any type of stone.

More specific medical therapy can be added depending on the response to the dietary changes and the particular composition of the stone. For patients with hypercalciuria, the potential for calcium stone formation can be further reduced by increasing potassium intake and urinary citrate levels.[12,13] Potassium citrate supplementation is easy to prescribe and reasonably well tolerated by children. In more severely affected children, urine calcium levels can be reduced further by treatment with hydrochlorothiazide (1 mg/kg/d). Long-term use of thiazides in children may be associated with electrolyte abnormalities and other potential side effects. Children should be followed carefully, preferably by a pediatric nephrologist, if this treatment is deemed necessary.

For certain stone types, a formed calculus can be dissolved by altering the urinary milieu. This process of stone chemolysis is particularly useful for cystinuria patients and those with uric acid stones. Cystine stones may be dissolved or prevented by maintaining a high urine output throughout the day and night (40–50 mL/kg/d) along with administration of potassium citrate to achieve persistent urinary alkalinization (to a pH of 7.5). Further reduction of urinary cystine may be required by prescribing sulfhydryl compounds such as D-penicillamine or α-mercaptopropionylglycine.

Uric acid stones are treated similarly by maintaining a high urine output (35 mL/kg/d) and administration of potassium citrate to achieve a urinary pH level of 6.5. Limiting meat intake is important to reduce purine metabolism and excretion of uric acid in affected patients. Allopurinol will further reduce the urinary uric acid level and may be needed in some patients with excessive hyperuricosuria. Because of the stringent nature of these protocols and the potential side effects of these medications, close surveillance by a pediatric nephrologist is required.

Because a significant number of children with stones will have an identifiable preexisting metabolic cause, a lifelong risk for stone recurrence with its attendant morbidity may be anticipated. As a result, children diagnosed with their first urinary stone should undergo a thorough metabolic evaluation to identify as specifically as possible any underlying metabolic causes so that treatment may be aimed at reducing the number of recurrences.[14] Generally, the metabolic evaluation is carried out by investigation of the stone composition and serum and urine parameters when the patient is nonacute. The most important initial information is the stone composition. Any spontaneously passed or surgically retrieved calculus should be sent for crystallographic evaluation to determine its exact composition. In most cases, the stone is composed of calcium oxalate or calcium phosphate and further evaluation

⁊ Pearl

Most patients with acute stone symptoms and no evidence of urinary infection can be managed as outpatients and referred to the pediatric urologist in 24 to 72 hours. Stones larger than 4 mm are more likely to require surgical intervention.

will be necessary. In some, however, such as uric acid, cystine, or struvite stones, the analysis will be conclusive.

In addition to the stone composition, baseline metabolic evaluation should be performed (see Box 19-2). Specific dietary and medical therapy can then be prescribed and the patient's course monitored for compliance and recurrences.

Prognosis

The prognosis for a child's recovery from an initial stone episode is generally excellent. With adequate support, acute stones may pass spontaneously within a few days. Even if surgical intervention is required, pediatric urologists can relieve obstruction and render the patient stone-free with minimally invasive procedures in most cases. However, because most stone occurrences in children are a result of some identifiable preexisting metabolic or urologic condition, failure to correctly identify these will put the child at risk for developing a new stone.

The patient who develops the first stone during childhood could potentially suffer multiple recurrences. Therefore, it is imperative that efforts be directed at discovering these preexisting conditions following the first stone episode. Urologic conditions such as chronic UTIs, congenital obstruction, or neurogenic bladder are usually apparent. Every effort should be made by the pediatric urologist to treat these problems to minimize the potential for new stones. Some patients with an underlying urologic problem, however, may also have hypercalciuria or some other metabolic condition.[1] As a result, a metabolic evaluation is important in all pediatric stone cases, not just those with normal urinary tract anatomy. Most of these patients will have hypercalciuria, although other, less common, conditions may be discovered. Management of these conditions is imperative to reduce the potential for new stone formation. The primary care physician can often manage these patients with dietary alterations, including hydration and modest salt restriction. Some patients, however, will require more intensive management with medication and close surveillance provided by a pediatric nephrologist.

✒ Pearl

Management of predisposing metabolic and anatomical causes is imperative to prevent recurrence.

References

1. Noe HN, Stapleton FB, Jerkins GR, Roy S. Clinical experience with pediatric urolithiasis. *J Urol.* 1983;129:1166–1168

2. Noe HN, Stapleton FB. Pediatric stone disease. In: Rous SN, ed. *Stone Disease: Diagnosis and Management.* Orlando, FL: Grune & Stratton, Inc.; 1987:347–376

3. Borgmann V, Nagel R. Urolithiasis in childhood—a study of 181 cases. *Urol Int.* 1982; 37:198–204

4. Coward RJM, Peters CJ, Duffy PG, et al. Epidemiology of paediatric renal stone disease in the UK. *Arch Dis Child.* 2003;88:962–965

5. Palmer JS, Donaher ER, O'Riordan MA, Dell KM. Diagnosis of pediatric urolithiasis: role of ultrasound and computerized tomography. *J Urol.* 2005;174:1413–1416

6. Strouse PJ, Bates DG, Bloom DA, Goodsitt MM. Non-contrast thin-section helical CT of urinary tract calculi in children. *Pediatr Radiol.* 2002;32:326–332

7. Frush DP, Donnelly LF, Rosen NS. Computed tomography and radiation risks: what pediatric health care providers should know. *Pediatrics.* 2003;112:951–957

8. Heneghan JP, McGuire KA, Leder RA, DeLong DM, Yoshizumi T, Nelson RC. Helical CT for nephrolithiasis and ureterolithiasis: comparison of conventional and reduced radiation dose techniques. *Radiology.* 2003;229:575–580

9. Pietrow PK, Pope JC IV, Adams MC, Shyr Y, Brock JW III. Clinical outcome of pediatric stone disease. *J Urol.* 2002;167:670–673

10. Lim DJ, Walker RD, Ellsworth PI, et al. Treatment of pediatric urolithiasis between 1984 and 1994. *J Urol.* 1996;156:702–705

11. Hill DE, Segura JW, Patterson DE, Kramer SA. Ureteroscopy in children. *J Urol.* 1990; 144:481–483

12. Osorio AV, Alon US. The relationship between urinary calcium, sodium, and potassium excretion and the role of potassium in treating idiopathic hypercalciuria. *Pediatrics.* 1997;100:675–681

13. Ettinger B, Pak CY, Citron JT, Thomas C, Adams-Huet B, Vangessel A. Potassium-magnesium citrate is an effective prophylaxis against recurrent calcium oxalate nephrolithiasis. *J Urol.* 1997;158:2069–2073

14. DeFoor W, Asplin J, Jackson E, Jackson, C, Reddy P, Sheldon C, et al. Urinary metabolic evaluations in normal and stone-forming children. *J Urol.* 2006;176:1793–1796

The Kidney in Systemic Disease

Eileen D. Brewer

Abbreviations

ACE	Angiotensin-converting enzyme
ANCA	Antineutrophil cytoplasmic antibody
ARB	Angiotensin receptor blockers
BUN	Blood urea nitrogen
C-ANCA	Cytoplasmic staining of anti-neutrophil cytoplasmic antibody
CKD	Chronic kidney disease
ESRD	End-stage renal disease
GBM	Glomerular basement membrane
GN	Glomerulonephritis
HSP	Henoch-Schönlein purpura
HUS	Hemolytic uremic syndrome
IgA	Immunoglobulin A
IgAN	Immunoglobulin A nephropathy
MPGN	Membranoproliferative glomerulonephritis
NS	Nephrotic syndrome
P-ANCA	Perinuclear antineutrophil cytoplasmic antibody
RBC	Red blood cell
RPGN	Rapidly progressive glomerulonephritis
SLE	Systemic lupus erythematosus
Stx	Shiga-like toxin

Introduction

A variety of systemic diseases may affect the kidney during childhood
(Box 20-1). Acute-onset renal disease may be associated with systemic vasculitis, such as HSP, SLE, or ANCA vasculitis. Remote infection elsewhere in
the body may lead to renal manifestations, such as HUS or chronic staphy-

lococcal bacteremia. Sometimes renal manifestations appear only after many years of chronic disease, such as sickle cell nephropathy or diabetic nephropathy. Malignancies or therapies used to treat malignancies also may lead to renal dysfunction. This chapter will review kidney abnormalities associated with common systemic diseases.

Vasculitis With Renal Disease in Children

Henoch-Schönlein Purpura

Henoch-Schönlein purpura is a small-vessel systemic vasculitis that typically affects children and presents as a combination of a lower extremity purpuric rash, crampy abdominal pain, bloody diarrhea, and joint pain. Another name given to HSP is *anaphylactoid purpura,* called so after a suggestion

---

Box 20-1. Systemic Diseases Affecting the Kidney

Systemic vasculitis
    Henoch-Schönlein purpura
    Systemic lupus erythematosus
    Antineutrophil cytoplasmic antibody vasculitis
    Wegener granulomatosis
    Goodpasture syndrome
Nonrenal infection
    Hemolytic uremic syndrome
    Chronic staphylococcal bacteremia and hypocomplementic nephritis
Late manifestation of chronic disease
    Sickle cell nephropathy
    Diabetic nephropathy
Malignancy
    Ureteral obstruction by tumor or uric acid stones
    Glomerular disease
        Hodgkin disease and minimal change nephrotic syndrome
        Solid tumors (carcinoma lung, colon, etc), leukemia, and membranous nephropathy
        Chronic lymphocytic leukemia and membranoproliferative glomerulonephritis
    Therapy-associated renal dysfunction
        Tumor lysis syndrome
        Cisplatinum, carboplatinum, and renal Fanconi syndrome; acute renal failure
        Ifosfamide and renal Fanconi syndrome
        Cytoxan-induced hemorrhagic cystitis
        Thrombotic microangiopathy/radiation nephritis with bone marrow transplant

in 1915 that hypersensitivity to food, drugs, or other inciting agents might play a pathogenetic role; no such agent has ever been identified.[1] Henoch-Schönlein purpura may be mediated by IgA, which is present in renal glomeruli and in skin biopsies from affected patients. The renal pathologic lesion is identical to that seen in IgAN, raising the question of whether IgAN and HSP may be a spectrum of the same disease.

Epidemiology

Children with HSP are most commonly boys (M/F 1.8:1) between the ages of 2 and 14 years, with peak ages of 4 to 6.[1-4] Peak seasonal incidence is in winter. Henoch-Schönlein purpura is uncommon in black children, both in the United States and Africa.[4] Two-thirds of patients report an upper respiratory tract infection 1 to 3 weeks before the onset of the characteristic rash.

Presenting Symptoms and Physical Examination Findings

Signs and symptoms of nephritis may not appear until days or weeks into the course of the disease. Henoch-Schönlein purpura usually begins with an erythematous macular rash on the lower extremities, buttocks and, occasionally, the ulnar surfaces of the arms that becomes purpuric within a day. The trunk is spared. The rash, present in all patients, may disappear in a few days to 2 weeks, but it may recur intermittently for weeks to years.[2,3] Joint pain with or without edema occurs in 60% to 80% of patients and may be the presenting symptom in 15%. Colicky abdominal pain with melena or bloody diarrhea occurs in about 50%, is the presenting symptom in about 10%, and mimics other gastrointestinal diseases. The incidence of abdominal pain is almost 90% in children with HSP nephritis. Severe vasculitis of the bowel may result in gastrointestinal hemorrhage, perforation, or intussusception. Scrotal pain and swelling occur in 2% to 40% of boys and is rarely a presenting symptom.

Renal disease occurs in 25% to 50% of patients with HSP, usually within 4 weeks of presentation.[2,3,5] The spectrum of renal disease in HSP is broad, ranging from asymptomatic microscopic hematuria and proteinuria to full-blown acute nephritis with gross hematuria.[5] Urinalysis must be checked periodically over the course of the disease to determine the occurrence of mild renal disease with only microscopic hematuria, proteinuria, and/or RBC casts. Nephrotic syndrome, renal failure, and hypertension are uncommon (1%–2%), but when present increase the risk for chronic renal disease.

Differential Diagnosis

The purpuric nature and distribution of the skin rash is characteristic of HSP. If the rash is atypical in distribution, other causes of purpura, such as leukemia, septicemia, HUS, SLE, or idiopathic thrombocytopenic purpura, must be considered. The abdominal symptoms mimic many infectious and inflammatory bowel diseases. Henoch-Schönlein purpura may cause an acute surgical emergency secondary to bowel perforation or intussusception. Pancreatitis is uncommon. Vasculitis of the testis may resemble torsion of the testis, orchitis, or incarcerated hernia. Distinguishing the joint symptoms of HSP from those seen in rheumatoid arthritis, SLE, and acute rheumatic fever is difficult at presentation. The clinical manifestations of HSP nephritis may appear identical to those seen in acute poststreptococcal GN, bacterial endocarditis, SLE, polyarteritis nodosa, or MPGN.

No laboratory test is diagnostic for HSP. Leukocytosis occurs early in the course. Hemoglobin, hematocrit, peripheral blood smear, platelet count, bleeding time, coagulation studies, serum C3 and C4, and antinuclear antibody are normal. Erythrocyte sedimentation rate and serum C-reactive protein level may be elevated. Urinalysis is essential to screen for microscopic hematuria, proteinuria, and RBC casts; gross hematuria occurs in 20% to 30%.[5] Elevation of serum creatinine occurs transiently in about 20% of patients and rarely persists (1%–2%). Serum electrolytes may be abnormal if serum creatinine is elevated or if diarrhea is significant.

If the clinical signs and symptoms of HSP are atypical or if the nephritis or NS is severe or persistent, the patient should be referred to a pediatric nephrologist. In addition, the diagnosis should be confirmed by microscopic examination of skin and/or renal biopsy specimens. Typically, skin lesions show a leukocytoclastic vasculitis[1] characterized by transmural and perivascular infiltration with polymorphonuclear leukocytes, histiocytes, and sometimes eosinophils. The renal lesion is identical to that seen in IgAN and ranges from no identifiable abnormalities by light microscopy to mesangial proliferation; focal, segmental, or diffuse proliferative glomerular lesions with or without crescents; and IgA deposits in the mesangium by immunofluorescence.

Treatment

Therapy is supportive, and acute dialysis is rarely needed. No specific drug therapy has been shown to be effective, including corticosteroids.[6] A combination of high-dose steroids and either azathioprine or cyclophosphamide may be useful for severe nephritis[7] or for unremitting NS.[8] When abdominal pain is severe and incapacitating, corticosteroids may provide relief, but care should be exercised not to miss symptoms of gastrointestinal perforation, which can be masked by this therapy.

Natural History and Prognosis

The clinical course varies from mild to severe. Most patients have several bouts of rash and abdominal pain during the first month of the disease. Recurrences during a longer period may be associated with a poorer prognosis. The main determinant of overall prognosis is the persistence and severity of the renal disease. Patients with severe crescentic nephritis, NS, or hypertension are most likely to develop chronic renal disease and even ESRD. Patients with persistent abnormalities on urinalysis should be followed long term until the urinalysis is normal for several years.

ࣙ Pearl

Renal disease occurs in 25% to 50% of patients with HSP.

Systemic Lupus Erythematosus

Systemic lupus erythematosus is a systemic inflammatory disease of uncertain etiology that involves many organs, including the kidney. Children initially may present with renal disease without extrarenal signs of SLE, but they usually rapidly develop other symptoms and fulfill the diagnostic criteria for SLE.

Epidemiology

Systemic lupus erythematosus is more common in young adult females (F/M, 8:1), but 20% to 25% of cases occur in childhood and even, rarely, in infancy.[9,10] Asian, black, and Hispanic children are more often affected than white children.[10,11] Nephritis is more common in childhood lupus, affecting up to 80% of patients at some point, usually within the first 6 months after diagnosis, so almost all children with SLE need to be referred for evaluation by a pediatric nephrologist.

Presenting Symptoms and Physical Examination Findings

Children often present with fever, malaise, arthritis, and anemia.[10,11] Less than half of children have a classic malar rash, but more than half have hematuria or proteinuria, and a few have edema, NS, or hypertension. The extent of the renal involvement may not be clinically apparent and usually requires referral to a pediatric nephrologist for full evaluation, including a kidney biopsy.[11]

Laboratory evaluation of SLE may reveal anemia, leukopenia, and thrombocytopenia, as well as severely decreased concentrations of serum C3 and C4. Antinuclear antibody and anti–double-stranded DNA antibody titers are elevated at diagnosis in 95% of patients with nephritis. Urine abnormalities include microscopic and gross hematuria, proteinuria, and casts (red cell, white cell, hyaline, and/or broad-waxy). Proteinuria may be mild, moderate, or in the nephrotic range. Heavy proteinuria is usually associated with more severe disease. One-half of children with SLE nephritis have elevated serum creatinine levels and decreased creatinine clearance during the initial course of their disease.[11]

Renal tubular disorders (eg, type IV renal tubular acidosis or glucosuria) may occur, especially in patients with evidence of tubulointerstitial disease by renal biopsy.[12] Ureteral vasculitis and noninfectious cystitis have been described and may be responsible for obstructive uropathy and lower urinary tract symptoms, respectively, in these patients.

Percutaneous renal biopsy is performed by a pediatric nephrologist to determine the extent of renal involvement.[11] Lupus nephritis has been divided into 6 classes by the appearance of the renal biopsy[13]; all classes occur in childhood (Table 20-1). Serial biopsies, especially after therapy, may reveal transformations between classes and will usually be needed to help guide therapy. Biopsies from about 5% of patients show minimal mesangial proliferation (class I).[11] Renal failure almost never occurs in these patients. Mesangial proliferative lupus nephritis (class II) accounts for 20% of biopsies. Clinically, only asymptomatic hematuria or proteinuria is seen in patients with class II disease.

Focal lupus nephritis (class III) occurs in about 25% of biopsies. Hematuria, proteinuria, edema, renal insufficiency, and hypertension may vary from mild to severe but are usually very responsive to therapy with corticosteroids.

Table 20-1. International Society of Nephrology/Renal Pathology Society Revision of World Health Organization Classification of Systemic Lupus Erythematosus Nephritis[13]

Class	Histopathology	Description
Class I	Minimal mesangial proliferative LN	Normal LM; mesangial immune deposits by IF
Class II	Mesangial proliferative LN	Mesangial hypercellularity with mesangial immune deposits by IF
Class III	Focal LN	Indicate proportion of glomeruli with active and with sclerotic lesions
Class IV	Diffuse LN	Indicate proportion of glomeruli with fibrinoid necrosis and cellular crescents
Class IV-S	Diffuse segmental	Diffuse segmental glomerular proliferation
Class IV-G	Diffuse global	Diffuse global glomerular proliferation
Class V	Membranous LN	Capillary walls diffusely thickened by subepithelial immune deposits by LM, IF, EM; may occur in combination with class III or IV
Class VI	Advanced sclerosing LN	≥90% glomeruli globally sclerosed

Abbreviations: LN, lupus nephritis; LM, light microscopy; IF, immunofluorescence; EM, electron microscopy.

Diffuse lupus nephritis (class IV) is found in 40% of biopsies. The lesion involves more than 50% of glomeruli and is associated with extensive deposits of all immunoglobulins and C3, C4, and C1q ("full house" immunofluorescence), especially in the subendothelial location of the glomerular capillary wall. When the deposits are circumferential, the capillary wall has a "wire loop" appearance. Crescent formation varies but may be severe, and it correlates with the clinical presence of RPGN. In class IV lupus nephritis, hematuria and proteinuria are present almost always. Most patients with renal failure and many with NS also have class IV disease. Class IV lupus nephritis is associated with progressive renal insufficiency and high mortality if not treated aggressively with cytotoxic drugs, such as cyclophosphamide and corticosteroids.

Membranous lupus nephritis (class V) accounts for 10% of renal biopsies, but in recent years the incidence appears to be increasing among pediatric patients. Class V lesions also may occur with class III or IV lesions. Membranous lupus nephritis occasionally may precede the extrarenal manifestations of SLE by years and may be diagnosed initially as idiopathic membranous nephritis.

A few patients have predominantly severe glomerulosclerosis (class VI), tubulointerstitial disease, or vascular disease. Tubulointerstitial disease often accompanies glomerular involvement in class III and IV nephritis but rarely occurs alone. When it does, the interstitial inflammatory infiltrates are focal and are associated with interstitial fibrosis and tubular atrophy. Vasculitis involving the larger blood vessels of the kidney sometimes leads to vascular necrosis, hypertension, and renal failure.

Differential Diagnosis

Lupus nephritis can mimic most other forms of acute and chronic GN, including MPGN, idiopathic membranous nephritis, and IgAN, especially if extrarenal symptoms are minimal. Lupus nephritis should always be considered when hematuria or proteinuria occurs with other systemic symptoms and multiorgan disease. Recurrent fever with leukopenia and thrombocytopenia may suggest infection, such as sepsis or occult abscess.

Treatment

Although the beneficial effect of corticosteroid therapy for the extrarenal manifestations of SLE is well accepted, no controlled trials of this therapy for lupus nephritis in children have been performed. Long-term controlled studies of adults with various classes of lupus nephritis have demonstrated that a combination of prednisone and a cytotoxic drug, such as cyclophosphamide, results in better control of class IV lupus nephritis, with fewer sclerotic lesions on follow-up renal biopsy and less progression to ESRD, compared with patients receiving prednisone alone.[14] Results suggest that intermittent bolus intravenous cyclophosphamide in combination with corticosteroids is associated with the fewest side effects in adults. The optimal frequency and duration of cyclophosphamide pulse therapy has not been determined, but monthly for 6 to 9 months and quarterly for a variable time thereafter has been effective clinically in many children.[15] The well-known oncogenic potential of cyclophosphamide and its gonadal toxicity render it a drug used only for the most serious forms of lupus nephritis, that is, class IV and severe class III. Recent studies in adults suggest mycophenolate mofetil may be useful in maintenance therapy after cyclophosphamide induction,[14] but no studies have been done yet in children and caution should be exercised when extrapolating from results for adult-onset lupus nephritis.[11,16] Rituximab, a chimeric anti-CD20 monoclonal antibody, also may be useful for treating resistant renal and extrarenal SLE, but its safety and efficacy are not proven in children.

Natural History and Prognosis

Overall, survival of children with SLE is good, with more than 80% alive at 10

years and 65% surviving 15 years after diagnosis. Most deaths are caused by infection or the neurologic complications of lupus. With early aggressive therapy of class IV lupus nephritis, progression to ESRD is uncommon.[15]

Antineutrophil Cytoplasmic Antibody Vasculitis, Wegener Granulomatosis, Goodpasture Syndrome, and Rapidly Progressive Glomerulonephritis

Rapidly progressive GN is a manifestation of several rare systemic diseases and is characterized by rapid deterioration in renal function to uremia and often ESRD within a few days to weeks of onset. The term *RPGN* has been used to describe both the clinical course and the renal biopsy lesion of diffuse glomerular crescent formation. Other pathologic lesions, such as the necrotizing glomerular lesion of Wegener granulomatosis and the linear deposition of antiglomerular antibody in the GBM of Goodpasture syndrome, also result in clinical RPGN and are associated with diffuse crescent formation.

Epidemiology

These diseases occur rarely, affect adolescents more often than young children, and affect adults more often than adolescents.[17]

Presenting Symptoms and Physical Examination Findings

Usually, RPGN presents with symptoms of acute nephritis, including gross hematuria, edema, hypertension, and oliguria or anuria.[17] Most patients have severe anemia out of proportion to their degree of renal failure or the apparent duration of their symptoms. Other symptoms may be those of the associated disorder, such as hemoptysis from pulmonary hemorrhage with Goodpasture syndrome or Wegener granulomatosis. Goodpasture syndrome includes the triad of nephritis (usually RPGN), pulmonary hemorrhage, and anti-GBM antibody in the circulation and deposited in renal or lung tissue.[18] Wegener granulomatosis is a systemic necrotizing vasculitis that involves the kidney, nasal mucosa, tracheobronchial tree, and lungs.[19] Vasculitic skin lesions, sinusitis, serous otitis media, epistaxis, saddle-nose deformity, cough, eye lesions, and cardiac and neurologic symptoms may be present.

Antineutrophil cytoplasmic antibody, with either cytoplasmic staining (C-ANCA) or perinuclear or nuclear staining (P-ANCA), is an important serologic marker for screening for the underlying disease and assessing the activity of clinical RPGN.[19-21] When ANCA is positive in the serum, the glomerular lesion always has few immune deposits but is necrotizing and is associated with crescent formation in the glomeruli. Ninety percent of patients with untreated active Wegener granulomatosis are C-ANCA positive, and 80% of patients with microscopic polyangiitis are either C-ANCA or P-ANCA positive, whereas patients with immune complex-mediated polyarteritis nodosa are ANCA negative. The diagnosis of ANCA vasculitis applies when other systemic symptoms of vasculitis are present along with ANCA-positive pauci-immune RPGN by renal biopsy.

Predominance of fibrous crescents, global glomerular sclerosis, interstitial fibrosis, and tubular atrophy in a renal biopsy specimen portends a poor clinical prognosis. Unpredictably, some cellular crescents may resolve without sclerosis and permanent injury.

Treatment

Therapy should be initiated as soon as possible if it is to be valuable in preventing further glomerular injury or progression of crescent formation to global sclerosis and ESRD. For this reason, RPGN is considered a medical emergency by nephrologists. Pulse intravenous corticosteroids may be started before diagnostic renal biopsy is performed or results are available.[19-21] Therapy can always be discontinued within a few days if the biopsy is not confirmative. Because RPGN is rare and is associated with many disorders of diverse etiology, no good, large, controlled therapeutic trials have been or ever might be performed to document the efficacy of a given drug regimen. However, high-dose steroids alone or in combination with cytotoxic agents such as cyclophosphamide have proved effective in improving renal function and reducing dialysis dependence in uncontrolled studies of adults and some children.[19-21] Plasmapheresis in combination with high-dose steroids and cytotoxic agents has been used to treat severely affected adults,[21] and also may be advantageous in the treatment of pediatric patients with anti-GBM disorders or vasculitis (ANCA, Wegener granulomatosis), especially in the presence of pulmonary hemorrhage.

Natural History and Prognosis

Hospitalization may be prolonged for children with RPGN. Most require acute dialysis and may have other severe complications such as pulmonary hemorrhage or hypertension. Approximately half of the children with crescentic GN and clinical RPGN progress to ESRD and require chronic dialysis and eventually renal transplantation. The recurrence rate of RPGN in the transplanted kidney is 10% to 30% depending on the underlying disorder, so renal transplantation usually is delayed for at least 1 year of dialysis therapy to allow the disease to become quiescent before transplant.

ᘎ Pearl

Rapidly progressive GN recurs in 10% to 30% of transplanted kidneys, depending on the underlying disorder.

Nonrenal Infection

Hemolytic Uremic Syndrome

Hemolytic uremic syndrome is characterized by the triad of microangiopathic hemolytic anemia, thrombocytopenia, and acute renal injury.[22-26] The typical disease follows a diarrheal prodrome, usually as a result of infection with enteropathogenic *Escherichia coli* (most commonly O157:H7), *Shigella*, or any bacteria that produce Stx. Shiga-like toxin translocates from the infecting bacteria into the circulation, where it binds to neutrophils, erythrocytes, and platelets and is carried to the small capillaries of the kidney and other organs, such as the brain, pancreas, and heart. In the kidney, Stx binds to globotriaosylceramide receptors on the vascular endothelial cells and renal tubular cells. Once Stx is internalized, it triggers a chain of events that leads to inflammation, endothelial cell injury, and microvascular thrombosis within the kidney.

Non-Stx HUS is often called *atypical HUS,* may be sporadic or familial, and is caused by bacteria such as *Streptococcus pneumoniae* infecting the lungs, viruses, medications including cyclosporine, systemic diseases such as SLE with antiphospholipid syndrome, and genetic defects in factors H or

I or membrane cofactor protein. All atypical HUS should be immediately referred to a specialist. This chapter will focus on diarrhea-positive Stx HUS.

Epidemiology

More than 90% of children with HUS have Stx-associated HUS, which commonly occurs in the summer months between June and September and has a peak incidence in children younger than 5 years. The source of entero-pathogenic *E coli* is often contaminated, undercooked meat or milk from endemically infected cattle, but also exposure to infected petting zoo animals, unpasteurized apple cider, sprouts or lettuce grown with contaminated animal manure, swimming in water contaminated with feces, or just person-to-person spread by hand contamination during diarrhea outbreaks.[22] Only 5% to 20% of patients with hemorrhagic colitis and diarrhea from entero-pathogenic *E coli* develop HUS. Treatment with antimicrobial and antimotility drugs increases the risk of HUS. In developing countries in Asia and Africa, *Shigella dysenteriae* serotype 1 is more commonly the infecting agent causing Stx HUS.

Presenting Symptoms and Physical Examination Findings

Most children have a prodrome of bloody diarrhea (70%), abdominal cramps, vomiting (30%–60%), and fever (30%) for 5 to 10 days before the abrupt onset of pallor, oliguria, and listlessness.[22–24,26] Initial laboratory evaluation, including complete blood count, peripheral smear, and blood chemistries will reveal microangiopathic hemolytic anemia with schistocytes (Figure 20-1), thrombocytopenia (platelet count usually <60,000) and acute kidney injury with elevated serum creatinine and BUN, hyperkalemia, acidosis, hypocalcemia, and/or hyperphosphatemia. Most patients also have leukocytosis and extremely elevated serum lactate dehydrogenase levels. Some patients have gross hematuria, but those with yellow urine usually have hematuria and proteinuria seen on urinalysis. The anemia, thrombocytopenia, and acute kidney injury of HUS usually get progressively worse during several days. About half the patients progress to oligoanuria. Hypertension may occur from volume overload in the presence of oligoanuria as well as from intrinsic renal injury. Some patients with severe disease have central nervous system involvement manifested by seizures, coma, hemiparesis from cerebrovascular accidents, and/or cortical blindness. Retinal microangiopathy can also lead to blindness. Cardiac dysfunction related to

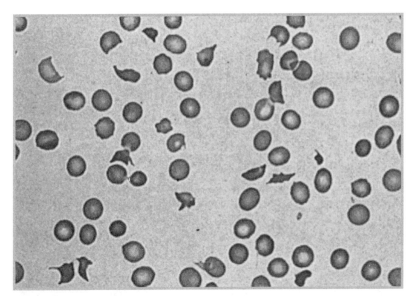

Figure 20-1.
Microangiopathic hemolytic anemia with multiple schistocytes.

volume overload or ischemic heart disease from microthrombi also occurs. Colitis can progress to bowel necrosis, bowel perforation, and/or intussusception. The liver may be enlarged and serum liver enzymes elevated. Some patients develop pancreatic microthrombi with transient diabetes mellitus that rarely persists after recovery from the acute illness. Some also develop adrenal insufficiency.

Differential Diagnosis

Severe gastrointestinal infections with bloody diarrhea and dehydration because of *Salmonella, Campylobacter,* or rotavirus can mimic the early stages of HUS, especially if dehydration is severe enough to cause hypovolemia and elevated serum creatinine and BUN. The absence of microangiopathic hemolytic anemia and thrombocytopenia distinguish these infections from HUS. Systemic vasculitis, such as SLE, ANCA, or HSP, may be difficult to differentiate from HUS, but microangiopathic anemia is not a feature of vasculitis, and HUS is not associated with skin rash or purpura. Rarely, renal biopsy showing characteristic glomerular thrombotic microangiopathy may be needed to definitively diagnose HUS. Thrombocytopenia often limits the performance of diagnostic renal biopsy. Disseminated intravascular coagulation may be suggested by thrombocytopenia, but it is associated with decreased blood levels of fibrinogen and prolonged prothrombin and partial thromboplastin times, which are not features of HUS. Thrombotic thrombocytopenic purpura is similar to HUS, but usually occurs in adults and has a predominance of central nervous system manifestations rather than renal disease.[23]

Treatment

No specific treatment has been shown to be effective, including heparin, plasma infusion, and steroids, so therapy remains symptomatic.[21,23,26] About 75% of patients eventually need packed RBC transfusions. Platelet transfusions should be avoided except for active bleeding because platelets may increase active formation of microthrombi. About 40% of hospitalized children with HUS have acute renal failure severe enough to require dialysis. If colitis is still active and patients are at risk of bowel necrosis and perforation, hemodialysis or continuous renal replacement therapy may be preferable to peritoneal dialysis. Hypertension should be controlled with dietary sodium and fluid restriction, and fluid removal should be controlled by dialysis and antihypertensive medications. A pediatric nephrologist should always be consulted in cases of hypertension and oligoanuria with progressive renal failure.

Natural History and Prognosis

Patients usually start to improve when the platelet count begins to rise, indicating cessation of active formation of microthrombi. Anemia usually does not improve until several days after the platelet count normalizes. Acute kidney injury may completely resolve, but about 25% of children have persistent renal sequelae, including proteinuria, hypertension, and CKD.[27] About 10% to 20% of children with HUS develop ESRD. Prolonged oligoanuria and severe central nervous system disease are associated with poorer prognosis. Mortality has decreased to 3% to 5% with advances in acute dialysis therapy for even the smallest children at specialized pediatric centers.

> ### ❧ Pearl
>
> About 10% to 20% of children with HUS develop ESRD.

Nephritis of Chronic Bacteremia

An immune complex–mediated proliferative GN may occur in the course of acute and subacute bacterial endocarditis, chronically infected ventriculoatrial shunts, and osteomyelitis.[28-30] All have in common the presence of chronic bacteremia, usually with coagulase-positive or coagulase-negative staphylococci or streptococci. Rarely, patients with visceral abscesses (pulmonary, sinus, intraabdominal), with and without documented bacteremia, may present with a similar picture. Bacterial pathogens causing bacteremia in these patients usually are coagulase-positive staphylococci, but occasionally are Gram-negative organisms.

Presenting Symptoms and Physical Examination Findings

The diagnosis should be suspected in patients who have a source of chronic bacteremia and develop hematuria, proteinuria, and/or RBC casts in the course of their disease.[28] Hydrocephalic children with "shunt nephritis" from chronically infected ventriculoatrial shunts have NS at presentation in 30% to 50% of cases.[29]

Blood cultures are the best source for identification of the inciting organism. Most patients have decreased serum C3 concentrations, positive rheumatoid factor, and circulating cryoglobulins and immune complexes. The serum levels of other components of complement (C4 and C1q) also may be depressed. Acute kidney injury with oliguria may occur, especially with bacterial endocarditis or a visceral abscess that is occult for a long time before diagnosis. The incidence of acute kidney injury is high in intravenous drug abusers, who present late for treatment and may be infected with resistant organisms or have right-sided heart valvular disease with initially negative blood cultures.

Kidney biopsy may be needed for diagnosis.[28,30] The renal lesion in affected patients is mesangial or membranoproliferative, such as MPGN type I. The lesion may be focal or diffuse, and is more severe when the underlying illness is unsuspected and goes untreated for a long time. Affected patients may develop focal or diffuse scarring of the glomeruli and CKD. Extensive crescent formation and the clinical course of RPGN occur rarely. Immunofluorescence staining shows granular deposits of immunoglobulin G, immunoglobulin M, and C3 in the mesangium and capillary loops. Soluble antigens of the infecting organism, with or without their specific antibodies, have been demonstrated in glomeruli on renal biopsy, suggesting a direct role for immune complexes in the pathogenesis of this lesion.

Treatment and Prognosis

Specific antibiotic therapy for the underlying infection results in resolution or inactivation of the GN in a few weeks. In some cases, GN persists years after apparent eradication of the infection. As part of therapy, infected ventriculoatrial shunts should be removed and replaced at a later date. Visceral abscesses should be drained surgically. If an infection is treated ineffectively, the GN may progress to chronic renal failure and ESRD, but this is rare with currently available antibiotic therapy.

> ### ₴ Pearl
> The diagnosis of nephritis of chronic bacteremia may require a kidney biopsy.

Late Manifestations of Chronic Disease

Sickle Cell Nephropathy

Renal disease is a late manifestation of sickle cell disease, likely the result of years of renal injury from chronic sickling in the acidic, hypertonic environment of the renal medulla, leading to progressive vasculopathy with obliteration of the medullary vasculature, segmental infarcts, papillary necrosis, interstitial fibrosis, and eventually ischemic glomerular sclerosis.[31-33] Progressive nephropathy is uncommon with sickle cell or combined hemoglobinopathies. The occurrence of progressive nephropathy is more likely with severe disease and chronically lower blood hemoglobin concentration. Other manifestations of sickle cell disease include hematuria and urine concentrating defects.

Epidemiology

The incidence of sickle cell nephropathy in children younger than 10 years is extremely rare, but 12% of adolescents already have proteinuria[34] and about 10% of adults have chronic renal failure before the age of 40.[33] Microalbuminuria, which may be a marker of early renal injury just as it is with diabetic nephropathy, has been documented in children younger than 10 years and in almost 50% of adolescents.[35] Long-term studies are needed to confirm the association of microalbuminuria and progressive renal failure.

Presenting Symptoms and Physical Examination Findings

Urinalysis is the key screening test for renal manifestations of sickle cell disease. Urine specific gravity may be persistently less than or equal to 1.010 because of decreased renal medullary concentrating ability. Microscopic or gross hematuria may occur in children with sickle cell disease or trait and is often predominantly from one kidney, usually the left. Painless gross hematuria is often a result of papillary necrosis. Hematuria and leukocytosis require further evaluation for occult urinary tract infection, which is more common in patients with autosplenectomy. Hematuria and flank pain in black children younger than 20 years with sickle cell trait or disease may be a result of a rare aggressive form of renal medullary carcinoma and should be evaluated by computed tomography of the abdomen.[36] Proteinuria is more common in patients with sickle cell disease, and NS with overt edema is the harbinger of progressive renal disease.[31,32] Serum creatinine, BUN, electrolytes, and albumin should be assessed regularly in patients with proteinuria to diagnose and follow the progression of renal disease.

Differential Diagnosis

In children with known sickle cell disease who develop acute onset of NS, hypertension, and renal failure, a renal biopsy may be necessary to exclude other forms of GN.

Treatment

No specific therapy for sickle cell nephropathy is known, but the use of ACE inhibitors or ARBs has been suggested for patients with proteinuria, even in the absence of hypertension,[31,37] to try to retard the onset of progressive renal failure, as has been done successfully in diabetic nephropathy. The use of ACE inhibitors and ARBs may be limited by the development of hyperkalemia, especially in the presence of elevated serum creatinine and chronic renal insufficiency. Whether optimizing hemoglobin levels and reducing the percentage of sickle cells through frequent blood transfusions might prevent further kidney injury is

> **Pearl**
>
> Urinalysis is the key test to screen for renal manifestations of sickle cell disease.

not known but needs further investigation. Patients who progress to ESRD should be offered chronic dialysis and renal transplantation because outcomes of these therapies are not adversely affected by sickle cell disease.

Prognosis

Heavy proteinuria, NS, and hypertension portend the development of pro-gressive renal failure.[31,33] When renal failure occurs, it usually progresses to ESRD within a few years, despite efforts to retard the progression of disease.

Diabetic Nephropathy

Diabetic nephropathy results from ongoing injury to the microvasculature of the kidney from decades of disease, so the incidence is uncommon in childhood.[38-40] Poor glycemic control is associated with worse vascular injury, but the mechanism is still uncertain.[39] Diabetic nephropathy is pro-gressive and will eventually lead to ESRD and the need for chronic dialysis or renal transplant without intervention. The earliest marker of diabetic renal injury is microalbuminuria, 30 to 300 mg/d. Microalbuminuria has been identified in as many as 5% to10% of adolescents with type 1 diabetes for 10 years, so annual screening of microalbu-minuria is now recommended by the American Diabetes Association for children 10 years or older and with diabetes for 5 years or more.[41]

> **Pearl**
>
> Diabetic nephropathy is uncommon in childhood.

Early identification of microalbuminuria allows early treatment with ACE inhibitors, which has been shown to reverse microalbuminuria and retard the progression of diabetic nephropathy. Blood pressure should also be screened yearly, and if high, treated to main-tain pressure at less than the 90th percentile for age and height to prevent further renal injury. The epidemic of type 2 diabetes is already exponentially increasing the number of adults progressing to chronic dialysis, and the same outcome can be expected for type 2 diabetes diagnosed in childhood and adolescence, likely within 20 years of diagnosis of their disease.[42] Chil-dren with type 2 diabetes also have an increased incidence of primary hyper-tension, another risk factor for progression of CKD.

Malignancy and Its Treatment

A variety of renal disorders are associated with childhood malignancies[43] (see Box 20-1). Unilateral or bilateral ureteral obstruction occurs with large abdominal lymphomas, such as Burkett lymphoma. If the tumor rapidly regresses in response to chemotherapy, the patient is at risk for postobstructive diuresis and the need for massive fluid replacement and close monitoring of fluids and serum electrolytes. Acute obstruction may also occur with uric acid nephropathy, but rarely occurs now with protocols for hydration and alkalinization of urine and newer drugs to lower blood uric acid.[44]

Lymphoproliferative malignancies have been associated with several forms of GN. Rarely, pediatric patients with Hodgkin disease present with NS that appears to be minimal change disease by renal biopsy and remits with successful therapy of the Hodgkin disease.[45] In adults, NS and membranous glomerulopathy have been associated with non-Hodgkin lymphoma, but mostly with solid tumors, such as lung or colon carcinoma, which are often occult at the time of the onset of NS. Membranoproliferative GN has been associated with chronic lymphocytic leukemia in adults,[46] but not in children.

Renal dysfunction may also occur with therapy of childhood malignancies.[43] Most common in children is tumor lysis syndrome, with acute kidney injury, hyperkalemia, hyperphosphatemia, hypocalcemia, and hyperuricemia that result from the rapid response to chemotherapy of patients with a large tumor burden from acute leukemia or lymphoma. As the tumor cells rapidly break down, intracellular potassium, phosphorus, and other toxic substances are released into the circulation and overwhelm the kidneys' capacity for removal. Acute hemodialysis followed by continuous renal replacement may be lifesaving in this circumstance. Leukemic infiltration of the kidney may also lead to nephromegaly and acute renal failure that improves with treatment of the leukemia.[43]

Some of the agents used to treat malignancies also are nephrotoxic, including the acute renal failure and proximal tubular dysfunction of renal Fanconi syndrome from cisplatinum, carboplatinum, and ifosfamide, as well as hemorrhagic cystitis from cyclophosphamide[43] (see Box 20-1).

ஜ *Pearl*

Some chemotherapeutic agents are nephrotoxic.

References

1. Willard RJ, Montemarano AD. Henoch-Schönlein purpura (anaphylactoid purpura). E-medicine from Web MD. 2007. http://www.emedicine.com/derm/topic177.htm. Accessed September 2007

2. Saulsbury FT. Henoch-Schönlein purpura in children. Report of 100 patients and review of the literature. *Medicine.* 1999;78:395–409

3. Trapani S, Micheli A, Grisolia F, et al. Henoch Schönlein purpura in childhood: epidemiological and clinical analysis of 150 cases over a 5-year period and review of literature. *Semin Arthritis Rheum.* 2005;35:143–153

4. Gardner-Medwin JMM, Dolezalova P, Cummins C, Southwood RT. Incidence of Henoch-Schönlein purpura, Kawasaki disease, and rare vasculitides in children of different ethnic origins. *Lancet.* 2002;360:1197–1202

5. Chang WL, Yang YH, Wang LC, Lin YT, Chiang BL. Renal manifestations in Henoch-Schönlein purpura: a 10-year clinical study. *Pediatr Nephrol.* 2005;20:1269–1272

6. Bayrakci US, Topaloglu R, Soylemezoglu O, et al. Effect of early corticosteroid therapy on development of Henoch Schonlein nephritis. *J Nephrol.* 2007;20:406–409

7. Singh S, Devidayal, Kumar L, Joshi K, Minz RW, Datta U. Severe Henoch-Schönlein nephritis: resolution with azathioprine and steroids. *Rheumatol Int.* 2002;22:133–137

8. Flynn JT, Smoyer WE, Bunchman TE, Kershaw DB, Sedman AB. Treatment of Henoch-Schönlein purpura glomerulonephritis in children with high-dose corticosteroid plus oral cyclophosphamide. *Am J Nephrol.* 2001;21:128–133

9. Lehman TJ, McCurdy KD, Bernstein BH, King KK, Hanson V. Systemic lupus erythematosus in the first decade of life. *Pediatrics.* 1989;83:235–239

10. Benseler SM, Silverman ED. Systemic lupus erythematosus. *Pediatr Clin North Am.* 2005; 52:443–467

11. Stichweh D, Arce E, Pascual V. Update of pediatric systemic lupus erythematosus. *Curr Opin Rheumatol.* 2004;16:577–587

12. Kozeny GA, Barr W, Bansal VK, et al. Occurrence of renal tubular dysfunction in lupus nephritis. *Arch Intern Med.* 1987;147:891–895

13. Weening JJ, D'Agnati V, Schwartz MM, et al. The classification of glomerulonephritis in systemic lupus erythematosus revisited. *J Am Soc Nephrol.* 2004;15:241–250

14. Houssiau F. Thirty years of cyclophosphamide: assessing the evidence. *Lupus.* 2007; 16:212–216

15. Askenazi D, Myones B, Kamdar A, et al. Outcomes of children with proliferative lupus nephritis: the role of protocol renal biopsy. *Pediatr Nephrol.* 2007;22:981–986

16. Paredes A. Can mycophenolate mofetil substitute cyclophosphamide treatment of pediatric lupus nephritis? *Pediatr Nephrol.* 2007;22:1077–1082

17. Bolton WK. Rapidly progressive glomerulonephritis. *Semin Nephrol.* 1996;16:517–526

18. Bolton WK. Goodpasture's syndrome. *Kidney Int.* 1996;50:1753–1766

19. Akikusa JD, Schneider R, Harvey EZ, et al. Clinical features and outcome of pediatric Wegener's granulomatosis. *Arthritis Rheum.* 2007;57:837–844

20. Bakkaloglu A, Ozen S, Baskin E, et al. The significance of antineutrophil cytoplasmic antibody in microscopic polyangitis and classic polyarteritis nodosa. *Arch Dis Child.* 2001;85:427–430

21. Seo P, Stone JH. The antineutrophil cytoplasmic antibody-associated vasculitides. *Am J Med.* 2004;117:39–50

22. Tarr PI, Gordon CA, Chandler WL. Shiga-toxin-producing *Escherichia coli* and haemolytic uraemic syndrome. *Lancet.* 2005;365:1073–1086

23. Hosler GA, Cusumano AM, Hutchins GM. Thrombotic thrombocytopenic purpura and hemolytic uremic syndrome are distinct pathologic entities. *Arch Pathol Lab Med.* 2003;127:834–839

24. Moake JL. Thrombotic microangiopathies. *N Engl J Med.* 2002;347:589–600

25. Kavanagh D, Goodship TH, Richards A. Atypical haemolytic uraemic syndrome. *Br Med Bull.* 2006;77–78:5–22

26. Noris M, Remuzzi G. Hemolytic uremic syndrome. *J Am Soc Nephrol.* 2005;16:1035–1050

27. Garg AX, Suri RS, Barrowman N, et al. Long-term renal prognosis of diarrhea-associated hemolytic uremic syndrome. *JAMA.* 2003;290:1360–1370

28. Kim Y, Michael AF. Chronic bacteremia and nephritis. *Ann Rev Med.* 1978;29:319–325

29. Haffner D, Schindera F, Aschoff A, Matthias S, Waldherr R, Schärer K. The clinical spectrum of shunt nephritis. *Nephrol Dial Transplant.* 1997;12:1143–1148

30. Griffin MD, Bjornsson J, Erickson SB. Diffuse proliferative glomerulonephritis and acute renal failure associated with acute staphylococcal osteomyelitis. *J Am Soc Nephrol.* 1997;8:1633–1639

31. Pham P-TT, Pham P-CT, Wilkinson AH, Lew SQ. Renal abnormalities in sickle cell disease. *Kidney Int.* 2000;57:1–8

32. Guasch A, Navarrete J, Nass K, Zayas CF. Glomerular involvement in adults with sickle cell hemoglobinopathies: prevalence and clinical correlates of progressive renal failure. *J Am Soc Nephrol.* 2006;17:2228–2235

33. Powars DR, Chan LS, Hiti A, Ramicone E, Johnson C. Outcome of sickle cell anemia: a 4-decade observational study of 1056 patients. *Medicine.* 2005;84:363–376

34. Wigfall DR, Ware RE, Burchinal MR, Kinney TR, Foreman JW. Prevalence and clinical correlates of glomerulopathy in children with sickle cell disease. *J Pediatr.* 2000;136:749–753

35. Dharnidharka VR, Dabbagh S, Atiyeh B, Simpson P, Saraik S. Prevalence of microalbuminuria in children with sickle cell disease. *Pediatr Nephrol.* 1998;12:475–478

36. Vargas-Gonzalez R, Sotelo-Avila C, Coria AS. Renal medullary carcinoma in a six-year-old boy with sickle cell trait. *Pathol Oncol Res.* 2003;9:193–195

37. Aoki RY, Saad ST. Enalapril reduces the albuminuria of patients with sickle cell disease. *Am J Med.* 1995;98:432–435

38. Svensson M, Nystrom L, Schon S, Dahlquist G. Age at onset of childhood-onset type 1 diabetes and the development of end stage renal disease: a nationwide population-based study. *Diabetes Care.* 2006;29:538–542

39. Svensson M, Eriksson JW, Dahlquist G. Early glycemic control, age at onset and development of microvascular complications in childhood-onset type 1 diabetes: a population-based study in northern Sweden. *Diabetes Care.* 2004;27:955–962

40. Karavanaki K, Baum JD. Coexistence of impaired indices of autonomic neuropathy and diabetic nephropathy in a cohort of children with type 1 diabetes mellitus. *J Pediatr Endocrinol Metab.* 2003;16:79–90

41. Silverstein J, Klingensmith G, Copeland K. Care of children and adolescents with type 1 diabetes: a statement of the American Diabetes Association. *Diabetes Care.* 2005;28: 186–212

42. Krakoff J, Lindsay RS, Looker HC, Nelson RG, Hanson RL, Knowler WC. Incidence of retinopathy and nephropathy in youth-onset compared with adult-onset type 2 diabetes. *Diabetes Care.* 2003;26:76–81

43. Rossi R, Kleta R, Ehrich JHH. Renal involvement in children with malignancies. *Pediatr Nephrol.* 1999;13:153–162

44. Wossmann W, Schrappe M, Meyer U, Zimmermann M, Reiter A. Incidence of tumor lysis syndrome in children with advanced stage Burkitt lymphoma/leukemia before and after introduction of prophylactic use of urate oxidase. *Ann Hematol.* 2003;82:160–165

45. Mallouk A, Pham PT, Pham PC. Concurrent FSGS and Hodgkin lymphoma: case report and literature review on the link between nephrotic glomerulopathies and hematological malignancies. *Clin Exp Nephrol.* 2006;10:284–289

46. Ronco PM. Paraneoplastic glomerulopathies: new insights into an old entity. *Kidney Int.* 1999;56:355–377

Prevention of Kidney Disease

Amin J. Barakat

Abbreviations

CKD	Chronic kidney disease
DMSA	Dimercaptosuccinic acid
ESRD	End-stage renal disease
GN	Glomerulonephritis
MMR	Measles, mumps, rubella
RPGN	Rapidly progressive glomerulonephritis
UTI	Urinary tract infection
VCUG	Voiding cystourethrogram

Introduction

Renal disease is a major cause of morbidity and mortality.[1] The overall incidence of kidney and urinary tract abnormalities is approximately 5% and may reach up to 10% in males younger than 18 years. Urinary tract abnormalities represent 25% of the total ultrasonographically diagnosed malformations, occurring in 0.25% to 0.7% of fetuses. These abnormalities, along with hereditary diseases of the kidney and UTIs, account for 50% to 90% of cases of ESRD. The annual incidence of ESRD is about 9.8 patients per million children.

The best available treatment for ESRD at the present time is renal transplantation, and as a temporary measure, chronic dialysis (see Chapter 14). Renal transplantation yields excellent results, but it is expensive and can be complicated by rejection and, sometimes, recurrence of the original disease in the transplanted kidney. In addition, the available facilities and number of renal grafts are not adequate to cover all patients requiring this treatment. Chronic dialysis is not the ideal treatment and is also expensive. Furthermore, technical problems are encountered in obtaining arterial access in children, thus making chronic hemodialysis difficult to maintain in the pediatric age group. Peritoneal dialysis may be complicated by metabolic derangements and infection, often interfering with adequate peritoneal exchange. The incidence of renal replacement therapy (dialysis and transplantation) is 9.9 per million age-related populations.

❧ Pearl

The best "treatment" of ESRD is prevention. Once children with CKD are identified, primary care physicians should refer them to a pediatric nephrologist.

The best "treatment" for ESRD in children, therefore, is prevention. In this chapter, the role of early diagnosis and intervention in the prevention, or the favorable alteration of, the natural course of kidney disease is briefly discussed. The role of primary care physicians in the early diagnosis, treatment, and screening of children for renal disease is outlined.

The prevention of renal disease is divided into primary and secondary prevention. Although it is difficult to clearly separate the role of a primary care physician from that of a pediatric nephrologist, the responsibility of a primary care physician probably lies with primary prevention. The role of a pediatric nephrologist is to perform more advanced diagnosis and try to prevent the progression of renal disease to ESRD.

Primary Prevention—The Role of the Primary Care Physician

Primary care physicians should be able to diagnose and treat various renal conditions depending on their level of comfort. To make a prompt diagnosis, they should keep a high index of suspicion for kidney disease.

History and Physical Examination

Early diagnosis of renal disease requires a high index of suspicion because it may be overt or asymptomatic, escaping medical attention. Children with asymptomatic renal disease deserve the same attention as symptomatic and sick ones. A thorough prenatal, postnatal, and family history should be obtained and a complete physical examination performed (Chapter 2). Physicians should look for subtle signs and symptoms, which may often appear unrelated to the urinary tract. These include unexplained fevers, failure to thrive, anemia, acidosis, gastrointestinal symptoms, deafness, neonatal hypoxia, a single umbilical artery, the use of nephrotoxic drugs, the presence of ear lobe anomalies, and supernumerary nipples.

Family history of early deafness, renal failure, hypertension, diabetes, or urologic surgery should be obtained. Kidney disease should be suspected in children with family history of certain renal conditions (Alport syndrome, polycystic kidney disease, vesicoureteral reflux, and others). Kidney and urinary tract abnormalities should be looked for in children with congenital abnormalities of other organ systems (cardiovascular, gastrointestinal, central nervous system, genital), chromosomal aberrations, UTI, failure to thrive, and various genetic and systemic diseases. Vesicoureteral reflux, a major cause of renal scarring in children, may be familial in as high as 45% of patients. More than 300 genetic conditions may be associated with renal and urogenital abnormalities. Some of these are presented in Appendix IV.

Blood Pressure Measurement

Hypertension occurs in about 1% of children. The 3 most common symptoms of hypertension in children are headache, difficulty sleeping, and fatigue. Mass screening programs for hypertension in children are not cost-effective; however, blood pressure should be measured routinely in every child beginning at 3 years and when indicated. Hypertension in children is defined as an average systolic and/or diastolic blood pressure at the 95th percentile or above for age and sex measured on at least 3 separate occasions. It is usually renal, renovascular, or essential in etiology. There is evidence that primary hypertension in adults may be preceded by high blood pressure in childhood. If inadequately treated, elevated blood pressure may be complicated by arteriosclerosis, nephrosclerosis, retinopathy, and cerebral hemorrhage. Early diagnosis and control of hypertension, therefore, are important in preventing future morbidity from this disease.

Management of hypertension consists of pharmacologic and nonpharmacologic therapy, which includes weight reduction, dietary modification, salt restriction, and physical conditioning. Effective therapy is necessary to preserve renal function. Angiotensin-converting enzyme inhibitors and angiotensin II receptor antagonists preferentially lower intraglomerular pressure and reduce proteinuria. These agents, especially when combined, are more effective than others in preventing the progression of renal failure.

ᕦ Pearl

Effective therapy of hypertension is necessary to preserve renal function.

Children presenting with persistent, severe, or malignant hypertension require comprehensive evaluation and initiation of antihypertensive therapy and should be referred to a pediatric nephrologist. Public education should advocate routine blood pressure measurement, weight control, exercise, and avoidance of high salt intake. Hypertension is discussed in detail in Chapter 15.

Urinalysis and Urine Culture

Abnormal findings in the urine may be the first sign of renal disease; therefore, a routine urinalysis should be performed periodically on all children. Hematuria, proteinuria, and casts suggest glomerular disease. Pyuria is usually a sign of UTI, but it may also be present with inflammation, renal calculi, or urinary tract abnormalities. Pyuria may be absent in preschool children with UTI, and a urine culture is necessary to make the diagnosis. Any child with suspected UTI or unexplained fever should have a urinalysis and urine culture. A defect in the concentrating ability of the kidney can occur in diabetes mellitus, diabetes insipidus, renal failure, sickle cell disease, and other tubular disorders. Urinalysis is discussed in detail in Chapter 3.

Urinary Tract Infection

Urinary tract infection is a major cause of morbidity in children (see Chapter 6). Delay in the diagnosis and treatment of UTI may lead to pyelonephritis, renal scarring, and ESRD. Children may have subtle symptoms not related to the urinary tract, such as unexplained fevers, gastrointestinal symptoms, irritability, and failure to thrive. Often, urinalysis is normal, making the recognition of UTI more difficult. Successful treatment of UTI in children consists of suspecting the condition, prompt and accurate diagnosis, adequate therapy, imaging of the urinary tract, surgical correction of urologic abnormalities when necessary, and close follow-up with urine cultures. When pyelonephritis is suspected, a DMSA scan should be performed in addition to renal ultrasound and VCUG to rule out renal scarring. Prolonged suppressive antibiotic therapy also plays a role in the prevention of recurrence.

Imaging of the Urinary Tract

Developmental anomalies of the urinary tract are found in about one-third of children following the first attack of pyelonephritis. Vesicoureteral reflux occurs in about 35% (50% in the first year of life), and obstructive uropathy occurs in 10% of children with symptomatic or asymptomatic UTI. A renal ultrasound, a VCUG and, if indicated, a renal scan should be performed following the first documented UTI (see Chapters 5 and 6). A DMSA scan should be performed on patients with UTI associated with fever, sepsis, and systemic findings suggestive of pyelonephritis. The DMSA scan can detect cortical scarring when renal ultrasound and VCUG are normal.

Congenital Abnormalities of the Kidney and Urinary Tract

When a congenital urinary tract abnormality is discovered in a fetus, renal function should be assessed after birth, and anomalies of other organs and chromosomal aberrations should be looked for. Urinary tract obstruction before 15 weeks' gestation may result in renal dysplasia, whereas late obstruction may produce hydronephrosis and cystic changes with functionally normal kidneys at birth. With unilateral renal malformations, investigation and treatment may be started following term delivery. Fetuses with bilateral hydronephrosis should be followed up closely with sonograms. Fetuses with no evidence of impairment should be investigated at term, and those with severe reduction in renal function may undergo preterm delivery to institute early diagnosis and treatment. If this is not possible, fetal surgery may be attempted (see the following section). Fetuses with oligohydramnios and bilateral renal agenesis or cystic malformations carry a poor prognosis for life.

Affected newborns should be managed as early as possible. Various factors, including volume status, diet, and the timing of obstruction, affect the severity of renal failure in obstructive uropathy. Relief of obstruction in children younger than 6 months may be associated with improvement in renal function. Keep in mind that a diseased kidney is more vulnerable to infection, obstruction, hemorrhage, stone formation and, consequently,

> ## ≈ *Pearl*
>
> A diseased kidney is more vulnerable to infection, obstruction, hemorrhage, stone formation, and further deterioration in function.

morbidity and further deterioration in renal function. Early treatment of these complications will help prevent additional renal damage. Congenital anomalies of the kidney and urinary tract are discussed by Barakat and Drougas[2] and in Appendix IV and Chapter 18.

Prenatal Diagnosis of Renal and Urinary Tract Abnormalities

Various renal and urinary tract abnormalities, particularly obstructive uropathy, may be diagnosed prenatally by ultrasonography at 17 and 32 weeks' gestation. The test is sensitive but nonspecific. Magnetic resonance imaging may be a valuable additional method if resolution of ultrasound is impaired because of oligohydramnios or technical problems. Transvaginal sonography is another additional tool that may be used in certain cases.

Different conditions and syndromes associated with kidney and urinary tract abnormalities can be diagnosed by chromosomal karyotyping, enzyme determination in amniocytes, and alpha-fetoprotein determination in maternal blood and amniotic fluid. Because the mutation for autosomal dominant polycystic kidney disease was localized to the short arm of chromosome 16 more than 2 decades ago, gene mutations have been described in many renal diseases (see Table 16-1).

> ## ≈ *Pearl*
>
> Prenatal diagnosis of urinary tract abnormalities contributes to early neonatal intervention to save kidney function.

Prenatal diagnosis of various urinary tract abnormalities contributes to early neonatal intervention to save kidney function. Fetal surgery for obstructive uropathy is widely debated and should be performed only for carefully selected patients. Currently, surgery is inadequate and it raises complex ethical questions that must be dealt with, such as the accuracy of diagnosis and termination of pregnancy in conditions that are compatible with life. Prenatal diagnosis of kidney and urinary tract abnormalities is discussed in Chapter 17.

Screening for Renal Disease

Primary care physicians may screen children for renal disease by performing routine urinalysis on all children. Patients with positive findings on urinalysis may be studied according to the specific abnormality as described elsewhere in this book. A quick screen to exclude the presence of renal disease includes some or all of the following: (1) history and physical examination including blood pressure measurement; (2) a repeat clean, early morning urinalysis and urine culture; (3) serum urea nitrogen, creatinine, electrolytes, calcium, phosphorus, C3 complement; (4) 24-hour urine for creatinine, protein, volume, and calcium (urine protein/creatinine and urine calcium/creatinine ratios correlate well with timed collections); (5) creatinine clearance; (6) renal ultrasound, VCUG and, when indicated, a renal scan; and (7) other studies as necessary. Mass screening is discussed under secondary prevention because it requires a dedicated team approach.

Consultation With the Pediatric Nephrologist and Urologist

Early diagnosis of kidney and urinary tract disease allows timely intervention to prevent renal damage. Primary care physicians may manage patients with renal disease to the extent that they feel comfortable, such as treatment of UTI and investigation or follow-up of children with hematuria, proteinuria, and renal anomalies. Complicated diseases and abnormalities, such as acute kidney injury, CKD, severe abnormalities requiring surgery, and

ᔛ *Pearl*

Primary care physicians may manage patients with renal disease to the extent that they feel comfortable.

other abnormalities requiring advanced diagnostic and therapeutic skills, should be referred to a specialist.

Prevention of Disease

Pediatric patients with CKD and those on dialysis should receive all routine immunizations recommended by the American Academy of Pediatrics, as well as the influenza vaccine. Recipients of renal transplants should also be immunized, but live viral vaccines (MMR, oral polio, varicella) should be avoided during immunosuppressive therapy. It is recommended to wait 6 months after transplantation when immune suppression is less intense to resume immunization. Antibody response to MMR and varicella should be checked before transplantation, and unprotected patients should be immunized at least 1 month before transplantation. Patients with CKD do better with the 2-dose regimen of varicella vaccine. Household and health care contacts of transplant recipients should have immunity or be immunized against polio, MMR, varicella, hepatitis A, and influenza. When needed, inactived polio vaccine and not oral polio should be used in patients and their household contacts. There are ongoing studies on Epstein-Barr virus and *Staphylococcus aureus* vaccines that will be important for patients who need dialysis or transplantation; however, vaccines for hepatitis C and *Pneumocystis carinii,* when available, will be of great help to patients with CKD. Oral health and hygiene are of utmost importance in patients with CKD.

> **꙳ Pearl**
>
> Pediatric patients with CKD and those on dialysis should receive all routine immunizations recommended by the American Academy of Pediatrics, as well as the influenza vaccine.

Secondary Prevention

Mass Screening

Asymptomatic bacteriuria occurs in 1.2% of schoolgirls, 0.03% of schoolboys, and 2% of young women. The cumulative incidence of UTI in schoolgirls followed over a 10-year span is about 5% (see Chapter 6). The prevalence of urinary abnormalities is about 0.5% among elementary schoolchildren and 0.75% among junior high students. The morbidity rate of chronic glomerular disease is about 40 to 50 per 100,000 hospitalized schoolchildren, and 2 to 4 times more than that when asymptomatic patients are picked up by mass screening for hematuria and proteinuria. Children with isolated asymptomatic hematuria tend to have minor histologic changes, whereas those with both hematuria and proteinuria have diffuse proliferative lesions. Severe lesions are more common in those with heavy proteinuria and hematuria. More than 70% of patients with IgA nephropathy and 65% to 80% with membranoproliferative GN may be detected by mass urine screening of schoolchildren.[3,4]

Although it is debatable whether mass urine screening programs are cost-effective, they can definitely contribute to the diagnosis of many asymptomatic children who do not have access to routine medical care.[3,4] The presence of urinary abnormalities on routine urinalysis leads to the early diagnosis and treatment of kidney disease, adequate follow-up and, when indicated, investigation of other members of the family.

Screening programs should be accurate, practical, and economical. They should be performed by individuals capable of interpreting the results and following up children with positive results, and they should be backed up by an institution to ensure continuity. Efforts should be made to get the support and cooperation of the local departments of health and education, as well as the school board,

☙ Pearl

Although it is debatable whether mass urine screening programs are cost-effective, they can contribute to the diagnosis of asymptomatic children who do not have access to routine medical care.

students, families of students, and the community as a whole. Public education to explain the signs and symptoms of renal disease and the benefits obtained from these screening programs through the use of the news media is also effective.

The automated urinary flow cytometer can differentiate between glomerular (dysmorphic red blood cells) and nonglomerular hematuria more accurately, thus making mass screening more cost-effective.

Primary care physicians may do their own screening by performing urinalyses (and other studies as needed) as a part of routine checkups (see previous section on screening for renal disease).

Kidney Disease Prevention Program

Early diagnosis and treatment of renal disease may be achieved by establishing kidney disease prevention programs, which, in collaboration with a pediatric nephrology service, should promote: (1) public education, (2) school screening programs, (3) genetic screening and family counseling, and (4) prenatal diagnosis of obstructive uropathy and genetic diseases of the kidney. The programs can be tailored according to specific needs of the population, and their practicality and cost-effectiveness should be considered. Although this may seem to be out of their realm, primary care physicians should be familiar with such programs available in their community.

Genetic Screening

Genetic markers and gene mutations have been identified in various renal diseases and syndromes associated with renal disease.[5,6] This contributes to early treatment of certain kidney diseases to reduce the risk of developing ESRD (see Chapter 16). Genetic markers also help in genetic counseling and avoiding transplanting an affected kidney from an asymptomatic donor. Some conditions with known gene mutations are presented in Table 16-1.

೩♥ Pearl

Genetic markers and gene mutations have been identified in various renal diseases and syndromes associated with renal disease.

Intervention

Once children with CKD are identified, primary care physicians should refer them to a pediatric nephrologist who will direct their treatment and intervention toward preventing progression of the disease to ESRD. Identifying reversible causes of renal failure and avoiding nephrotoxic drugs are paramount in the prevention of renal failure. Cardiovascular disease and infection are the major causes of death in children with ESRD.

It is not well known whether treatment of glomerulopathies can prevent progression of the disease to CKD.[7-10] Because these diseases are heterogeneous, they may represent similar end-organ responses to different pathologic processes, and some of them may have spontaneous recovery. There is some evidence, however, that treatment of some of these conditions, such as membranoproliferative disease, anti–glomerular basement membrane disease, and RPGN may prevent or delay the development of renal failure.[11] Methylprednisolone pulse therapy and plasma exchange, for example, may be effective in RPGN. Limiting protein intake and the use of essential amino acid or ketoacid supplements may have some beneficial effect on slowing the rate of progression of renal failure, although the effect on renal histology has not been confirmed.

Phosphate and sodium restriction, altering lipid intake and composition, controlling acidosis, antihypertensive treatment, and the use of oral adsorbents may also help delay progression of renal failure. A nutritionist should be involved early in the course of CKD to help patients maintain proper caloric and protein intake to slow the progression of renal failure and avoid malnutrition. If linear growth is not maintained on adequate energy, protein, and micronutrient intake and after correction of acidosis, hyperphosphatemias and secondary hyperparathyroidism, then growth hormone treatment should be considered (see Chapter 14).

Angiotensin-converting enzyme inhibitors and angiotensin receptor blockers may reduce proteinuria and attenuate the magnitude of injury from hyperfiltration and glomerulosclerosis. Correction of anemia with erythropoietin improves growth, energy levels, psychosocial development, and cardiac function of patients; limits the progression of CKD; and may reduce mortality. Growth hormone increases growth velocity.

☙ Pearl

Identifying reversible causes of renal failure and avoiding nephrotoxic drugs are paramount in the prevention of renal failure.

Uncontrolled diabetes mellitus produces diabetic nephropathy, which is the most common cause of CKD in adults. Glycated hemoglobin (A1C) control (<7%), screening for microalbuminuria, and control of blood pressure with an angiotensin-converting enzyme inhibitor or angiotensin II receptor antagonist reduce the progression of renal disease.

Other less understood and experimental treatment modalities for chronic GN and CKD include cytokine modulation, antifibrotic therapy, endothelin receptor antagonists, nitric oxide modulation, vasopeptidase inhibition, antioxidant therapy, statin therapy, and others.[9,10]

Gene Therapy

Although gene therapy has a great potential in the treatment of renal disease, the technology is too preliminary for clinical application. Potential applications of gene therapy in renal disease include Alport syndrome, renal tumors (replacement of tumor suppressor genes), genetic renal disease, acute kidney injury, glomerular and tubulointerstitial disease (delivery of antagonists of cytokines of cell adhesion molecules), transplant rejection, stone disease, and others. Before this mode of therapy becomes clinically applicable, gene delivery must be improved, renal cell–specific genes developed, and side effects minimized.

> **ဆ Pearl**
>
> Although gene therapy has great potential in the treatment of renal disease, technology at the present time is too preliminary for clinical application.

Research

Systematic collection of information on patients who have or are at risk for having renal disease and identifying research priorities is crucial in the prevention of CKD. A more complete knowledge is needed concerning the etiology, pathogenesis, epidemiology, and treatment of renal disease, as well as molecular mechanisms of the disease, growth factors, renal hormones, molecular genetics of renal dysgenesis, and renal disease genes. New markers of kidney damage, new treatments to slow progression of CKD, and new health care policies are needed.

Summary

Prevention of renal disease can be achieved by early diagnosis and treatment, clinical and genetic screening, prenatal diagnosis, and early intervention to prevent the progression of CKD to ESRD. Primary care physicians can contribute significantly to this process. Although these measures will have a considerable impact on reducing morbidity and mortality from renal disease, certain limitations still exist and further research in the fields of pathogenesis and treatment of renal disease is needed before more effective prevention can be achieved.

References

1. Barakat AY, ed. *Renal Disease in Children: Clinical Evaluation and Diagnosis.* New York, NY: Springer-Verlag; 1990

2. Barakat AY, Drougas JG. Occurrence of renal and urinary tract abnormalities in 13,775 autopsies. *Urology.* 1991;38:347–350

3. Murakami M, Hayakawa M, Yanagihara T, Hukunaga Y. Proteinuria screening for children. *Kidney Int Suppl.* 2005;94:S23–S27

4. Kitagawa T. Lessons learned from the Japanese nephritis screening study. *Pediatr Nephrol.* 1988;2:256–263

5. Milunsky A. *Genetic Disorders and the Fetus: Diagnosis, Prevention, and Treatment.* 5th ed. Baltimore, MD: Johns Hopkins University Press; 2004

6. McKusick-Nathans Institute for Genetic Medicine, Johns Hopkins University (Baltimore, MD), and National Center for Biotechnology Information. Online Mendelian Inheritance in Man (OMIM). Bethesda, MD: National Library of Medicine; 2000. http://www.ncbi. nlm.nih.gov/omim/. Accessed March 20, 2008

7. Coppo R, Amore A. New perspectives in treatment of glomerulonephritis. *Pediatr Nephrol.* 2004;19:256–265

8. Jeber BL, Madias NE. Progression of chronic kidney disease: can it be prevented or arrested? *Am J Med.* 2005;118:1323–1330

9. Levey AS, Andreoli SP, DuBose T, Provenzano R, Collins AJ. Chronic kidney disease: common, harmful and treatable—World Kidney Day 2007. *Pediatr Nephrol.* 2007;22:321–325

10. Chesney RW, Brewer E, Moxey-Mims M, et al. Report of an NIH task force on research priorities in chronic kidney disease in children. *Pediatr Nephrol.* 2006;21:14–25

11. Klahr S, Schreiner G, Ichikawa I. The progression of renal disease. *N Engl J Med.* 1988;318:1657–1666

Reference Range

*Amin J. Barakat and Coni Evans**

This appendix presents the reference range of laboratory tests performed to help in the diagnosis of renal disease. Also, please refer to Chapter 4. Values may vary according to the methodology used. Laboratory values are given in conventional and international units. Key references have been used in the formulation of this table.[1-4] Some values have been obtained from specific studies and reports, and the references may be found elsewhere.[4] The prefixes for units are the standard ones approved by the Conference Generale des Poids et Mesures (1964), the International Union of Pure and Applied Chemistry, and the International Federation of Clinical Chemistry. Few other abbreviations are used in the table; for these, please see the table footnote.

---

*Director, Clinical Laboratory, Northern Virginia Pediatric Associates, Falls Church, VA.

Test	Specimen		Conventional Units, g/dL	International Units, g/L
Albumin	S	Premature	1.8–3.0	18–30
		NB	2.5–3.4	25–34
		Infant	3.9–5.0	39–50
		Thereafter	4.0–5.3	40–53
	U	See urine protein		
			ng/dL	nmol/L
Aldosterone	S	3 d	7–184	0.19–5.1
		1 wk	5–175	0.14–4.8
		1–12 mo	5–90	0.14–2.5
		1–2 y	7–54	0.19–1.5
		2–10 y	3–35	0.1–0.97
		10–15 y	2–22	0.1–0.6
		Adult		
		Average sodium diet		
		Supine	3–10	0.08–0.3
		Upright		
		F	5–30	0.14–0.8
		M	6–22	0.17–0.61
			U/L	
Alkaline phosphatase	S	Infant	150–420	Same
		Child, 2–10 y	100–320	
		11–18 y, M	100–390	
		11–18 y, F	100–320	
		Adult	30–120	
Angiotensin I	P (EDTA)	Peripheral vein	11–88 pg/mL	11–88 ng/L
Angiotensin II	P (EDTA)	Arterial	1.2–3.6 ng/dL	12–36 ng/L
		Venous	50%–75% of arterial conc	Fraction of arterial conc 0.50–0.75
Anion gap ($[Na^+ + K^+] - [Cl^- + HCO_3^-]$)	P (heparin)		7–16 mmol/L	Same

		Plasma, mOsmol/kg	Plasma ADH, pg/mL	Plasma ADH, ng/L
Antidiuretic hormone (ADH vaso-pressin)	P (EDTA)	270–280	<1.5	Same
		280–285	<2.5	
		285–290	1–5	
		290–295	2–7	
		395–300	4–12	
Anti-nDNA antibody		<1:20		
Antinuclear antibody (ANA) titer		Not significant <1:80		
		Significant >1:320		
Antistreptolysin S (ASO) titer		2–5 y	120–160 Todd units	
		6–8 y	>240 Todd units	
		10–12 y	>329 Todd units	
			mmol/L	
Base excess	B (heparin)	NB	–10 to –2	Same
		Infant	–7 to –1	
		Child	–4 to +2	
		Thereafter	–2 to +3	
			mEq/L	**mmol/L**
Bicarbonate (HCO$_3$)	S	Premature	18–26	Same
		Infant	17–24	
		2 mo–2 y	16–24	
		1–2 y	20–25	
		2 y	22–26	
Blood volume	B (heparin)	M	52–83 mL/kg	0.052–0.083 L/kg
		F	50–75 mL/kg	0.050–0.075 L/kg

			pg/mL	pmol/L
Calcitonin (hCT)	S, P (heparin, EDTA)	M	3–26	0.8–7.2
		F	2–17	0.6–4.7
		Higher in NBs		
			mg/dL	**mmol/L**
Calcium, ionized (iCa)	S, P, B	3–24 h	4.3–5.1	1.07–1.27
		24–48 h	4.0–4.7	1.00–1.17
		Thereafter	4.48–4.92	1.12–1.23
			mg/dL	**mmol/L**
Calcium, total	S	Cord	9.0–11.5	2.25–2.88
		Premature	6.1–11.6	1.52–2.90
		3–24 h	9.0–10.6	2.3–2.65
		24–48 h	7.0–12.0	1.75–3.0
		4–7 d	9.0–10.9	2.25–2.73
		Child	8.8–10.8	2.2–2.70
		Thereafter	8.4–10.2	2.1–2.55
	U	See urine calcium		
			mm Hg	**kPa**
Carbon dioxide, partial pressure pCO$_2$)	B (heparin)	NB	27–40	3.6–5.3
		Infant	27–41	3.6–5.5
		Thereafter		
		M	35–48	4.7–6.4
		F	32–45	4.3–6.0
			mmol/L	
Carbon dioxide, total (tCO$_2$)	S, P (heparin)	Cord	14–22	Same
		Premature	4–27	
		NB	13–22	
		Infant	20–28	
		Child	20–28	
		Thereafter	23–30	

			pg/mL	pmol/L
Catecholamines, fractionated	P (EDTA)	**Norepineph-rine**		
		Supine	100–400	591–2,364
		Standing	300–900	1,773–5,320
		Epinephrine		
		Supine	<70	<382
		Standing	<100	<546
		Dopamine (no postural change)	<30	<196
			ug/d	**mmol/d**
	U, 24 h	**Norepineph-rine**		
		0–1 y	0–10	0–59
		1–2 y	0–17	0–100
		2–4 y	4–29	24–171
		4–7 y	8–45	47–266
		7–10 y	13–65	77–384
		Thereafter	15–80	87–473
		Epinephrine		
		0–1 y	0–2.5	0–13.6
		1–2 y	0–3.5	0–19.1
		2–4 y	0–6.0	0–32.7
		4–7 y	0.2–10	1.1–55
		7–10 y	0.5–14	2.7–76
		Thereafter	0.5–20	2.7–109
		Dopamine		
		0–1 y	0–85	0–555
		1–2 y	10–140	65–914
		2–4 y	40–260	261–1,697
		Thereafter	65–400	424–2,611
			µg/d	
Catecholamines, total free	U, 24 h	0–1 y	10–15	Same
		1–5 y	15–40	
		6–15 y	20–80	
		Thereafter	30–100	

			mg/dL	mg/L
Ceruloplasmin	S	0–5 d	5–26	50–260
		1–19 y	20–46	200–460
			mmol/L	
Chloride	S, P (heparin)	Cord	96–104	Same
		Premature	100–117	
		NB	97–110	
		Thereafter	98–106	
	U	Look under urine chloride		
			mmol/L	
	Sweat	Normal	<40	Same
		Marginal	45–60	
		Cystic fibrosis	>60	
			mg/dL	
Cholesterol, total	S, P (EDTA or heparin)	Child	<170	
		Adult	<200	
Complement, total hemolytic	P (EDTA)		75–160 U/mL or <33% of plasma CH$_{50}$	Same
			mg/dL	**mg/L**
C3	S	Cord	57–116	570–1,160
		1–3 mo	53–131	530–1,130
		3 mo–1 y	62–180	620–1,800
		1 y–10 y	77–195	770–1,950
		Adult	140–250	1,400–2,500
		At birth, conc is 50%–75% of adult values		
			mg/dL	**mg/L**
C4	S	Cord	7–23	70–230
		1–3 mo	7–27	70–270
		3 mo–10 y	7–40	70–400
		Adult	15–45	150–450

			µg/dL	µmol/L
Copper	S	0–5 d	9–46	1.4–7.2
		1–9 y	80–150	12.6–23.6
		10–14 y	80–121	12.6–19.0
		15–19 y	64–160	11.3–25.2
	U, 24 h		0–30 ug/d	0–0.47 µmol/d
			µg/dL	nmol/L
Cortisol	S, P (heparin)	NB	1–24	28–662
		Adult: 08:00 h	5–23	138–635
		16:00 h	3–15	82–413
		20:00 h	50% of 08:00 h	Same
			µg/d	nmol/d
Cortisol, free	U, 24 h	Child	2–27	5.5–74
		Adolescent	5–55	14–152
		Adult	10–100	27–276
			mg/dL	mol/L
Creatinine Jaffe, kinetic or enzymatic	S, P	Cord	0.6–1.2	53–106
		NB	0.3–1.0	27–88
		Infant	0.2–0.4	18–35
		Child	0.3–0.7	27–62
		Adolescent	0.5–1.0	44–88
		Adult		
		M	0.6–1.2	53–106
		F	0.5–1.1	44–97
Jaffe, manual	S, P		0.8–1.5	70–133
			mg/kg/d	µmol/kg/d
	U, 24 h	Premature	8–20	71–180
		Full term	10–16	90–144
		Infant	8–20	71–180
		Child	8–22	71–195
		Adolescent	8–30	71–265
		Adult		
		M	14–26	124–230
		F	11–20	97–177

			ng/mL	nmol/L
Cyclic AMP	P (EDTA)	M	5.6–10.9	17–33
		F	3.6–8.9	11–27
	U, 24 h		<3.3 mg/d or <1.64 mg/g creatinine	1,000–11,500 nmol/d; <6,000 nmol cAMP/g creatinine
			mU/mL	U/L
Erythropoietin	S			
RIA			<5–20	Same
Hemagglutination			25–125	
Bioassay			5–18	
			ng/mL	
α-Fetoprotein	S		Fetal peak of 200–400 mg/dL in first trimester	
		Premature	134,734 ± 41,444	
		NB	48,406 ± 34,718	
		2–4 wk	2,654 ± 3,080	
		2 mo	323 ± 278	
		3 mo	88 ± 87	
		4 mo	74 ± 56	
		5 mo	46.5 ± 19	
		6 mo	12.5 ± 9.8	
		7 mo	9.7 ± 7.1	
		8 mo	8.5 ± 5.5	
		1 y	<30	
		Adult	<40	
		weeks	mg/dL	mg/L
	Amniotic fluid	10–12	0.5–3.3	5–33
		13–14	0.3–3.7	3–37
		15–16	0.4–2.7	4–27
		17–18	0.1–2.6	1–26
		19–20	<0.1–1.14	<1–11.4
		21–22	<0.1–1.1	<1–11
		23–24	<0.1–0.7	<1–7

		weeks	mg/dL	mg/L
Fibrin, degradation products	B (thrombin and proteolytic p[c] inhibitor in tube)		68–494 µg/L	
	U (2 mL in similar tube)		<0.25 g/mL	<0.25 mg/L
Agglutination (Thrombo-Wellco test)				
Fibrinogen	B (sodium citrate)	NB	125–300 mg/dL	1.25–3.00 g/L
		Adult	200–400	2.00–4.00

Functions, renal

Age	GFR[a] (mL/min/ 1.73 m²)	PAH Clearance[b] (mL/min/ 1.73 m²)	TmPAH[c] (mg/min/ 1.73 m²)			Concentrating Capacity mOsm/kg H₂O
				Basal	Dehydration	Pitressin
Preterm						
27 wk	2–10			190–300	370–680	
32	4–12					
34	5–15					
36	6–40					
37	12–26					
Term						
NB	8–42	33–162	6–26	180–400	210–650	
4–7 d	20–53	38–162				
8–12 d	40–60	120–188				
15–30 d	30–90	103–260	3.7–22	776	780–1,100	
2 mo	42–90	203–321	13.3–93		870–1,200	400–960
3 mo	46–125	154–345	41–58			450–1,030
4 mo	56–120	204–327			950–1,260	500–1,060
6 mo	89–144	392–601	57–68			550–1,120
8 mo	58–160	262–781	46			600–1,160
12 mo	63–150	332–557	21–88		1,000–1,310	640–1,220
18 mo	105–235	503–724	52		1,020–1,330	700–1,280

Functions, renal, continued

Age	GFR[a] (mL/min/ 1.73 m²)	PAH Clearance[b] (mL/min/ 1.73 m²)	TmPAH[c] (mg/ min/ 1.73 m²)	Basal	Dehydration	Concen-trating Capacity mOsm/kg H₂O — Pitressin
2 y	105–172	503–724	77–84		1,040–1,390	
3 y	101–179	624–754				820–1,340
4 y	100–184	632–723	84			1,060–1,410
5 y	120–184					
6 y	79–170	497–872	65			
7 y	110–156		31–100			
8 y	90–148	680–711	75		1,100–1,420	820–1,340
9 y	88–166	490–744	88			
10 y	95–162	566–704	95			
11 y	110–146	562–784	82			
12 y	110–136	55–747	95		1,110–1,430	820–1,340
Adult						
M	110–152	561–833	80 ± 12	800–1,400	1,200–1,500	
F	101–133	92–696	77 ± 11	800–1,400	1,200–1,500	

[a]Glomerular filtration rate, > age 40 y, decreases ~6.5 mL/min/1.73 m²/decade.
[b]Para-aminohippurate (renal plasma flow), age 40 yr, decreases ~75 mL/min/1.73 m²/decade.
[c]Maximum tubular excretory capacity.

Test	Specimen		Conven-tional Units mg/dL	International Units mmol/L
Glucose	S	Fasting cord	45–96	2.50–5.33
		Premature	20–60	1.1–3.3
		Neonate	30–60	1.7–3.3
		1 d	40–60	2.2–3.3
		>1 d	50–80	2.8–5
		Child	60–100	3.3–5.5
		Adult	70–105	3.9–5.8
	U	See urine glucose		
Glucose, 2 h postprandial	S		<120 mg/dL	<6.7 mmol/L

Test	Specimen		Conventional Units	International Units
			mg/dL	mmol/L
Hematocrit	B	1 d (capillary)	48%–69%	
		2 mo	28%–42%	
		6–12 y	35%–45%	
		Adult, M	41%–53%	
		Adult, F	36%–46%	
			g/dL	mmol/L
Hemoglobin (Hb)	B (EDTA)	Cord	14.5–22.5	2.25–3.49
		1–3 d (capillary)	14.5–22.5	2.25–3.49
		2 mo	9.0–14.0	1.40–2.17
		6–12 y	11.5–15.5	1.78–2.09
		12–18 y, M	13.0–16.0	2.02–2.48
		12–18 y, F	12.0–16.0	1.86–2.48
		18–49 y, M	13.5–17.5	2.09–2.71
		18–49 y, F	12.0–16.0	1.86–2.48
			mg/dL	mg/L
Immunoglobulin A (IgA)	S	Cord	1.4–3.6	14–36
		1–3 mo	1.3–53	13–530
		4–6 mo	4.4–84	44–840
		7 mo–1 y	11–106	110–1,060
		2–5 y	14–159	140–1,590
		6–10 y	33–236	330–2,360
		Adult	70–312	700–3,120
Immunoglobulin D (IgD)		NB	None detected	None detected
		Thereafter	0–8 mg/dL	0–80 mg/L
Immunoglobulin E (IgE)		M	0–230 IU/mL	0–230 kIU/L
		F	0–170	0–170

Test	Specimen		Conventional Units	International Units
			mg/dL	**g/L**
Immunoglobulin G (IgG)		Cord	636–1,606	6.36–16.06
		1 mo	251–906	2.51–9.06
		2–4 mo	176–601	1.76–6.01
		5–12 mo	172–1,069	1.72–10.69
		1–5 y	345–1,236	3.45–12.36
		6–10 y	608–1,572	6.08–15.72
		Adults (higher in blacks)	639–1,349	6.39–13.49
			mmol/L	
Ketone bodies	S	1–12 mo	0.1–1.5	
		1–7 y	0.15–2.0	
		7–15 y	<0.1–0.5	
			mg/dL	**mmol/L**
Lactate	B capillary	NB	<27	0.0–3.0
		Child	5–20	0.56–2.25
	Venous		5–20	0.5–2.2
	Capillary		5–14	0.5–1.6
			mEq/L	**mmol/L**
Magnesium		NB	1.5–2.3	0.75–1.15
		Adult	1.4–2.0	0.7–1
			mOsm/kg H_2O	
Osmolality	S	Child, Adult	275–295	
	U	Look under urine osmolality		
Osmolality ratio	U/S		1.0–3.0	
			>3.0 after 12 h fluid restriction	

Test	Specimen		Conventional Units mm Hg	International Units kPa
Oxygen, partial pressure (pO₂)	B, arterial (heparin)	Birth	8–24	1.1–3.2
		5–10 min	33–75	4.4–10.0
		30 min	31–85	4.1–11.3
		>1 h	55–80	7.3–10.6
		1 d	54–95	7.2–12.6
		Thereafter (decreases with age)	83–108	11–14.4
				Fraction saturated
Oxygen saturation	B, arterial (heparin)	NB	85%–90%	0.85–0.90
		Thereafter	95%–99%	0.95–0.99
Parathyroid hormone (IRMA)	S	Cord	<3.0 pq/mL	<0.32 pmol/L
		2 y–adult	9–65 pq/mL	<0.95–6.8 pmol/L
				H⁺ concentration
pH	B (arterial, heparin)	Premature (48 h)	7.35–7.50	31–44 nmol/L
		NB, full term	7.11–7.36	43–77
		5–10 min	7.09–7.30	50–81
		30 min	7.32–7.38	41–61
		>1 h	7.26–7.49	32–54
		1 d	7.29–7.45	35–51
		Thereafter (must be corrected to body temperature)	7.35–7.43	35–44
	U	See urine pH		

Test	Specimen		Conventional Units	International Units
			mg/dL	**mmol/L**
Phosphorus, inorganic	S	0–5 d	4.8–8.2	1.55–2.65
		1–3 y	3.6–6.5	1.25–2.10
		4–11 y	3.7–5.6	1.20–1.80
		12–15 y	2.9–5.4	0.95–1.75
		16–19 y	2.7–4.7	0.90–1.50
	U, 24 h		Adults on diet with 0.9–1.5 g P and 10 mg Ca/kg	Adults on diet with 29–45 mmol P and 0.25 mmol Ca/kg
			<1.0 g/d; on nonrestricted diet 0.4–1.3 g/d	<32.3 mmol/d; on nonrestricted diet 12.9–42.l mmol/L
Plasma volume	P (heparin)	M	25–43 mL/kg	0.025–0.043 L/kg
		F	28–45	0.028–0.045
			mmol/L	
Potassium	S	Premature	4.6–6.7	Same
		Full-term NB	3.9–5.9	
		Infant	4.1–5.3	
		Child	3.4–4.7	
		Thereafter	3.5–5.1	
	P, heparin		3.5–4.5	
	U	See urine potassium		
			ng/h/1.73 m²	
Prostaglandin E₂		Premature	16.4–21.4	
		NB	20.6–41.2	
		3–12 mo	31.1–43.9	
		Adult	227–295	
Protein selectivity index (CI ratio of IgG/albumin)	<10% highly selective			
	>20% poorly selective			

Test	Specimen		Conventional Units	International Units
			g/dL	**g/L**
Protein, serum total	S	Premature	4.3–7.6	43–76
		NB	4.6–7.4	46–74
		Child	6.2–8.0	62–80
		Adult		
		Recumbent	6.0–7.8	60–78
		Ambulatory	~0.5 g higher	~5 g higher
			g/dL	**g/L**
Electrophoresis		**Albumin**		
		Premature	3.0–4.2	30–42
		NB	3.6–5.4	36–54
		Infant	4.0–5.0	40–50
		Thereafter	3.5–5.0	35–50
		α_1-Globulin		
		Premature	0.1–0.5	1–5
		NB	0.1–0.3	1–3
		Infant	0.2–0.4	2–4
		Thereafter	0.2–0.3	2–3
		α_2-Globulin		
		Premature	0.3–0.7	3–7
		NB	0.3–0.5	3–5
		Infant	0.5–0.8	5–8
		Thereafter	0.4–1.0	4–10
		β-Globulin		
		Premature	0.3–1.2	3–12
		NB	0.2–0.6	2–6
		Infant	0.5–0.8	5–8
		Thereafter	0.5–1.1	5–11
		γ-Globulin		
		Premature	0.3–1.4	3–14
		NB	0.2–1.0	2–10
		Infant	0.3–1.2	3–12
		Thereafter (higher in blacks)	0.7–1.2	7–12

Test	Specimen		Conventional Units	International Units
			g/dL	g/L
Protein, urine total	U, 24 h	See urine protein		
			Average % of Total Protein	**Fraction of Total**
Electrophoresis		Albumin	37.9	0.379
		Globulin		
		α1	27.3	0.273
		α2	19.5	0.195
		β	8.8	0.088
		γ	3.3	0.033
			ng/mL/h	g/L/h
Renin activity; PRA	P (EDTA)	Premature (17)	18.2 ± 5.1	Same
		0–3 y	<16.6	
		3–6 y	<6.7	
		6–9 y	<4.4	
		9–12 y	<5.9	
		12–15 y	<4.2	
		15–18 y	<4.3	
		Normal-sodium diet		
		Supine	0.2–2.5	
		Upright	0.3–4.3	
		Low-sodium diet		
		Upright	2.9–24	
			ng/mL/h	
	or	Premature, 1–3 d	61.3–67.30	
		Full term, 1–3 d	9.95–13.45	
		3–12 mo	5.02–7.48	
		Adult		
		Supine	0.15–1.65	
		Upright	0.66–8.10	

Size, kidney				
	Age		Kidney weight (g)	Kidney Length (cm)
	Preterm			
	27 wk		10.5	
	28 wk		11	
	32 wk		16	
	34 wk		19	
	36 wk		22	
	Full-Term NB		24	4.6
	15–30 d		26	5
	2 mo		29	
	4 mo			5.3
	6 mo		40	
	8 mo		60	5.9
	12 mo		72	6
	2 y		85	7
	3 y		93	7.5
	4 y		100	8
	5 y		106	8.5
	6 y		112	8.9
	7 y		120	9.3
	8 y		128	9.7
	9 y		132	10.1
	10 y		150	10.44
	11 y		164	10.81
	12 y		178	11.19
	13–19 y		196–282	11.19
	Adult			
	M		290	13.4
	F		248	13.4

Test	Specimen		Conventional Units	International Units
			mmol/L	
Sodium	S, P (heparin)	NB	134–146	Same
		Infant	139–146	
		Child	138–145	
		Thereafter	136–146	
	U	See urine sodium		
	Sweat	Normal	10–40	
		Cystic fibrosis	>70	
			mg/dL	**mmol urea/L**
Urea nitrogen	S, P	Cord	21–40	7.5–14.3
		Premature (1 wk)	3–25	1.1–9
		NB	3–12	1.1–4.3
		Infant/child	5–18	1.8–6.4
		Thereafter	7–18	2.5–6.4
Urea nitrogen/ creatinine	S		10–15	
			mg/dL	**umol/L**
Uric acid	S	0–2 y	2.4–6.4	0.14–0.38
		2–12 y	2.4–5.9	0.14–0.35
		12–14 y	2.4–6.4	0.14–0.38
		Adult		
		M	3.5–7.2	0.20–0.43
		F	2.4–6.4	0.14–0.38

Urine acidifying capacity				
Age	pH		H⁺ Excretion (µEq/min/1.73 m²)	
	Control	After NH₄Cl or CaCl₂	Control	After NH₄Cl or CaCl₂
Full-term NB	4.9–6.8			
4–7 d	5.7–7.4			
2 mo	4.9–6.3	5.02–5.4	54–168	67–230
3 mo	5.4–6.6	4.6–6.4	30–113	
4 mo	5.2–7.3	4.7–6.4	8–68	83–172
5 mo	5.0–5.4	5.0–5.1	86–125	165–197
6 mo	6.5–7.2	4.9–5.0		
8 mo	5.5–6.8	4.6–5.0	43–73	109–113
2–5 y	5.3–6.7	4.7–5.6	9–48	62.1–164
6–11 y	5.67–6.83	4.7–5.04	23–58	108.7–150.8
12–16 y	5.23–5.90	4.80–5.0	59–111	89–148
Adult (M and F)	5.40–7.02	4.5–7.0	10–50	60–130
Acidity, titratable		Premature	0–12 µM/min/m²	
		Full term	0–11	
		Child	20–50 mEq/d	
Addis count (12-h specimen)		Red cells	<1 million	
		White cells	<2 million	
		Casts	10,000	
		Protein	<55 mg	
Ammonia			500–1,200 mg N/24 h	36–86 mmol/24 h
Amount		Preterm	1–3 mL/kg/d	
		Full-term NB, 1–2 d	15–60 mL	
		Neonate, 4–12 d	100–300	
		Infant, 6–12 mo	400–600	
		Child, 2–4 y	500–750	

Urine acidifying capacity				
Age	pH		H⁺ Excretion (μEq/min/1.73 m²)	
	Control	After NH₄Cl or CaCl₂	Control	After NH₄Cl or CaCl₂
		6–7 y	650–1,000	
		8–19 y	700–1,500	
		Adult	1,000–1,600	
		Varies with intake and other factors: extreme dehydration, 0.2–0.3 mL/min; extreme hydration, 16 mL/min		
Bladder capacity		32 × age in y + 73 (mL)		2 + age in y (oz)
		mg/24 h	mmol/24 h	
Calcium		Ca⁺²-free 5–40	Ca⁺²-free 0.13–1.0	
		Low to average 50–150	Low to average 1.25–3.8	
		Average 100–300	Average 2.5–7.5	
Calcium/creatinine		Preterm NB	0.3–2.3	
		Full-term NB	0.05–1.2	
		Infant and child	<0.21	
Catecholamines		See catecholamines		
Chloride		Infants	2–10 mmol/24 h	
		Children	15–40	
		Adults	110–250	
		Varies with chloride intake		
Citrate			439 + 49 mg/g creatinine	
Copper			See copper	
Cortisol			See cortisol	
Creatinine			See creatinine	

H^+

		mg/24 h	mmol/ 24 h	
Cyclic AMP			See cyclic AMP	
Cystine			<75 mg/g creatinine	
Frequency		3–6 mo	20 times/d	
		6–12 mo	16	
		1–2 y	12	
		2–4 y	9	
		12 y	4–6	
		Qualitative	**Negative**	
Glucose			Dip stick detects 75–125 mg/ dL	
		Quantitative		
		Full-term NB	12–32 mg/ dL	
		Preterm	60–130 mg/ dL	
		Adult	<15 mg/dL or 30–300 mg/1.73 m²/d	
			mg/min/ 1.73 m²	
Glucose, maximal tubular reabsorption of (TmG)		Infant	142–284	
		Child	266–458	
		Adult	289–361	

			mg/mL	
Glucose, renal threshold		Premature	2.21–2.84	
		Infant	2.20–3.68	
		Child	2.36–3.30	
		Adult	1.98–2.78	
Hemoglobin			Negative	
Hypoxanthine			5.9–13.2 mg/d	
Ketone bodies		Qualitative: negative		
			µg/mg	
Lysozyme/creatinine (tubular proteinuria)		Neonate	1.2–19	
		1 y	0.1–23	
		2–12 y	0.1–5	
		Adult	0.1–14	
Magnesium			1.3–2.0 mEq/L	0.65–1.0 mmol/L
Magnesium/calcium			1.56	
			mosm/L	
Osmolality		Infant	50–600	
		Child	50–1,400	
		12-h restriction	>850	
		24-h urine	~300–900	
		Malnourished children	201–275	
Oxalate			<50 mg/ 1.73 m²/d	
pH		NB/neonate	5–7	
		Thereafter	4.5–8	
		Average	~ 6	
Phosphorus			See phosphorus	
Phosphorus, tubular			78%–97% reabsorption	

			mosm/L	
Potassium			26–123 mmol/L	
			0.4–5.2 mEq/kg/d	
			Varies with diet	
Fractional excretion			<30% (normal renal function and regular diet)	
	NB		18.5–32.9	
	1–12 mos		7.5–25.7	
	2–20 y		7.0–23.8	
Protein, 24 h			1–14 mg/dL	
			50–80 mg/24 h (at rest)	
			<250 mg/ 24 h (intense exercise)	
Proteins, Bence Jones			Negative	
Protein/creatinine ratio			<0.2 (>3.5 in nephrotic syndrome)	
Sediment		Casts		
		Hyaline	Occasional (0–1) casts/ hpf	
		RBC	Not seen	
		WBC	Not seen	
		Tubular epithelial	Not seen	
		Transitional and squamous epithelial	Not seen	
		RBC	0–2/hpf	
		WBC, M	0–3/hpf	

			mosm/L	
		F and children	0–5/hpf	
		Epithelial cells	Few, more frequent in NB	
		Bacteria, unspun	No organisms/oil immersion field	
		Spun	<20 organisms/hpf	
Sodium	U, 24 h		40–220/hpf (diet-dependent)	
Sodium/potassium		Premature and NBs	1.4–7.9 mmol/d	
		Infants 1–12 mo	1.1 + 1.5 mmol/d	
		Children	0.5–2.5 mmol/d	
		Infants on milk	0.7 mmol/d	
		Generally	>1 mmol/d	
Specific gravity, random		NB	1.006–1.008	
		Adult	1.002–1.030	
		After 12 h of fluid restriction	>1.025	
Uric acid			5–12 mg/kg/d	
		Child	520±147 mg/d	
		Adult	250–750 mg/d	
Urobilinogen			1–4 mg/d	
Vanillylmandelic	U, 24 h	0–1 y	<18.8 mg/g Cr	<11 µmol/mol Cr
Acid (VMA)		2–4 y	<11 mg/g Cr	<8 µmol/mol Cr
		5–19 y	<8 mg/g Cr	<5 µmol/mol Cr

			mosm/L	
Xanthine			4.1–8.6	
			pg/mL	
Vasopressin	P	Full term, 1–3 d	5.0	
		Adult, supine	0.8–3.2	
		Upright	1.9–10.5	
			ng/24 h	
	U, 24 h	NB	1.0–1.4	
		3–12 mo	4.8–6.0	
		Adult	32.5–39.5	
Vitamin D	S	25(OH) D	30 ± 5 ng/mL	
		1,25(OH)2 D	20–80 pg/mL	
		24,25(OH)2 D	1–5 ng/mL	

Abbreviations: 1,25(OH)$_2$ D,1, 25 dihydroxyvitamin D (calcitriol); 24,25(OH)$_2$ D, 24,25 dihydroxyvitamin D; 25(OH) d, 25 hydroxyvitamin D (calcidiol); ADH, antidiuretic hormone; AMP, adenodine monophosphate; B, blood; Ca, calcium; Ca$^+$2, calcium; CaCl$_2$, calcium chloride; CH$_{50}$, total hemolytic complement; conc, concentration; Cr, creatinine; d, day; EDTA, ethylenediaminetetraacetate (edetic acid); F, female; GFR, glomerular filtration rate; h, hour; H$^+$, hydrogen; hpf, high-power field; M, male; min, minute; mo, month; NB, newborn; nDNA, native DNA; P, plasma; PAH, para-aminohippurate; PRA, plasma rennin activity; NH$_4$Cl, ammonium chloride; RBC, red blood cell; RIA, radioimmunoassay; S, serum; TmPAH, maximum tubular excretory capacity; U, urine; VMA, vanillylmandelic acid; WBC, white blood cell; wk, week; y, year.

References

1. Robertson J, Shilkofski N, eds. *The Harriet Lane Handbook.* 17th ed. Philadelphia, PA: Elsevier Mosby; 2005

2. Nicholson JF, Pesce MA. Reference ranges for laboratory tests and procedures. In: Behrman RE, Kliegman RM, Jenson HB, eds. *Nelson Textbook of Pediatrics.* 17th ed. Philadelphia, PA: Saunders; 2004:1,535–1,5585-1

3. Henry JB. *Clinical Diagnosis and Management by Laboratory Methods.* 20th ed. Philadelphia, PA: WB Saunders; 2001

4. Barakat AY. Appendix I: reference intervals. In: Barakat AY, ed. *Renal Disease in Children: Clinical Evaluation and Diagnosis.* New York, NY: Springer Verlag; 2001:413–4313-

Appendix II

Charts

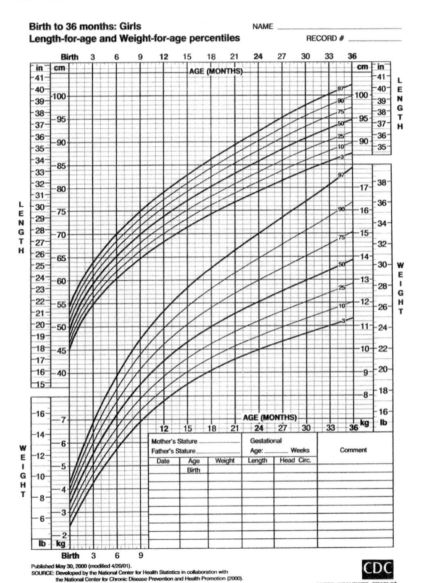

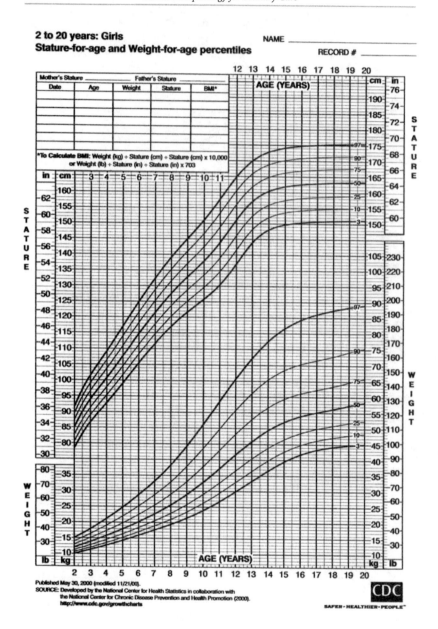

2 to 20 years: Girls
Stature-for-age and Weight-for-age percentiles

NAME _____

RECORD # _____

Published May 30, 2000 (modified 11/21/00).
SOURCE: Developed by the National Center for Health Statistics in collaboration with
the National Center for Chronic Disease Prevention and Health Promotion (2000).
http://www.cdc.gov/growthcharts

CDC
SAFER · HEALTHIER · PEOPLE™

Developed by the National Center for Health Statistics in collaboration with the National Center for
Chronic Disease Prevention and Health Promotion (2000)

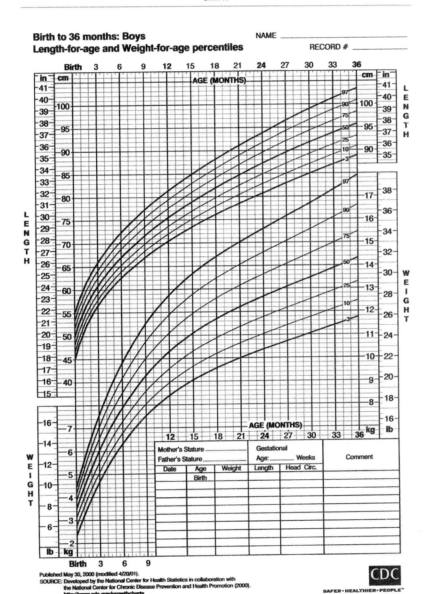

Birth to 36 months: Boys
Length-for-age and Weight-for-age percentiles

NAME _____

RECORD # _____

Published May 30, 2000 (modified 4/20/01).
SOURCE: Developed by the National Center for Health Statistics in collaboration with
the National Center for Chronic Disease Prevention and Health Promotion (2000).
http://www.cdc.gov/growthcharts

Developed by the National Center for Health Statistics in collaboration with the National Center for
Chronic Disease Prevention and Health Promotion (2000)

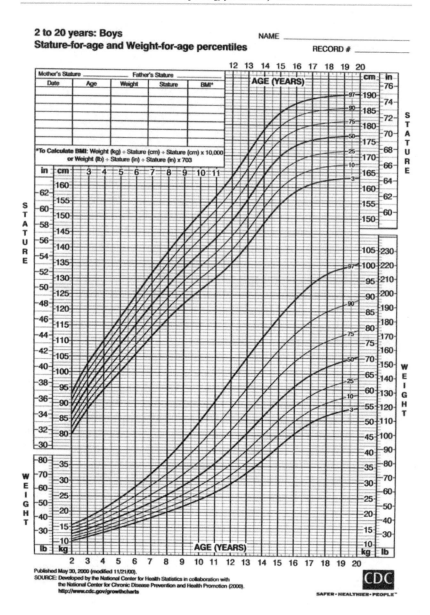

2 to 20 years: Boys
Stature-for-age and Weight-for-age percentiles

NAME _____

RECORD # _____

Published May 30, 2000 (modified 11/21/00).
SOURCE: Developed by the National Center for Health Statistics in collaboration with
the National Center for Chronic Disease Prevention and Health Promotion (2000).
http://www.cdc.gov/growthcharts

SAFER · HEALTHIER · PEOPLE™

Developed by the National Center for Health Statistics in collaboration with the National Center for
Chronic Disease Prevention and Health Promotion (2000)

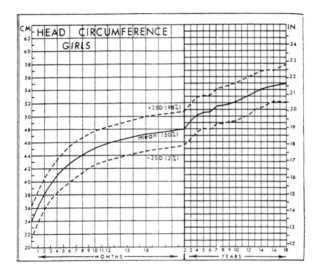

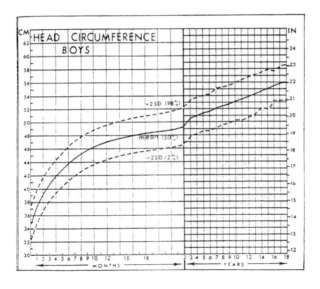

Head circumference for girls and boys from birth through 18 years. Reprinted from Nellhaus G. Head circumference from birth to eighteen years. *Pediatrics.* 1968;41:106–114, with permission from the American Academy of Pediatrics.

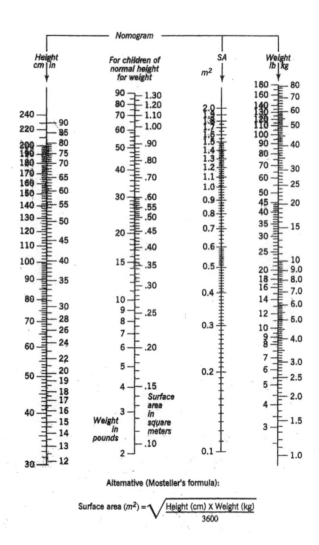

Body surface area nomogram and equation. From Briars GL, Bailey BJ. Surface area estimation: pocket calculator v nomogram. *Arch Dis Child* 1994;70:246–247.

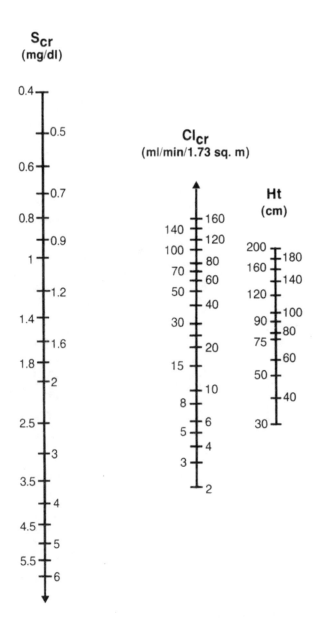

Nomogram used to estimate creatinine clearance in patients 1 to 18 years of age. A straight line connecting the child's serum creatinine value (S_{cr}) and height (Ht) will intersect the center line at a value approximating creatinine clearance (Cl_{cr}). Originally published in Traub SI, Johnson CE. Comparison of methods of estimating creatinine clearance in children. *Am J Hosp Pharm.* 1980;37:195–201. Copyright 1980, American Society of Health System Pharmacists, Inc. All rights reserved. Reprinted with permission. (R0706)

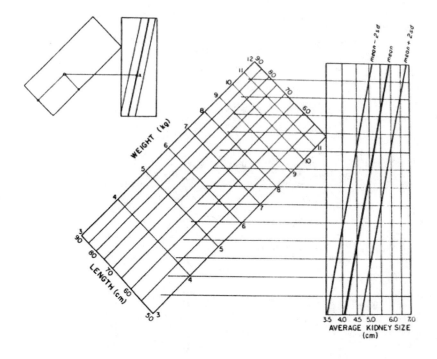

Nomogram used to determine normal infant kidney length. The infant's weight and length determine 2 oblique lines on the left of the plot. The intersection should then be extended parallel to the horizontal rulings to its intersection with the heavy (mean) line on the right graph. The predicted kidney length is indicated on the abscissa. From Blane CE, Bookstein FL, DiPietro MA, Kelsch RC. Sonographic standards for normal infant kidney length. *AJR Am J Roentgenol.* 1985;145:1289–1291. Reprinted with permission from the *American Journal of Roentgenology.*

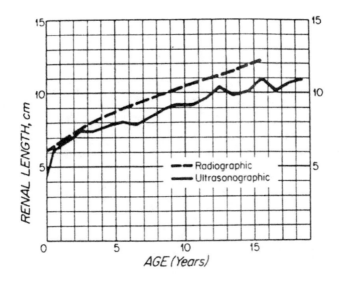

Sonographic and radiographic renal length as function of age. From Rosenbaum DM, Korngold E, Teele RL. Sonographic assessment of renal length in normal children. *AJR Am J Roentgenol.* 142:467–469. Reprinted with permission from the *American Journal of Roentgenology.*

Formulas

Amin J. Barakat

The following conversions and formulas are commonly used in nephrology to assist in the clinical workup of a patient. The clinician should keep in mind that these are estimates, and the results should be interpreted in the context of the clinical picture.[1-4]

I. Conversions

MW: molecular weight; Eq W: equivalent weight

$$mEq/L = \frac{mg/dL \times 10 \times valence}{MW} \text{ or } \frac{mg/dL \times 10}{Eq\,W}$$

$$mg/dL = \frac{mEq/L \times Eq\,W}{10}$$

$$Eq\,W = \frac{Atomic\,weight}{valence}$$

Temperature: ºC, centigrade; ºF, Fahrenheit

$$ºC = \frac{5(ºF - 32)}{9} \qquad ºF = \frac{(ºC \times 9)}{5} + 32$$

1 in = 2.54 cm; 1 cm = 0.3973 in

1 oz = 28.350 g

1 lb = 16 oz = 0.454 kg; 1 kg = 2.204 lb

1 L =1.06 qt = 33.81 oz

1 dL = 100 mL

mm Hg × 1.36 = cm water; cm water × 0.735 = mm Hg

Compound	mEq/g salt	mg salt/mEq
NaCl	17	58
NaHCO$_3$	12	84
KCl	13	75
CaCO$_3$	20	50
NH$_4$Cl	19	54

Element	mEq/L to mg/dL		mg/dL to mEq/L	
Na	1	2.30	1	0.4348
K	1	3.91	1	0.2558
Cl	1	3.55	1	0.2817
HCO$_3$	1	6.10	1	0.1639
Ca	1	2.005	1	0.4988
P (valence 1)	1	3.10	1	0.3226
P (valence 1.8)	1	1.72	1	0.5814
Mg	1	1.215	1	0.8230

II. Measurements

Ideal body mass (5)

<5 feet (males and females): $\dfrac{\text{height}^2\,(\text{cm}) \times 1.65}{1,000}$

>5 feet, males, kg = 39 + 2.27 (height in inches − 60)
lb = 86 + 5 (height in inches − 60)

females, kg = 42.2 + 2.27(height in inches − 60)
lb = 93 + 5 (height in inches − 60)

Body surface area (m²), approximation to weight (kg)

1–5 kg	0.05 × weight + 0.05
6–10 kg	0.04 × weight + 0.10
11–20 kg	0.03 × weight + 0.20
21–70 kg	0.02 × weight + 0.40
10 kg	0.5 m²
30 kg	1.0 m²

Kidney size in normal children (6)

Length (cm) (5–13 y) = 0.379 × age (y) + 6.65 ± 1.45
Sectional area (cm²) = 1.0126 × height (in) − 9.272 ± 10.24
or 7.23 × kidney length (cm) − 29.37 ± 9.8
or 28.47 × body surface (m²) + 12 ± 9.94

Urinary bladder capacity (values level off after age 9 years) (7)

mL = 32 × age in years + 73
oz = 2 + age in years

III. Clearance (C)

$C_k = \dfrac{Uk\,V}{Sk}$ (k is any substance; U, urine; S, serum; V, volume)

$C_{H_2O} = V(1 - U/S\ \text{Osm})$

GFR

Full-term infants (mL/min/1.73 m²) = 1.1 × body length (cm) (8)

Children (mL/min/1.73 m²) = $\dfrac{k \times \text{body length (cm)}}{S\ Cr\ (\text{mg/dL})}$ (Cr, creatinine) (9)

k in low birth-weight infants <1 y	0.33 (0.2–0.5)
term infants <1 y	0.45 (0.3–0.7)
children (2–12 y)	0.55 (0.4–0.7)
females (13–21 y)	0.55 (0.4–0.7)
males (13–21 y)	0.70 (0.5–0.9)

Adolescent boys = $1.5 \times \text{age (y)} + \dfrac{0.5 \times \text{length (cm)}}{S\ Cr\ (\text{mg/dL})}$ (10)

Adults (18–92 y), males (mL/min) = $\dfrac{(140 - \text{age in years}) \times \text{weight (kg)}}{72 \times S\ Cr\ (\text{mg/dL})}$ (11)

females, 85% of male values

IV. Fluids and Electrolytes

Total body water	60% body weight
Intracellular fluid	40%
Extracellular fluid	20%
Interstitial fluid volume	15%
Plasma volume	~50 mL/kg
Blood volume	~75 mL/kg

Potassium

Total body potassium   55 mEq/kg

Falls ~ 370 mEq for each 1 mEq/L fall in measured serum potassium

Serum K concentration increases by 0.6 mEq/L for every 0.1 decrease in serum pH

Chloride

Decrease in 1 mEq/L of chloride = decrease of 1% of total body chloride

Correction of electrolyte abnormality

mEq needed = (desired level - actual level) × distribution factor × baseline weight in kg

Distribution factor:	HCO_3	0.4–0.5
	Cl	0.2–0.3
	Na	0.6–0.7

Correction of serum Na^{+2}

Hyperlipidemia: Reduction of Na (mEq/L) = plasma lipids (mg/dL) × 0.002

Hyperproteinemia: Reduction of Na (mEq/L = amount of protein >8 (gm/dL) × 0.25

Hyperglycemia: Expected Na (mEq/L) = measured Na + 0.028 (glucose − 100)

Hyperglycemia with insulin treatment: Expected Na (mEq/L) = measured Na + 0.16
   (glucose −100)

Total CO_2 exhaled

3.2 mL/kg/min; 7% increase/°C of fever

$pH = \log 1/H^+$

$pH = 6.1 + \dfrac{\log (HCO_3^-)}{0.03\ PCO_2}$

$H^+ = \dfrac{24\ (PaCO_2)}{HCO_3^-}$

Metabolic acidosis

pCO_2 decreases 1–1.5 mm Hg per mEq/L decrease in HCO_3^-

pCO_2 = last 2 digits of pH

$pCO_2 = 1.5\ HCO_3^- + 8$

$HCO_3^- + 15$ = last 2 digits of pH

Metabolic alkalosis

pCO_2 increases 0.5–1 mm Hg/mEq/L increase in HCO_3^-

pCO_2 = last 2 digits of pH

Respiratory acidosis

HCO_3^- increases 0.35 mEq/L/mm Hg increase in pCO_2

Respiratory alkalosis

HCO_3^- decreases 0.5 mEq/L/mm Hg decrease in pCO_2

Prediction of compensatory response in simple acid-base disturbances (12)

Metabolic acidosis $\qquad$ $PaCO_2 = (1.5 \times HCO_3^-) + 8 \pm 2$

Metabolic alkalosis $\qquad$ $PaCO_2 = (0.9 \times HCO_3^-) + 9 \pm 2$

Respiratory alkalosis $\qquad$ $\Delta HCO_3^- = \dfrac{\Delta PaCO_2 \times 4}{10}$

Respiratory acidosis $\qquad$ $\Delta HCO_3^- = \dfrac{\Delta PaCO_2 \times 2.5}{10}$

Osmolality

Estimated serum osmolality (mOsm/kg water)

$$2\,Na\,(mEq/L) + \frac{glucose}{18} + \frac{BUN}{2.8} + \frac{mannitol}{18} + \frac{ethyl\ alcohol}{4.6}\ (all\ in\ mg/dL)$$

Normal ~ 290 mOsm/kg water

Osmolar gap (mOsm/kg water) = measured osmolality − caculated osmolality
    (normal < 10)

V. Tubular

$FE_{(K)} = U\ K/S\ K \times S\ Cr/U\ Cr \times 100$ (FE, fractional excretion; K, HCO_3^-, PO_4, Na, etc)

Tubular reabsorption of phosphate (TRP%) = $(1 - FE_{PO_4}) \times 100$

$Tm_{PO_4} = P_{PO_4}$ (threshold) $\times$ GFR $\qquad\qquad$ (13)

P_{PO_4} (threshold) = Tm_{PO_4}/GFR

TP/GFR: $\qquad$ (13)

Newborn	6.9 ± 1.2
1 mo–12 y	4.4 ± 0.6
12–16 y	4.0 ± 0.6
>16 y	3.2 ± 0.4

% Na (or water) delivery = $\dfrac{V \times 100}{GFR}$

% distal Na reabsorption = $\dfrac{C_{H_2O} \times 100}{C_{H_2O} + C_{Na}}$

VI. Renal Failure Indices

FE_{Na} (%) = $U_{Na}/S_{Na} \times S_{Cr}/U_{Cr} \times 100$ $\qquad\qquad$ (14)

Acute tubular necrosis	>3 (adults)
Prerenal and others	<1 (adults); <2 (neonates)

In small premature infants, may normally reach as high as 5%

$\dfrac{U\ urea\ (mg/dL)}{S\ urea\ (mg/dL)}$ $\qquad$ Acute tubular necrosis, <14 $\qquad$ (15)
$\qquad\qquad\qquad\quad$ Prerenal failure, > 14

Renal failure index (RFI) = $\dfrac{UNa\ (mEq/L) \times PCr\ (mg/dL)}{UCr\ (mg/dL)}$ $\qquad$ (16,17)

Acute tubular necrosis:	adults	>1.98
	infants	>3
	neonates	>2
Prerenal		<1.5

VII. Others

Creatinine, serum (age 1–20 y) (mg/dL)   (18)
Males, $0.35 + (0.025 \times$ age in years)
Females, $0.37 + (0.018 \times$ age in years)

Creatinine, urine
Children (mg/kg/24 h) $= 15 + (0.5 \times$ age, y) $+ 3$ (19)
Adults (mg/kg/24 h) $= 28 - (0.2 \times$ age, y)   (11)

Protein selectivity index (PSI) =
(U IgG $\times$ P IgG/U albumin x S albumin) x 100   (20)
<10%, selective
>20%, non-selective

Calcium
Corrected serum calcium in hypoalbuminemia:
Serum calcium (mg/dL) − serum albumin (g/dL) + 4, or
Each g/dL of albumin binds ~ 0.8 mg/dL calcium
% calcium bound = 8 (albumin) + 2 (globulin) + 3

Uric acid
Acute uric acid nephropathy suspected if spot urine uric acid/creatinine ratio >1

References

1. Barakat AY, ed. *Renal Disease in Children: Clinical Evaluation and Diagnosis.* New York, NY: Springer-Verlag; 1990

2. Behrman RE, Kliegman RM, Arvin AM, eds. Nelson *Textbook of Pediatrics.* 15th ed. Philadelphia, PA: WB Saunders Co.; 1996

3. Holliday MA, Barratt TM, Avner ED. *Pediatric Nephrology.* 3rd ed. Baltimore, MD: Williams & Wilkins; 1994

4. Rollings RC. *Facts and Formulas.* Nashville, TN: Rollings and Rollings; 1984

5. Rowe PC, ed. *The Harriet Lane Handbook.* 11th ed. Chicago, IL: Year Book Medical Publishers; 1987

6. DuBose TD. Clinical approach to patients with acid-base disorders. *Med Clin North Am.* 1983;67:799–813

7. Stark H, Eisenstein B, Tieder M. TP/GFR as a measure of normal PO_4 handling in children. *Eur J Pediatr.* 1983;140:181

8. Soothill JF. The estimation of eight serum proteins by gel diffusion precipitation technique. *J Lab Clin Med.* 1962;59:859–870

9. Traub SL, Johnson CE. Comparison of methods of estimating creatinine clearance in children. *Am J Hosp Pharm.* 1980;37:195–201

10. Hodson CJ, Drewf JA, Karn MN, et al. Renal size in normal children. A radiographic study during life. *Arch Dis Child.* 1962;37:616–622

11. Berger RM, Maizels M, Moran GC, et al. Bladder capacity (ounces) equals age (years) plus 2 predicts normal bladder capacity and aids in diagnosis of abnormal voiding patterns. *J Urol.* 1983;129:347–349

12. Schwartz GJ, Feld LG, Langford DJ. A simple estimate of glomerular filtration rate in full-term infants during the first year of life. *J Pediatr.* 1984;104:849–854

13. Espinel CH. The FENa test. Use in the differential diagnosis of acute renal failure. *JAMA.* 1976;236:579–581

14. Luke RG, Linton AL, Briggs JD, et al. Mannitol therapy in acute renal failure. *Lancet.* 1965; 1:980–982

15. Mathew OP, Jones AS, James E, et al. Neonatal renal failure: usefulness of diagnostic indices. *Pediatrics.* 1980;65:57–60

16. Handa SP, Morrin PAF. Diagnostic indices in acute renal failure. *Can Med Assoc J.* 1967; 96:78–82

17. Schwartz GJ, Haycock GB, Spitzer A. Plasma creatinine and urea concentration in children: normal values for age and sex. *J Pediatr.* 1976;88:828–830

18. Ghazali S, Barratt TM. Urinary excretion of calcium and magnesium in children. *Arch Dis Child.* 1974;49:97–101

19. Schwartz GJ, Gauthier B. A simple estimate of glomerular filtration rate in adolescent boys. *J Pediatr.* 1985;106:522–526

20. Schwartz GJ, Brion LP, Spitzer A. The use of plasma creatinine concentration for estimating GFR in infants, children and adolescents. *Pediatr Clin North Am.* 1987;34:571–590

21. Cockcroft DW, Gault MH. Prediction of creatinine clearance from serum creatinine. *Nephron.* 1976;16:31–4

Some Conditions and Syndromes Associated With Renal and Urinary Tract Abnormalities

Amin J. Barakat

Abbreviations			
AD	Autosomal dominant	HDR	Hyperparathyroidism, sensorineural deafness, renal dysplasia
AR	Autosomal recessive	Ig	Immunoglobulin
ATN	Acute tubular necrosis	NS	Nephrotic syndrome
CNS	Central nervous system	RTA	Renal tubular acidosis
CV	Cardiovascular	UTI	Urinary tract infection
DIC	Disseminated intravascular coagulation	UPJ	Ureteropelvic junction
		UVJ	Ureterovesical junction
ESRD	End-stage renal disease	VSD	Ventricular septal defect
GFR	Glomerular filtration rate	VUR	Vesicoureteral reflux
GN	Glomerulonephritis	XL	X-linked
HBsAg	Hepatitis B surface antigen	XLR	X-linked recessive

This section is intended to help primary care physicians to suspect and diagnose renal disease and urinary tract abnormalities associated with various diseases and syndromes, and help them initiate diagnosis and genetic counseling, or refer patients to the appropriate specialist. The syndromes/diseases are presented alphabetically with a brief presentation of the main features, associated renal and urinary tract abnormalities and inheritance. The mode of inheritance and gene map locus of the genetic disorders can be found on OMIM "Online Mendelian Inheritance in Man"[1] which is a continuously updated database. It is recommended to review the updated mode of inheritance and genetic information since this is a fast growing field and this information may change.

A more comprehensive list of conditions associated with renal abnormalities is available.[1-9]

Syndrome/Disease	Main Features	Renal/Urinary Tract Abnormalities	Inheritance
Acro-osteolysis with osteoporosis and changes in skull and mandible (Hajdu-Cheney)	Acro-osteolysis, generalized osteoporosis, joint laxity, small stature, skeletal dysplasia, early loss of teeth	Polycystic, dysplastic, hypoplastic kidneys; GN; chronic renal failure; VUR	AD
Adrenal hyperplasia III (21-OH-ase deficiency)	Virilization, adrenal insufficiency	Unilateral renal agenesis, UPJ obstruction, double collecting system	AR
AIDS (HIV)	Abnormality in cellular immunity, infections, Kaposi sarcoma	Proteinuria, focal glomerular sclerosis, GN, acute and chronic renal failure, type IV RTA, interstitial nephritis, nephrocalcinosis	—
Alagille (arteriohepatic dysplasia)	Unusual facies, vertebral and eye anomalies, chronic cholestasis, peripheral pulmonary stenosis	Unilateral renal agenesis, proteinuria, tubular acidosis, renal insufficiency, mesangial lipidosis with foam cells, horseshoe kidney	AD?
Alcohol embryopathy (fetal alcohol syndrome)	Prenatal and postnatal growth retardation, microcephaly, short palpebral fissures, joint contractures, mental retardation	Unilateral renal agenesis and hypoplasia, hydronephrosis, duplication of urinary tract	—
Aldrich (Wiskott-Aldrich)	Congenital thrombocytopenia, bloody diarrhea, eczema, recurrent infections, elevated serum IgA	Hematuria, proteinuria, NS, renal failure	XL
Amyloidosis	Macroglossia, peripheral polyneuropathy, hepatosplenomegaly	Renal involvement in 87%, glomerular amyloid deposition, proteinuria, hypertension, nephrosis	AD? Sporadic
Angiokeratoma, diffuse (Fabry disease, alpha-galactosidase A deficiency)	Pain; skin lesions; cerebral, ocular, cardiac, and renal manifestations	Abnormal lipid deposition in epithelial and endothelial cells of kidney	XL

Syndrome/Disease	Main Features	Renal/Urinary Tract Abnormalities	Inheritance
Asphyxiating thoracic dystrophy	Hypoplastic thorax, respiratory difficulty, protruding abdomen, polydactyly, tapetoretinal degeneration	Proteinuria, hypertension, renal failure, Fanconi-like syndrome, cystic dysplasia, nephronophthisis, UVJ stenosis	AR
Bacterial endocarditis	Fever, heart and renal disease	60%–80% of patients are affected. Hematuria (90%), proteinuria (35%–88%), renal infarcts (57%), focal or diffuse GN, renal failure	—
Barakat (HDR)	Hypoparathyroidism, sensorineural deafness, renal disease	Proteinuria; hematuria; nephrosis; renal failure; cystic, dysplastic, and hypoplastic kidneys	AD ?
Bartter (hypokalemic alkalosis)	Hypokalemic alkalosis, hyperaldosteronism, normal blood presure	Hyperplasia of juxtaglomerular apparatus	AR?
Beckwith-Wiedemann	Omphalocele, macroglossia, nephromegaly, increased birth weight, facial flame nevus, characteristic ear helix anomaly, hypoglycemia	Renal medullary dysplasia, Wilms tumor, hydronephrosis, hydroureter, ectopic and double kidney, cortical cysts	AD?
Behçet	Recurrent inflammatory lesions of mouth, genitalia, and eyes	Proteinuria, hematuria, nephrosis, renal failure, GN, amyloidosis	AD?
Biliary atresia, extrahepatic	Biliary atresia, renal and cardiac malformations	Renal aplasia or hypoplasia, nephrosis, polycystic kidneys, megaloureter, atresia of ureter	AR?
Bloom	Growth failure, facial telangiectasia, defective immunity	Wilms tumor	AR
Blue diaper	Bluish discoloration of diapers, failure to thrive, hypercalcemia, infections	Azotemia, nephrocalcinosis, interstitial nephritis	AR, XL?

Syndrome/Disease	Main Features	Renal/Urinary Tract Abnormalities	Inheritance
Brachio-oto-renal dysplasia (BOR)	Preauricular pits, cervical fistulae, hearing loss	Ectopic, aplastic, hypoplastic, dysplastic, and polycystic kidneys; chronic interstitial nephropathy; renal failure	AD?
C (Opitz trigonocephaly)	Trigonocephaly, polysyndactyly, abnormal ears, joint dislocations	Unilateral renal agenesis, hypospadias	AR
Campomelic dysplasia	Congenital bowing of long bones, abnormal facies, dwarfism	Hydronephrosis, hydroureter, hypoplastic and cystic kidneys	AR?
Cerebro-costo-mandibular	Cerebral maldevelopment, micrognathia, costovertebral abnormalities	Renal ectopia, medullary cysts	AD?
Cerebro-oculo-facio-skeletal	Microcephaly, ocular, facial and skeletal abnormalities	Horseshoe kidney, bilateral renal agenesis, double collecting system	AR?
Chloride diarrhea, familial	Defective intestinal transport of Cl⁻; diarrhea, salt, and water wasting	Juxtaglomerular hyperplasia, nephrocalcinosis	AR?
Chromosome aberrations	See page 493.		
Collagen, type III glomerulopathy	Renal disease, anemia, elevated serum type III procollagen peptide	GN, hypertension, fibrillar collagen in glomeruli, proteinuria, NS, acute and chronic kidney disease	?
Coloboma, cardiac defect, other anomalies	Same	Unilateral renal agenesis, ectopia, double collecting system, posterior urethral valves, UPJ obstruction, hypospadias	?
Connective tissue disease, mixed	Arthritis, sclerodactyly, Raynaud phenomena, lymphadenopathy, anemia	Proteinuria, membranous and proliferative GN, renal failure	—
Cornelia de Lange	Prenatal and postnatal growth deficiency, dysmorphic facies, hirsutism, mental retardation	Renal cystic dysplasia and hypoplasia, hydronephrosis, hypospadias	AD? Sporadic

Syndrome/Disease	Main Features	Renal/Urinary Tract Abnormalities	Inheritance
Cystic fibrosis	Failure to thrive, respiratory and gastrointestinal involvement	Microscopic nephrocalcinosis, hypercalciuria	AR
Cushing disease, adrenal	Obesity, osteoporosis, growth retardation, hypertension	Urolithiasis, renal dysplasia	Sporadic AR?
Cytomegalovirus (CMV)	Jaundice, hepatosplenomegaly, encephalitis, thrombocytopenia	Renal CMV, inclusions, GN, proteinuria, hematuria, nephrosis, renal failure	—
Denys-Drash (Drash)	Pseudohermaphroditism, nephropathy, and Wilms tumor	Wilms tumor, NS, GN, diffuse mesangial sclerosis	?
Dermatomyositis	Myositis, muscle weakness, skin lesions, edema, low-grade fever	Proteinuria, arteriolar fibrosis, GN, vasculitis, nephrosis, renal failure	—
Diabetes mellitus	Hyperglycemia, polyuria, polydipsia, diabetic ketoacidosis	7% of cases affected, proteinuria, clinical diabetic nephropathy develops 10–20 years after diagnosis	Multifactorial AD, AR?
Diabetic embryopathy	Infants of diabetic mothers, skeletal, cardiac, GI and other malformations	Hydronephrosis, renal agenesis, double ureter	—
Diaphragmatic hernia, congenital	Congenital diaphragmatic hernia, respiratory distress at birth	Aplastic, polycystic, horseshoe, double and ectopic kidney; hydronephrosis, hydroureter	Multifactorial
DiGeorge syndrome	Absence of thymus and parathyroid glands, immunodeficiency, congenital heart defect, characteristic facies	Hydronephrosis, malrotation of kidney	AD
Dystrophia myotonia 1	Myotonia, muscle wasting, cataract, hypogonadism	Polycystic kidneys	AD

Syndrome/Disease	Main Features	Renal/Urinary Tract Abnormalities	Inheritance
Ectrodactyly-ectodermal dysplasia and cleft lip/palate (EEC 1)	Ectrodactyly, ectodermal dysplasia, cleft lip/palate	Unilateral renal agenesis, hypospadias	AD
Ehlers-Danlos	Hyperelasticity and fragility of skin and blood vessels, hypermobility of joints	UPJ abnormality, dissected or hypoplastic renal artery, polycystic/medullary sponge kidney, RTA, bladder neck obstruction	AD AR XL Sporadic
Elliptocytosis	Mild anemia, if any	RTA	AD
Ellis-van Creveld	Acromelic dwarfism, polydactyly, hypoplasia and dystrophy of nails and teeth, cardiac malformation	Nephrocalcinosis, glomerulosclerosis, unilateral renal agenesis, megaureter	AR
Faciocardiorenal	Characteristic facies, severe mental retardation, cardiac and renal defects	Horseshoe kidney, hydroureter	AR?
Faciooculoacoustico-renal	Ocular and craniofacial anomalies, deafness	Proteinuria, aminoaciduria, VUR	AR?
Familial cold auto-inflammatory syndrome	Cold urticaria, pain and swelling of joints, fever	Renal failure, amyloid nephropathy	AD
Fanconi anemia	Pancytopenia, hyperpigmentation, skeletal deformities, absent or hypoplastic thumb	1/3 of patients are affected. Aplastic, ectopic, and horseshoe kidney; duplication of urinary tract; hydronephrosis; renal cysts	AR
Fanconi renotubular	Retarded growth, rickets, aminoaciduria, hypophosphatemia	Renal tubular defect with aminoaciduria, glucosuria, proteinuria, acidosis, renal failure	AD
Femoral-facial	Femoral hypoplasia, unusual facies, cleft palate	Hemangioma of urinary tract, polycystic kidneys, renal agenesis, abnormal collecting system	?

Syndrome/Disease	Main Features	Renal/Urinary Tract Abnormalities	Inheritance
Fructose intolerance, hereditary	Hypoglycemia, liver cirrhosis	RTA, proteinuria, aminoaciduria	AR
Fungus infections	Systemic involvement with fever, rash, sepsis, hepatosplenomegaly. Most commonly *Candida*	UTIs, micro-abcesses of kidney, acute renal failure	—
Galactosemia	Cataracts, hepatosplenomegaly, failure to thrive, variable mental retardation	Proteinuria, aminoaciduria	AR
Gitelman	Muscle cramps, weakness, abdominal pain	Hypokalemia, hypomagnesemia, hypocalciuria, metabolic alkalosis	AR?
Glycogen storage disease I	Short stature, hepatomegaly, hypoglycemia, hyperuricemia	Enlarged kidneys, Fanconi-like syndrome, vacuolated renal tubular cells	AR
Gout	Hyperuricemia, arthritis, tophi	Uric acid urolithiasis, nephropathy, acute renal failure, chronic urate nephropathy with nephrosclerosis and hypertension	?
Heart, congenital malformations	Cardiac murmur and other findings depending on nature of malformation	Renal agenesis, dysgenesis, ectopia, and hypoplasia. 25% of patients with VSD have renal abnormalities, particularly renal hypoplasia	?
Heart disease, congenital cyanotic	Cyanosis and hypoxia secondary to cardiac malformation	Glomerular enlargement, proteinuria, decreased renal plasma flow, proximal RTA, glomerular sclerosis	?
Heart failure, congestive	Tachypnea, tachycardia, hepatomegaly, edema, poor perfusion	Proteinuria (85%), hematuria, pyuria, infarcts, arteriolar sclerosis, inability to concentrate urine (27%–77%), prerenal azotemia, GN	—

Syndrome/Disease	Main Features	Renal/Urinary Tract Abnormalities	Inheritance
Hemihypertrophy	Total or partial asymmetry, hemihyperesthesia, hemi-areflexia, scoliosis	Wilms tumor, enlarged kidneys, nephrocalcinosis, medullary sponge kidneys, hypospadias	AR?
Hemolytic uremic	Coombs negative hemolytic anemia, thrombocytopenia	Renal microangiopathy, acute renal failure	?
Hemophilia A and B	Factor VIII or factor IX deficiency, bleeding episodes	Filling defects, calculi, papillary necrosis, hydronephrosis	XL
Hemorrhagic fevers	Fever, hemorrhage, shock, rash, arthralgia, GI and neurologic manifestations. Caused by Dengue, yellow, Lassa, and other fevers	Acute renal failure, ATN, interstitial nephritis, GN	—
Henoch-Schönlein purpura	Purpuric skin rash, arthralgia, abdominal pain, GN (20%–30%)	Hematuria, proteinuria, nephritis of variable severity and histology	—
Hepatic fibrosis, congenital	Hepatic fibrosis, congenital heart disease	Cystic, dysplastic kidneys	AR
Hepatitis, viral	Jaundice, abnormal liver functions, positive hepatitis antigens	Proteinuria, hematuria, cylindruria, decreased GFR, immune complex glomerular disease with HBsAg	—
Herpes simplex	Vesicular rash, fever, encephalitis, multisystem involvement	Acute GN, NS, focal glomerulosclerosis	—
Hirschsprung disease (megacolon, aganglionic)	Congenital megacolon	Obstructive uropathy	AD?
Hypereosinophilic	Eosinophilia with multi-organ involvement, especially heart	20% of patients. Hematuria, proteinuria, interstitial nephritis, renal infarct, eosinophilic infiltration, renal failure	—
Hyperoxaluria, primary	Renal colic	Hematuria, nephrocalcinosis, oxalate urolithiasis	AR

Syndrome/Disease	Main Features	Renal/Urinary Tract Abnormalities	Inheritance
Hyperparathyroidism 1	Hypercalcemia, osteitis fibrosa, medullary sponge kidney	Nephrocalcinosis, urolithiasis, salt wastage	AD
Hypertension, essential	Asymptomatic elevation in blood pressure, atherosclerotic organ damage	Proteinuria, nephrosclerosis	AD?
Hypoaldosteronism, congenital	Hypoaldosteronism, hyporeninemia, hyperkalemia	Distal RTA, renal insufficiency	AD
Hypomagnesemia, primary	Tetany, hypocalcemia, acidosis, seizures, polyuria	Renal magnesium wasting, hypercalciuria, nephro-calcinosis, RTA, renal calculi, glomerulosclerosis, inter-stitial nephritis, chronic kidney disease	AR
Ichthyosis, mental retarda-tion, dwarfism, and renal impairment	Same, hypogonadism, spasticity	Chronic pyelonephritis, glomerulosclerosis, double kidney and ureter, vacuolization of proximal tubular cells, renal insufficiency	AR?
Infectious mononucleosis (Epstein-Barr virus)	Fever, lymphadenopathy, splenomegaly	Hematuria (common), proteinuria and acute GN (rare), nephrosis, acute renal failure, tubular necrosis, interstitial nephritis	—
Inflammatory bowel disease 1 (Crohn)	Abdominal pain, diarrhea, weight loss, growth retardation	Nephrosis, nephrolithiasis, hydronephrosis, hydroureter, ileovesical fistulae	AR
Kawasaki (mucocutaneous lymph node)	Fever, desquamation of skin, rash, lymph-adenopathy, arthritis, urethritis	Urethritis, renal artery involvement in 50% of cases, interstitial nephritis, acute renal failure, renal insuffi-ciency, renal scarring	—
Laurence-Moon	Retinitis pigmentosa, mental retardation, obesity, short stature, hypogonadism, polydactyly	Pyelonephritis; GN; cystic, dysplastic, hypoplastic, hydro-nephrotic kidneys; VUR; nephrosclerosis	AR

Syndrome/Disease	Main Features	Renal/Urinary Tract Abnormalities	Inheritance
Legionella pneumophilia (Legionnaires' disease)	Fever, pneumonia, leukocytosis, shock	Rare. Acute renal failure, tubular necrosis, interstitial nephritis. Organism detected in kidney	—
Leishmaniasis	Chronic protozoan infection with fever, hepatosplenomegaly, anemia, leukopenia	Mild and resolves after treatment. Pyuria (50%), proteinuria, hematuria, GN (mesangial, proliferative, others)	—
Leptospirosis	Headache, fever, chills, myalgias, jaundice, rash	Affects 80% of patients. Proteinuria, pyuria (65%), hematuria, cylindruria (5%–10%), tubulo-interstitial nephritis, acute renal failure	—
Lesch-Nyhan	Self-mutilation, extra-pyramidal signs, delayed motor development, excessive uric acid production	Uric acid urolithiasis, nephropathy, shrunken kidneys	XLR
Lowe oculocerebrorenal	Growth and mental retardation, general-ized aminoaciduria, proteinuria, rickets, eye changes	Aminoaciduria, proteinuria, hypotonia, metabolic acidosis, hematuria, pyuria, decreased tubular absorption of phosphate, renal failure	XL
Lupus erythematosis, systemic	Collagen disease with multisystem involve-ment, arthritis, fever, malar rash, autoanti-body abnormality	Proteinuria, abnormal urine sediment, lupus nephritis, NS, hypertension, chronic kidney disease	?
Malaria	Paroxysmal fevers, anemia, splenomegaly	NS, membranous and, rarely, proliferative immune complex GN	—
Malignancy, disease	Depends on the type and site of disease	Acute renal failure secondary to renal parenchymal involvement, obstruction or urate nephropathy, immune complex glomerulopathy	?
Malignancy, therapy	Tumor lysis syndrome, creatinine, drug nephrotoxicity	Increased serum urate and creatinine, drug nephrotoxicity	—

Syndrome/Disease	Main Features	Renal/Urinary Tract Abnormalities	Inheritance
Marfan	Musculoskeletal abnormalities, hypotonia, excessive length of limbs, CV abnormalities, ectopia lentis and other eye changes	Hydronephrosis, polycystic, ectopic, and medullary sponge kidney; unilateral renal agenesis; nephrolithiasis; duplication of urinary tract	AD?
Measles	Rash, fever, Koplik spots	Acute GN	—
Meckel, type I	Occipital encephalocele, microcephaly, abnormal facies, cleft lip/palate, polydactyly	Dysplastic, polycystic, hypoplastic, horseshoe, hydro-nephrotic, and medullary sponge kidney; dilated ureters; renal vascular abnormalities	AR
Mediterranean fever, familial	Fever, pleuritis, peritonitis, arthritis	Amyloid nephropathy	AD
Megaduodenum and/or megacystis	Megacystis, dilated small bowel, malrota-tion	Megacystis, hydronephrosis, hydroureter	AD
Mumps	Fever, parotitis	Hematuria and proteinuria (1/3 of cases), acute nephritis with deposits of IgA, IgM, C3 and mumps virus antigen, abnormal renal function	—
Mycoplasma pneumoniae	Fever, pneumonia, arthritis, hemolysis	Acute, membranoproliferative, and interstitial nephritis	—
Nail patella	Dystrophic nails, hypoplastic/absent patella, dysplastic elbows, iliac horns	Nephropathy in 30%–55% of patients, proteinuria, renal insufficiency	AD
Neurofibromatosis, type 1	Café au lait spots, cutaneous neurofibromas, CNS tumors	Neurofibromatosis of urinary tract, renal vascular changes, renal artery involvement with hypertension	AD
Neuropathy, hereditary sensory and autonomic, type III (Riley-Day)	Reduced or absent tear production, postural hypotension, excessive perspiration, relative indifference to pain, emotional lability	Glomerulosclerosis secondary to renal vascular denervation	AR

Syndrome/Disease	Main Features	Renal/Urinary Tract Abnormalities	Inheritance
Nevus sebaceous of Jadassohn	Linear sebaceous nevus, epilepsy, mental retardation	Renal hamartomas, nephroblastoma, renal artery stenosis	AD?
Niemann-Pick disease type A (sphingo-myelinase deficiency)	Hepatosplenomegaly, retarded mental and physical growth, severe neurologic disturbances	Rare vacuolated glomerular cells, swollen glomerular epithelial cells	AR
Nipples, supernumerary	Accessory nipples, and sometimes breast tissue	Double collecting system; hypoplastic, microcystic, and polycystic kidneys; hydronephrosis; UPJ stenosis; ureteral prolapse; Wilms tumor	AD
Noonan syndrome 1	Short stature, webbed neck, pulmonary stenosis, mental retardation	Polycystic, malrotated, and hydronephrotic kidneys; double collecting system	AD
Oculorenocerebellar	Tapetoretinal degeneration, choreo-athetosis of upper limbs, spastic diplegia, mental retardation, glomerulopathy	Glomerulosclerosis, renal failure	AR
Orofaciodigital I	Malformation of oral cavity, face, and digits; anomalies of anterior teeth; mental retardation	Polycystic kidney disease	XL
Osteogenesis imperfecta	Short, broad long bones; multiple fractures; blue sclerae	Aminoaciduria, cystinuria	AD, AR
Polyarteritis nodosa	Fever, myalgia, arthralgia, abdominal pain, hypertension	Proteinuria, hematuria, fibrinoid arterial necrosis, renal failure	—
Prune-belly	Congenital absence of abdominal musculature, urinary tract abnormalities, cryptorchidism	Dilated urinary tract; dysplastic, aplastic, multicystic, and hydronephrotic kidneys	AD?

Syndrome/Disease	Main Features	Renal/Urinary Tract Abnormalities	Inheritance
Pyloric stenosis, infantile	Hypertrophic pylorus, vomiting	Polycystic, horseshoe, and hypoplastic kidney; double collecting system; hydronephrosis	Multi-factorial
Q fever (*Coxiella burnetii*)	Fever, pneumonia, other organ involvement	Proteinuria, hematuria, acute GN, acute renal failure, hypertension, nephrosis	—
Radial-renal	Radial ray aplasia, short stature, renal anomalies	Unilateral renal agenesis, crossed ectopia	AD?
Renal, genital, and middle ear anomalies	Abnormal facies, low folded ears, renal abnormalities, vaginal atresia, middle ear anomalies with deafness	Renal agenesis or hypoplasia, hemiatrophy of urinary bladder	AR?
Rheumatic fever	Fever, arthritis, carditis, other systemic involvement	Hematuria, focal or diffuse GN, rheumatic arteritis	—
Rheumatoid arthritis	Polyarthritis, joint stiffness, fever, organo-megaly	Proteinuria (40%), hypertension (30%), hematuria (25%), UTI (20%), amyloidosis, GN, nephrosclerosis	?
Rocky mountain spotted fever	Fever, rash, headache, heart failure, thrombocytopenia	Acute renal failure, acidosis	—
Rokitansky-Kuster-Hauser	Vaginal atresia, rudimentary uterus, primary amenorrhea	Renal agensis and hypoplasia, double renal pelvis and ureters, pelvic and solitary fused kidney	Sporadic AR?
Rubella, congenital	Small for age, microcephaly, cataracts, heart defects, hepatosplenomegaly	Polycystic and unilateral agenetic kidney, glomerulosclerosis, double collecting system, hypospadias	—
Rubinstein-Taybi	Broad thumbs and great toes, characteristic facial abnormalities, mental retardation	Renal calculi, non-functioning aplastic or extra kidney, double renal pelvis, dilated ureter, posterior urethral valves, VUR	AD?

Syndrome/Disease	Main Features	Renal/Urinary Tract Abnormalities	Inheritance
Sarcoidosis	Fever, arthralgias, pulmonary hilar adenopathy	Interstitial granulomas and inflammation, nephrocalcinosis, renal failure	?
Schistosomiasis	Cercarial forms attack body through skin and involve every organ	Mostly *Schistosoma mansoni*. Terminal hematuria. Granulomatous inflammation of ureters and bladder, urinary obstruction, hydronephrosis, bladder cancer, urinary infection, renal failure	—
Scleroderma, familial progressive	Morphea, progressive systemic sclerosis, system involvement	Proteinuria, hematuria, renal failure	—, AD?
Seckel syndrome 1 (bird-headed dwarfism)	Severe short stature, microcephaly, narrow face, beak-like nose	Renal ectopy and hypoplasia, nephritis	AR
Sepsis	Fever, hypotension, organ under-perfusion, shock	Oliguria, acute renal failure, pyuria, proteinuria, hematuria	—
Sickle cell disease	Characteristic anemia, fever, pain, infection	Papillary necrosis, cortical infarcts, nephrosis, hematuria, proteinuria	AR
Smith–Lemli–Opitz	Growth retardation, microcephaly, mental retardation, abnormal facies, hypospadias, microphallus	Rotated, hypoplastic, dysplastic or multicystic kidney; cortical cysts; hypospadias	AR
Sotos (cerebral gigantism)	Acceleration of growth, acromegalic appearance, characteristic facies, variable mental retardation	Urethral stricture, Wilms tumor	AD
Spherocytosis	Anemia, intermittent jaundice splenomegaly	Polycystic kidneys	AD, AR

Syndrome/Disease	Main Features	Renal/Urinary Tract Abnormalities	Inheritance
Spina bifida	Asymptomatic or neurologic symptoms, urinary incontinence	Ureteral duplication, neurogenic bladder	AD?
Syphilis	Rhinitis, rash, bone involvement, other protean and latent manifestations	Occurs in 0.3% of patients. Nephrosis, rarely acute and interstitial nephritis, gumma of kidney	—
Testicular regression (XY gonadal agenesis)	Absence of gonads in an XY person	Interstitial nephritis, ESRD	AR?
Thalassemia B	Anemia, growth retardation, hepatomegaly	Distal RTA	AR
Townes-Brocks (imperforate anus; hand, foot, and ear anomalies)	Anal stenosis; dysgenetic ears; digital, renal, and cardiac abnormalities	Renal hypoplasia, aplasia, dysplasia, proteinuria, VUR, posterior urethral valves	AD
Toxic shock syndrome	Fever, rash, shock, DIC, encephalopathy	Acute renal failure, GN	—
Toxoplasmosis (*Toxoplasma gondii*)	Microcephaly, seizures, hepatosplenomegaly, rash, fever (congenital) lymphadenopathy resembling mononucleosis (acquired)	Nephrosis, especially affects transplant kidney	—
Tuberculosis	Systemic manifestations or those related to specific site of infection	Sterile pyuria, hematuria, renal necrosis and caseating granulomas with destruction of collecting system, diffuse miliary renal parenchymal lesions, GN, nephrosis	—
Tuberous sclerosis	Epilepsy, mental retardation, adenoma sebaceum, retinal phakomas	40%–80% of patients have renal angiomyolipomas, cystic kidneys, adenomas, or renal cell carcinoma	AD
Typhoid fever (*Salmonella typhi*)	Fever, stupor, rose spots, splenomegaly, symptoms of other organ involvement	Occur in 2%–3% of patients. Tubulo-interstitial disease, oliguric renal failure, immune complex nephritis	—

Syndrome/Disease	Main Features	Renal/Urinary Tract Abnormalities	Inheritance
Ulcerative colitis	Bloody diarrhea, abdominal cramps, weight loss	Nephrolithiasis	— AD?
Uterine anomalies	Uterovaginal duplication, hematocolpos	Unilateral renal agenesis	Sporadic, AD?
Varicella-zoster	Fever, vesicular skin rash	Rare. Nephritis with IgG, IgM, IgA, and C3 deposition; tubular necrosis; NS; acute renal failure; rapidly progressive GN	—
VATER association	Vertebral anomalies, <u>a</u>nal atresia, <u>t</u>racheo-<u>e</u>sophageal fistula, <u>r</u>enal dysplasia	Renal agenesis or ectopia; hydronephrosis; UPJ stenosis; hypospadias; recto-urethral, vaginal, and vesical fistulae	AD?
Viruses (other)	Fever, rash, diarrhea, other symptoms	Hemorrhagic cystitis (20%–50% adenovirus, acute GN and acute renal failure (influenza, enterovirus), tubular necrosis, glomerular fibrin deposition (Ebola)	—
Wegener granuloma	Fever; cutaneous vasculitis; arthralgia; renal, cardiac, and CNS involvement	Segmental necrotizing and crescentic GN, renal granulomas	—
Wilson disease (hepatolenticular degeneration)	Ceruloplasmin deficiency; severe neurologic abnormalities	Nephrocalcinosis, RTA, aminoaciduria	AR
Zellweger (cerebro-hepato-renal)	Failure to thrive; cerebral, renal, and skeletal abnormalities; severe hypotonia; liver disease; distinctive facies; death in early infancy	Renal cysts and dysplasia	AR?

Chromosomal Aberrations	Renal and Urinary Tract Abnormalities
Autosomal trisomies	
Trisomy 8	75% of patients are affected. Hydronephrosis, horseshoe and non-functioning kidney, bifid pelvis, VUR
Trisomy 13	50%–60% of patients are affected. Cystic, aplastic, horseshoe, and hydronephrotic kidney; duplication of urinary tract; megacystis, UV obstruction, bladder neck stenosis
Trisomy 18	Duplication of urinary tract (33%–70%); horseshoe, cystic, hydronephrotic, ectopic, aplastic, and hypoplastic kidney. Glomerulosclerosis, rarely, Wilms tumor, hamartoma, fetal lobulation, and rotational anomalies of the kidney
Trisomy 21	7% of cases are affected. Aplastic, hypoplastic, dysplastic, cystic, and horseshoe kidney; hydronephrosis; hydroureter; ureteral stenosis; persistent fetal lobulation; hypoplastic or large bladder; urethral valves and stricture; renal artery stenosis; GN
Autosomal monosomies	
4p-	1/3 of patients are affected. Agenetic, hypoplastic, hydronephrotic, and non-functioning kidney; VUR; pyelonephritis; dilated collecting system; hypospadias
5p- (Cri-du-chat)	40% of patients are affected. Ectasia of distal tubules, cystic and horseshoe kidney, duplication of urinary tract
18 q-	40% of patients are affected. Polycystic, aplastic, ectopic, and horseshoe kidney; hydronephrosis; hydroureter
17p11.2 monosomy	22% of patients may be affected. Enlarged or solitary kidney, hydroureter, hydropelvis, malpositioned UVJ
Sex chromosomes	
Turner Syndrome (XO)	60%–80% of patients are affected. Horseshoe kidney (commonest); duplications and rotational anomalies; hydronephrotic, ectopic, ptotic, aplastic, hypoplastic, and cystic kidney; urethral meatal stenosis; hypertension; double renal artery; UPJ and UVJ stenosis
Klinefelter syndrome (XXY)	Renal cysts, hydronephrosis, hydroureter, ureterocele, chronic GN
Fragile X syndrome	UPJ stenosis
Other chromosomal aberrations	
Triploidy (69 chromosomes)	Cystic renal dysplasia and hydronephrosis (50%) fetal lobulations, pelvic kidney
Tetraploidy (92 chromosomes)	50% of patients are affected. Renal hypoplasia or dysplasia, pyelonephritis, megaureter, VUR, urethral stenosis
Cat-eye syndrome	60%–100% of patients affected. Renal agenesis, hypoplasia; and cystic dysplasia; horseshoe and pelvic kidney; UPJ obstruction; vesicoureteral stenosis and VUR; hypoplastic urinary bladder; chronic pyelonephritis

References

1. Online Mendelian Inheritance in Man. http://www.ncbi.nlm.nih.gov/omim/

2. McKusick VA, ed. *Mendelian Inheritance in Man. A Catalog of Human Genes and Genetic Disorders.* 12th ed. Baltimore, MD: Johns Hopkins University Press; 1998

3. Jones KL, Smith DW. *Smith's Recognizable Patterns of Human Malformation.* 5th ed. Oxford, UK: Elsevier; 2005

4. Barakat AY, ed. *Renal Disease in Children: Clinical Evaluation and Diagnosis.* New York, NY: Springer-Verlag; 1990

5. Barakat AY, Butler MG. Renal and urinary tract abnormalities associated with chromosome aberrations. *Int J Pediatr Nephrol.* 1987;8:215–226

6. Barakat AY, Der Kaloustian VM, Mufarrij AA, et al. *The Kidney in Genetic Disease.* Edinburgh, UK: Churchill Livingstone; 1986

7. Barakat AY, Seikaly MG, Der Kaloustian VM. Urogenital abnormalities in genetic disease. *J Urol.* 1986;136:778–785

8. Avner ED, Harmon WE, Niaudet P. *Pediatric Nephrology.* 5th ed. Baltimore, MD: Lippincott, Williams & Wilkins; 2003

9. Rimoin D, Connor JM, Pyeritz R, Korf B, Emery A, eds. *Emery and Rimoin's Principles and Practice of Medical Genetics.* Oxford, UK: Elsevier; 2001

Index

A